Workbook for

McCurnin's Clinical Textbook for Veterinary Technicians

Seventh Edition

Workbook for

McCurnin's Clinical Textbook for Veterinary Technicians

Seventh Edition

Joanna M. Bassert, VMD

Professor and Director
Program of Veterinary Technology
Manor College
Jenkintown, Pennsylvania

Dennis M. McCurnin, DVM, MS, Dipl ACVS

Professor of Surgery and Management
Director of Continuing Education
Veterinary Clinical Sciences
School of Veterinary Medicine
Louisiana State University
Baton Rouge, Louisiana

SAUNDERS

ELSEVIER

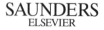

11830 Westline Industrial Drive
St. Louis, Missouri 63146

Workbook for McCurnin's Clinical Textbook for Veterinary Technicians   978-1-4160-5702-4

Notice

Knowledge and best practice in this field are constantly changing. As new research and experience broaden our knowledge, changes in practice, treatment, and drug therapy may become necessary or appropriate. Readers are advised to check the most current information provided (i) on procedures featured or (ii) by the manufacturer of each product to be administered, to verify the recommended dose or formula, the method and duration of administration, and contraindications. It is the responsibility of the practitioner, relying on their own experience and knowledge of the patient, to make diagnoses, to determine dosages and the best treatment for each individual patient, and to take all appropriate safety precautions. To the fullest extent of the law, neither the Publisher nor the Editors assumes any liability for any injury and/or damage to persons or property arising out of or related to any use of the material contained in this book.

The Publisher

ISBN: 978-1-4160-5702-4

Vice President and Publisher: Linda Duncan
Publisher: Penny Rudolph
Managing Editor: Teri Merchant
Publishing Services Manager: Catherine Jackson
Project Manager: Rachel E. McMullen
Design Direction: Paula Catalano
Cover Designer: Paula Catalano

Printed in the United States of America

Last digit is the print number: 9 8 7 6 5 4 3 2

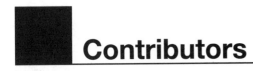

Contributors

Paige A. Allen, MS, RVT
Instructional Technologist
Veterinary Administration
Purdue University
West Lafayette, Indiana

Allen Balay, DVM
Veterinary Technology Program
Ridgewater College
Willmar, Minnesota

Susan A. Berryhill, BS, RVT, VTS (Dentistry)
Senior Veterinary Nursing Specialist
Pfizer Animal Health
Branson, Missouri

Regina Brotherton, CCRP, DVM
Professor/Program Director
Animal Health
Louisiana Technical College
Florida Parish, Louisiana

Mary Tefend Campbell, CVT, VTS (ECC)
Shorter, Alabama

Joann Colville, DVM
North Dakota State University, retired
Fargo, North Dakota

Markiva Contris, RVT
Pierce College at Fort Steilacoom
Lakewood, Washington

Harriet Doolittle, DVM*
Associate Professor of Biology and Animal Science, retired
Camden County College
Blackwood, New Jersey

Peggy Dorsey, BA, CVT
Director, Veterinary Technology
Camden County College
Blackwood, New Jersey

Lisa Martini-Johnson, DVM
Lehigh Carbon and Northampton Community College
Schnecksville, Pennsylvania

Stuart L. Porter, VMD
Professor, Veterinary Technology
Blue Ridge Community College
Weyers Cave, Virginia

Lori Renda-Francis, MA, BBA, LVT
Professor and Program Director
Veterinary Technician Department
Macomb Community College
Clinton Township, Michigan

Jill A. Richardson, DVM
Consultant, Technical Services and Marketing
Lloyd Labs, Inc.
Shenandoah, Iowa

Kathy Ruane, BS, RVT
Penn Foster College
Scottsdale, Arizona

Katie Samuelson, DVM, AHT
Adjunct Professor, Anatomy and Physiology
Penn Foster College
Scottsdale, Arizona

Sue Sanders, BS, RVT
Distance Learning Instructional Technologist
Veterinary Technology Program
Purdue University
West Lafayette, Indiana

Sara Sharp, CVT, VTS (Dentistry)
Denver, Colorado

Margi Sirois, EdD, MS, RVT
Program Director
Veterinary Technician Program
Penn Foster College
Scottsdale, Arizona

Marianne Tear, MS, LVT
Program Director
Veterinary Technology Program
Baker College
Clinton Township, Michigan

*Deceased

Preface

This workbook is intended to accompany the seventh edition of the textbook *McCurnin's Clinical Textbook for Veterinary Technicians*. Each chapter in the workbook relates to a corresponding chapter in the textbook and stresses the essential information of the chapter through the use of definitions, short essays (comprehension), photo quizzes, matching, completion, true and false, multiple choice questions, word searches, crosswords, and superclues.

Learning objectives are included at the beginning of each chapter to help you focus on the material and concepts that you are expected to learn and how this is to be applied in the veterinary clinical setting.

The following suggestions will help you use this workbook to identify strengths and weaknesses.

1. Review the contents of each chapter before you attempt to do the exercise. Do not treat the questions individually and then refer to the text for the correct answer. Deal with the chapter's subject matter as a whole, since many of the questions are interrelated. This is a learning exercise meant to help you learn the material presented in the textbook, not an examination for grades.
2. Remember that the same subject matter may be repeated in different question forms in each chapter or other chapters, since the material overlaps. The subjects of the questions are not in the same order as they appear in the textbook.
3. Read each question and study each illustration carefully before answering. You may know the answer or you may arrive at the correct answer by knowing which answers are incorrect.
4. This workbook is designed so that the pages can be easily removed, submitted if required, and placed in your notebook with the corresponding lecture notes.

The answers to all the exercises appear in the *TEACH Instructor Resource for McCurnin's Clinical Textbook for Veterinary Technicians,* both in the print resource and on the Evolve website.

Contents

2 | Laws, Regulations, and Ethics

LEARNING OBJECTIVES

When you have completed this chapter, you will be able to:
1. Name the laws and regulations that govern the practice of veterinary medicine
2. Differentiate between laws and regulations
3. Describe the components of veterinary practice acts
4. Describe the term specialty academy and explain the role of the academy in credentialing of veterinary professionals
5. List the specialty academies recognized by NAVTA
6. Describe the nomenclature used for credentialed veterinary technicians in various locales
7. Describe requirements for credentialing of veterinary technicians
8. Describe the roles of the state boards of veterinary medicine in credentialing of veterinary professionals
9. Define ethics and name the organizations that develop ethical guidelines for veterinary professionals
10. List the tasks that veterinary technicians are not permitted to perform

TRUE OR FALSE

1. _T_ A veterinary technicians' license can be revoked.
2. _T_ Veterinary technicians can become specialists in an area of interest.
3. _F_ A vet tech cannot be sued as a result of her or his actions.
4. _T_ The license of a vet tech can be revoked by NAVTA.
5. _T_ A veterinary technician can administer anesthesia.
6. _T_ The public may have input into laws and regulations of the vet tech.
7. _T_ In the United States, all vet techs are licensed, certified, or registered.
8. _T_ The practice act governs veterinarians and vet techs.
9. _T_ Veterinary state boards and specialty boards are the same entity.
10. _F_ Continuing education is part of the specialty certification.
11. _T_ Programs of study for the vet tech must be accredited by the AVMA.
12. _____ TVIA verifies all vet tech certification.
13. _____ Criminal history records must be submitted for licensure.
14. _____ The licensing board will provide the licensee a lawyer for hearings.
15. _____ The most severe sanction that may be imposed is revocation of a license.
16. _____ OSHA requires safety guidelines be followed in the workplace.
17. _____ A veterinary technician is required to have a bachelor's degree.
18. _____ The veterinary technician's license will automatically be renewed.
19. _____ Continuing education is a requirement for licensure.
20. _____ A notice of disciplinary action may be hand delivered to the licensee.
21. _____ A civil penalty is a fine paid to the licensing board.
22. _____ The most common reason for a disciplinary action is a traffic ticket.

23. _____ Ethical behavior is easy to define for all veterinary technicians.

24. _____ The veterinarian can impose sanctions on a vet tech.

25. _____ A vet tech must know the tasks that he or she may legally perform.

YES OR NO

Does each offense have to be reported when applying for a license?

(Y or N)

1. _____ Underage drinking

2. _____ Speeding

3. _____ Failure to yield

4. _____ DUI/DWI

5. _____ Disorderly conduct

MATCHING

Match the following acronyms:

1. _____ THE BOARD   A. Regulates safety in the workplace

2. _____ AVMA   B. National association for vet techs

3. _____ RACE   C. Continuing education registry

4. _____ OSHA   D. Associated with specialty boards

5. _____ NAVTA   E. Governs the practice act in the state

SHORT ANSWER

1. List crimes of moral turpitude:

    A. _____

    B. _____

    C. _____

    D. _____

    E. _____

2. List crimes of depravity:

    A. _____

    B. _____

    C. _____

    D. _____

    E. _____

3. List the sanctions that may be imposed by a board:

A. _Revocation_

B. _Suspension_

C. _Probation_

D. _Reprimand_

E. _Civil Penalty_

4. List three levels of defined veterinary supervision:

A. _____

B. _____

C. _____

5. List the states where vet techs are not currently credentialed by the state board:

A. _Arizona_

B. _Arkansas_

C. _Colorado_

D. _Idaho_

E. _Louisiana_

F. _Maine_

G. _Maryland_

H. _Minnesota_

I. _New Mexico_

J. _Oregon_

FILL IN THE BLANK

1. State laws are _____ (written and passed) by the legislature and signed into law by the governor.

2. _Practice Act_ _____ is the primary law that governs a profession.

3. The term adopted by NAVTA to refer to a group that has received recognition as a specialty.

   academy

4. The term _Specialist_ should not be used by a tech who is a member of a society.

5. A veterinary technician is considered _certified_ if an application is reviewed and approved by the state board.

6. State criminal history record checks are obtained from the _State_ police.

7. Federal criminal history record checks are obtained from the _Federal Bureau_.

8. Eluding a police officer is an example of _Interference_ with justice.

9. A vet tech in a substance abuse program will have their license put on _Probationary_ status.

10. _Distance_ learning education is done through computers and teleconferences.

11. Most states require continuing _Education_ for license renewal.

12. Practicing beyond the scope of license and _Malpractice_ are the two most important grounds for discipline.

13. _Notice_ means an authority is considering a professional license and contacts the member.

14. Hearings are a matter of _Public_ record.

15. The most severe sanction by a board is the _Revocation_ of a license.

16. _Suspension_ means the vet tech is limited in his or her practice of nursing.

17. A _Censure_ is a public reprimand of a licensee.

18. A fine paid to the licensing board is called a _Civil penalty_.

19. Violations of the practice act are called _Technical_ violations.

20. Conduct that disparages the profession in the eye of the public is called _Unprofessional conduct_.

21. Deviation from or failure to conform to acceptable standards is _Malpractice_.

22. _Incompetence_ is conduct that increases the risk that negligence will occur.

23. _Ethics_ is what is good or bad or right or wrong with moral duty or obligation.

24. _Conflicts_ will arise when the recommendations of the veterinary team is not followed by the client.

25. _____ is when an animal has been placed in life-threatening conditions.

WORD PUZZLE

Answer the following questions to reveal the hidden word:

Letter

1. M o (r) a l   ____

2. __ (__) __ __ __   ____

3. (g) o o d   ____

4. __ __ __ (__) __ __   ____

5. (__) __ __ __   ____

6. (__) __ __   ____

7. e f f e c (t)   ____

8. __ __ __ __ (__) __ __ __   ____

9. B (o) a r d   ____

10. (__) __ __ __ __ __   ____

Unscrambled word __ __ __ __ __ __ __ __ __ __

FILL IN THE BLANK

1. Veterinary technicians must practice good ___Moral___ conduct.

2. Medical records are considered a _____ document.

3. Veterinary technicians must have a ___good___ moral code.

4. To lie in a court of law is called _____.

5. State _____ are enacted.

6. The Veterinary Practice _____ governs state law regarding vet techs.

7. Laws are said to have "force and ___effect___."

8. _____ individuals have had or currently have addiction issues.

9. The committee that governs the practice of a profession is called the ___Board___.

10. Contacting a licensee of disciplinary actions is called _____.

CROSSWORD PUZZLE

Across

2. Practicing beyond the scope of the license granted by the state or negligence in carrying out the duties of the license

4. The administrative agency that governs the practice of veterinary medicine and technology in each state

6. Crimes of _Depravity_ include murder, rape, and distribution of drugs, but also include misdemeanor offenses, such as stalking, harassment, and assault

8. The process of pursuing formal charges against an offender to final judgment

Down

1. Statute

3. Making a false statement under oath

5. A grave crime

7. A wrong or injury for which a court will provide a remedy

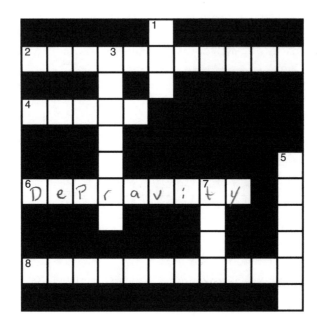

3 Veterinary Practice Management

LEARNING OBJECTIVES

When you have completed this chapter, you will be able to:
1. List the terms used to describe various types of veterinary facilities and describe each type of facility
2. Describe the components and management issues related to the inpatient, outpatient, surgical, and support areas of the small animal hospital
3. List and explain the requirements for maintenance in a veterinary facility
4. List the roles and responsibilities of each member of the veterinary health care team in a variety of practice settings
5. List and describe the steps in the hiring process and appropriate questions to ask potential employees during an interview
6. Describe the components of an effective inventory control program
7. Name the components to consider in setting fees for practice services
8. Describe procedures related to collections, billing, and cash flow
9. Describe the components of effective client communication and methods of handling difficult clients
10. List the components related to marketing of the veterinary practice services and products

TRUE OR FALSE

1. _____ It is important to check the parking lot of the veterinary hospital on a daily basis.
2. _____ Facility design must accommodate the client, staff, and patients.
3. _____ Veterinarians do not typically send problem cases to referral practices.
4. _____ The foundation for good management is online accessibility.
5. _____ Location is not important for a veterinary practice.
6. _____ Animals that escape are the legal responsibility of the hospital.
7. _____ The waiting room must be neat and clean, and free of debris.
8. _____ Well cared for plants help to create a feeling of warmth in the waiting room.
9. _____ The client will spend the most time in the reception area.
10. _____ The patient wards area should be insulated and quiet.
11. _____ The isolation ward has a separate ventilation system.
12. _____ An automatic dishwasher is not recommended for animal dishes.
13. _____ Animals should be discharged when clean and dry.
14. _____ Hot and cold water should be available in the necropsy room.
15. _____ A necropsy room is within the outpatient area of the hospital.
16. _____ It is a good idea to keep a file of warranties and repair information.
17. _____ It is better to have more inventory than not enough.
18. _____ The larger the practice, the more scheduling flexibility is needed.
19. _____ The clients will evaluate the level of care by the look of the building.
20. _____ A written job description should be available to all employees.
21. _____ A file must be kept for all MSDS.
22. _____ Pharmaceutical sales representatives are not a source of useful information.

23. _____ A business method of accounting was developed in 2002 by NVCEI.

24. _____ It is OK to judge a client's ability to pay and adjust the treatment as necessary.

25. _____ Pet insurance covers all services needed for animals.

26. _____ The goal of veterinary offices is to charge fair and equitable fees.

27. _____ Typically 20% of the initial payment is expected at the time of admission.

28. _____ A numbered fee slip can be tracked.

29. _____ Good communication skills will result in personalized services for the client.

30. _____ The main goal of dealing with a difficult client is to resolve their problem.

31. _____ The veterinary technician is not involved with marketing.

32. _____ Explaining hospital services will increase client awareness.

33. _____ A success strategy for practice management is vaccine reminders.

34. _____ Printed brochures can be purchased from AAHA.

35. _____ Clients find sympathy cards and newsletters a nuisance.

MATCHING

A. Match the following areas with the rooms:

1. _____ Wall mounted x-ray viewer   A. Outpatient

2. _____ Bathing/grooming   B. Surgical

3. _____ Public restroom   C. Support

4. _____ Employee lounge   D. Inpatient

B. Match the employee with the specific task performed:

1. _____ Diagnoses and prescribes   A. Receptionist

2. _____ Bookkeeping   B. Veterinarian

3. _____ Prevents nosocomial infections   C. Animal caretakers

4. _____ Facilitates client services   D. Ward nurse

5. _____ Clean and feed patients   E. Practice manager

SHORT ANSWER

1. List eight members of the veterinary health care team:

     A. _____

     B. _____

     C. _____

     D. _____

     E. _____

     F. _____

     G. _____

     H. _____

2. List 12 possible questions an employer could consider when preparing for an interview:

A. _____

B. _____

C. _____

D. _____

E. _____

F. _____

G. _____

H. _____

I. _____

J. _____

K. _____

L. _____

3. List four skills that the vet tech should have in a management position:

A. _____

B. _____

C. _____

D. _____

4. List seven points that should be considered at discharge:

A. _____

B. _____

C. _____

D. _____

E. _____

F. _____

G. _____

5. List four areas the veterinarian will be evaluated on by the client:

A. _____

B. _____

C. _____

D. _____

6. List the 12 major steps in the hiring process:

A. _____

B. _____

C. _____

D. _____

E. _____

F. _____

G. _____

H. _____

I. _____

J. _____

K. _____

L. _____

FILL IN THE BLANK

1. The practice is designed to accommodate the _____ and their

_____.

2. AAHA is an acronym for American Animal Hospital _____.

3. _____ is a primary factor in attracting new clients.

4. Animal _____ within the hospital is a high priority.

5. Grass, hay, and alfalfa should be protected from _____ and _____ in a dry area.

6. The large animal practice makes use of a _____ facility for farm visits.

7. Cattle _____ can be manual or hydraulic.

8. Necropsies in large animals are _____ frequently performed.

9. Major equipment items should have a specific documented _____ schedule.

10. The _____ approach to veterinary practice allows members of the practice to focus on areas of responsibility.

11. The greatest percentage of overhead is in _____.

12. Vet techs should be paid according to the _____ produced.

13. _____ meetings should be held at least once a month.

14. _____ management can best be described by the progress throughout the hospital.

15. _____ is the second largest expense area in the veterinary hospital.

16. The most important person in the practice is the _____.

17. One of the most contagious attitudes is _____.

18. _____ appointments can be scheduled when a 15-minute block is used for appointments.

19. The _____ fees should be increased by the inflation rate.

20. Billings charged by clients for future payments are called _____.

WORD PUZZLE

Answer the following questions and unscramble the letters in parenthesis to reveal the hidden word:

Letter

1. __ __ __ __ __ __ __ __ (__)   ____

2. __ __ __ (__) __   ____

3. __ __ __ (__) __ __   ____

4. __ __ __ __ __ (__) __ __ __   ____

5. __ (__) __ __   ____

6. (__) __ __ __ __ __ __ __ __ __   ____

7. (__) __ __ __   ____

8. __ __ __ __ __ (__)   ____

9. __ __ __ __ __ __ __ __ (__)   ____

10. (__) __ __ __ __ __ __ __ __   ____

Unscrambled word __ __ __ __ __ __ __ __ __ __

1. The area that includes the treatment and isolation rooms is the _____ area.

2. Livestock and horses are classified as _____ animals.

3. It is important to follow _____ guidelines in radiology.

4. Management of drugs, supplies, and pet food is called _____ control.

5. Fee slips in triplicate are a good way to control _____ flow.

6. A technician's _____ should be neat and professional.

7. As a rule, there should be two _____ rooms available for each veterinarian.

8. Assistants should be assigned the most non-_____ producing tasks.

9. The clients should only spend a short time in the _____ area.

10. Client education and product promotion is part of _____ skills.

CROSSWORD PUZZLE

Across

1. Small amounts of discretionary funds in the form of cash
4. Money that is due to the practice from the sale of goods or services
7. Commission that evaluates the economic status of the profession
9. First in, first out for inventory stock rotation
11. Specific period of time that the veterinarian meets with the client and patient for the purpose of diagnosis/treatment
15. Patient that comes into the practice and is treated and leaves without staying
16. A measurement of a practice's inflow and outflow of cash over a period of time
18. Those fees that clients call the practice to find out the charge before the visit
19. All forms of client communication

Down

2. A sheet of specific charges for a patient that follows the patient with them in the practice facility to capture all charges
3. Clients come into the practice at will with no appointment needed
5. The pattern of movement of patients through the practice
6. Clients call ahead and are given a specific time and date to come into the practice
8. Fees that clients do not call the practice to find out the cost. These make up the largest percentage of the fee schedule.
10. Made up of veterinarians, practice manager, veterinary technicians, veterinary assistants, ward attendants, and receptionists
12. Total income less all expenses and taxes
13. Patient that comes into the practice and is hospitalized for further treatment or work-up
14. Total income before expense
17. Reference to a large animal facility where animals are brought to the practice for examination or treatment

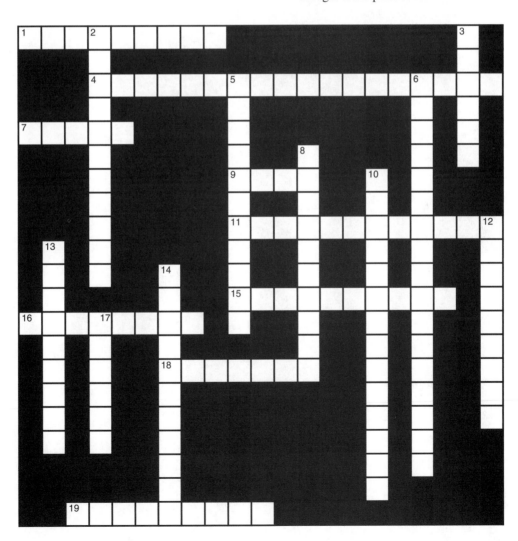

Chapter **3** **Veterinary Practice Management**

4 Computer Applications in Veterinary Practice

LEARNING OBJECTIVES

When you have completed this chapter, you will be able to:

1. Differentiate between operating software and application software
2. Describe methods to research, select, and purchase hardware and software
3. List routine maintenance needs for computer hardware
4. Define the terms server, network, and database
5. Describe the types of data included in the veterinary practice database
6. List the advantages of computerized scheduling and name common features of scheduling software programs
7. List the advantages of electronic medical records and describe common components of an electronic medical record
8. Describe common features of inventory software systems
9. Describe common features of billing software systems
10. List and describe computer applications and websites related to veterinary research and education

TRUE OR FALSE

1. _____ Computers were initially used in the veterinary office for invoices and bookkeeping tasks.
2. _____ As technology advances, so does the role of the computer in veterinary offices.
3. _____ A 32-bit program is a Macintosh program.
4. _____ Computers enable better time management.
5. _____ The monitor is part of the operating software.
6. _____ The operating system translates strikes on the keyboard to letters.
7. _____ Application software are programs that help the user perform tasks.
8. _____ 32-bit programs rely on DOS platforms.
9. _____ Terminals are not connected through a server.
10. _____ Tablet PC's are a type of notebook computer.
11. _____ A notebook computer requires a stylus.
12. _____ Computer technology makes client education obsolete.
13. _____ Cool air damages computer fans and slots.
14. _____ Compressed air is used to clean the inside of the computer case.
15. _____ A single hard drive is sufficient as a backup for information.
16. _____ Research of the software company is needed when considering purchase.
17. _____ Computers make it possible for staff members to add or delete appointments concurrently.
18. _____ Most office software will not identify clients that have missed appointments.
19. _____ Adding computers to the practice will decrease staff burnout.
20. _____ Data is pieces of information.
21. _____ Travel sheets are the best way to increase income.
22. _____ Hundreds of thousands of documents can be stored on 10 CD-ROMs.
23. _____ Deposit slips are automatically generated with computers.

24. _____ VIN is a network for vet techs.

25. _____ Digital radiology is computer generated.

MATCHING

Match each piece of equipment with the specific function:

1. _____ Video capture system   A. Adapted to microscopes for slide imaging

2. _____ Digital radiology   B. Scanner used for radiographs

3. _____ DICOM   C. Ultrasonography

4. _____ Flatbed   D. Transmit and store medical imaging

5. _____ Digital camera   E. Organized dental radiographs

SHORT ANSWER

1. List seven tasks the computer is capable of in the veterinary office:

   A. _____

   B. _____

   C. _____

   D. _____

   E. _____

   F. _____

   G. _____

2. Name six operating systems:

   A. _____

   B. _____

   C. _____

   D. _____

   E. _____

   F. _____

3. List five locations for printers:

   A. _____

   B. _____

   C. _____

   D. _____

   E. _____

4. List four initial questions to ask when deciding to purchase a computer:

A. _____

B. _____

C. _____

D. _____

5. List four parameters in which a patient record can be called up in a query:

A. _____

B. _____

C. _____

D. _____

WORD PUZZLE

Answer the following questions to reveal the hidden word:

	Letter
1. (___) ___ ___ ___ ___	____
2. ___ ___ ___ (___)	____
3. (___) ___ ___ ___ ___ ___	____
4. ___ (___) ___ ___	____
5. (___) ___ ___ ___ ___ ___ ___ ___	____
6. ___ ___ ___ ___ ___ ___ (___) ___ ___ ___ ___	____
7. ___ (___) ___ ___	____
8. (___) ___ ___ ___ ___ ___	____

Unscrambled word __ __ __ __ __ __ __ __ __ __

1. Manually moves the curser

2. Travel sheets have a list of _____ items.

3. _____ centers generate income.

4. The case will collect _____ and must be cleaned monthly.

5. In order to purchase a computer, you must _____ the type needed.

6. Some software synchronizes the _____ scheduler.

7. A password and membership number are needed for the AVMA _____ website.

8. Digital _____ captures images of teeth lesions.

FILL IN THE BLANK

1. _____ software tells different parts of the hardware how to communicate with each other.

2. _____ software are programs that help a user perform certain tasks.

3. A _____ manages the network.

4. It is important to back up information on _____ hard drives.

5. The current trend is for vets to practice as a _____.

6. A _____ menu will offer a link to the appointment scheduler.

7. _____% of all scheduled appointments is generated from reminders.

8. An _____ is created by the computer when the client enters the practice.

9. _____ are printed and mailed monthly.

10. The _____ has improved the quality of information.

5 Medical Records

When you have completed this chapter, you will be able to:

1. List and describe the primary and secondary purposes of the medical record
2. Differentiate between letter-size, card file, and carbonized sheet medical records
3. Differentiate between source-oriented and problem-oriented medical records
4. List and describe the components of a problem-oriented veterinary medical record
5. List the information recorded on a patient medical history
6. Define the SOAP process and explain the types of information included in each portion of the SOAP record
7. List and describe the types of forms and logs commonly used in veterinary practice
8. Describe the requirements of the Comprehensive Drug Abuse and Control Act
9. List and describe the types of filing systems commonly used in veterinary practices
10. Describe ethical and legal issues related to ownership of medical records, release of medical information, and maintenance of medical records

TRUE OR FALSE

1. _____ Veterinary medical records document the treatment of patients.
2. _____ Small animal hospitals use lengthy, extensive medical records.
3. _____ Primary purpose medical records are not clinically based.
4. _____ Medical records document communication with clients.
5. _____ Medical records are legal documents.
6. _____ Equine practitioners often use carbonized forms.
7. _____ Most veterinary hospitals use 5 × 8-size folders.
8. _____ Letter-size folders are stored horizontally.
9. _____ Card files are stored in file drawers.
10. _____ Card files are written in reverse chronological order.
11. _____ AAHA requires letter-size folders.
12. _____ Food animal veterinarians carry records on individual animals.
13. _____ Veterinary medical records are subject to federal and state regulations.
14. _____ SOMR is used in records that have limited space.
15. _____ Most companion animal practices use SOMR and POMR style records.
16. _____ In SOMR records, the most recent information is located last.
17. _____ Teaching hospitals use SOMR records.
18. _____ All veterinary hospitals have the same databases.
19. _____ The master problem list is a defining part of the problem-oriented record.
20. _____ The working problem list helps evaluate symptoms.
21. _____ The ongoing management of patients is in the progress notes.
22. _____ Medications should be stored away from the wards room.
23. _____ Discharge instructions should be reviewed with the client.

25

24. _____ Obtaining written consent before admittance is critical.

25. _____ A necropsy log lists data regarding animal death.

26. _____ The most addictive controlled drugs are schedule V.

27. _____ Alphabetical stickers are usually colored.

28. _____ Records that are 3 years or older can be shredded.

29. _____ Patient records are owned by the client.

30. _____ The only person who should release client information is the veterinarian.

MATCHING

Match each acronym with its description:

1. _____ O   A. Standing, panting, tail wagging

2. _____ S   B. Meds to be given

3. _____ P   C. Diabetes mellitus likely

4. _____ A   D. Temperature, pulse, respiration

SHORT ANSWER

1. List eight pieces of information included in the POVMR record:

A. _____

B. _____

C. _____

D. _____

E. _____

F. _____

G. _____

H. _____

2. List seven pieces of information included in a previous history report:

A. _____

B. _____

C. _____

D. _____

E. _____

F. _____

G. _____

3. List nine specialty departments in a teaching hospital:

A. _____

B. _____

C. _____

D. _____

E. _____

F. _____

G. _____

H. _____

I. _____

4. List eight items listed in a surgery log:

A. _____

B. _____

C. _____

D. _____

E. _____

F. _____

G. _____

H. _____

5. List four guidelines for generating clear, accurate records:

A. _____

B. _____

C. _____

D. _____

WORD PUZZLE

Answer the following questions to reveal the hidden word:

Letter

1. (___) ___ ___ ___ ___ ___ ___   ___

2. (___) ___ ___ ___ ___   ___

3. ___ ___ ___ (___) ___ ___   ___

4. ___ ___(___) ___ ___ ___ ___   ___

5. ___ ___ ___ ___ (___)   ___

6. ___(___) ___ ___   ___

7. ___ ___ ___ ___ ___ ___ ___ ___ ___(___) ___   ___

Unscrambled word ___ ___ ___ ___ ___ ___ ___

1. Before veterinary services rendered, a _____ form should be signed.

2. In the veterinary hospital, controlled _____ must be logged.

3. _____ oriented records are used in limited space records.

4. A complete medical _____ is needed for a justified diagnosis.

5. _____ coded tabs with year are convenient for the front desk staff.

6. _____ records can be embarrassing for a hospital.

7. Animals with reportable diseases must be _____ to reduce the threat of spread.

FILL IN THE BLANK

1. The primary purpose of medical records is to _____ excellent care.

2. The medical record documents _____ with the client.

3. The medical record is a _____ document, admissible in a court of law.

4. It is important to keep records _____ and _____.

5. To maintain _____, markers must be removed from medical records.

6. _____-size folders are 8 × 10 records.

7. 5 × 8 records are called _____ file system.

8. _____ large animal practices use carbonized sheets.

9. The _____ of a patient is the first bit of critical information that helps the veterinarian with problem solving.

10. The physical examination must be done _____ and carefully.

11. A _____ forms the foundation of information for a diagnosis.

12. The ongoing management of patients is documented on _____ notes.

13. The _____ portion of the SOAP includes temperature, pulse, and respiration.

14. A treatment _____ may be used in the ward area.

15. A common source of miscommunication is in regards to the _____ of services.

16. The _____ Drug Abuse Act is a federal law regulating the possession of drugs.

17. The _____ file system generates fewer filing mistakes.

18. VMDB is a _____ data bank located at Purdue University.

19. _____ guidelines for medical records vary from state to state.

20. A separate _____ record must be kept for each controlled drug.

6 Occupational Health and Safety in Veterinary Hospitals

LEARNING OBJECTIVES

When you have completed this chapter, you will be able to:

1. Describe the role of OSHA in veterinary practice safety
2. List the general requirements of the federal laws related to workplace safety
3. Explain proper methods for lifting objects and animals
4. List common workplace hazards in a veterinary facility
5. Describe the requirements and the OSHA "Right To Know" law
6. Explain the acronym MSDS and describe the components of an MSDS
7. List the hazards associated with the use of ethylene oxide, formalin, glutaraldehyde, anesthetic gases, and compressed gases
8. Define the term zoonotic disease and list common zoonotic diseases encountered in the veterinary clinic
9. List methods to minimize hazards associated with animal handling
10. Describe proper handling of hazardous and medical wastes

TRUE OR FALSE

1. _____ As a staff member of the veterinary hospital, technicians are exposed to hazards.
2. _____ The purpose of safety programs is to reduce or eliminate injury.
3. _____ OSHA enforces only local laws that ensure compliance.
4. _____ Educating employees is a requirement of OSHA.
5. _____ In the veterinary office, all hazards must be eliminated.
6. _____ Radiation exposure reports must be shared with the employee.
7. _____ The employee is responsible for learning the rules of safety.
8. _____ The employer cannot set rules of conduct for the staff.
9. _____ The practice owner has the right to be present during an OSHA inspection.
10. _____ Employees should know where the Hospital Safety Manual is kept.
11. _____ Open toed shoes are safe in the veterinary hospital.
12. _____ Heavy equipment should be stored on lower shelves.
13. _____ Eating on the job should be limited to the employee lounge.
14. _____ Equipment with grounded plugs can be used with extension cords.
15. _____ The first responsibility during a fire is to alert others.
16. _____ Working bottles of hazardous chemicals should be stored with screw-on lids.
17. _____ Ethylene oxide can be used to sterilize rubber gloves.
18. _____ The most common form of injury in the veterinary hospital is animal-related.
19. _____ All zoonotic diseases are easily passed to humans.
20. _____ Scatter radiation is not harmful to humans.
21. _____ It is acceptable to use kitty litter to absorb spilled anesthetic agent.
22. _____ Anesthesic agents are metabolized completely during surgery.
23. _____ Removing the needle from the syringe is not required for disposal.

24. _____ Cytotoxic drugs are not used to treat cancer patients.

25. _____ Thorough hand washing is important to deter the spread of disease.

SHORT ANSWER

1. List five employee responsibilities required by OSHA regulations:

   A. _____

   B. _____

   C. _____

   D. _____

   E. _____

2. List four conditions under which you should not attempt to fight a fire.

   A. _____

   B. _____

   C. _____

   D. _____

3. List five of the most common chemicals used in the veterinary office:

   A. _____

   B. _____

   C. _____

   D. _____

   E. _____

4. List five precautions you must take when using EtO:

   A. _____

   B. _____

   C. _____

   D. _____

   E. _____

5. List five guidelines for a pregnant woman to avoid exposure to toxoplasmosis:

   A. _____

   B. _____

C. _____

D. _____

E. _____

WORD PUZZLE

Answer the following questions to reveal the hidden word:

Letter

1. __ __ __ __ (__) __ __ __ __ __   ____

2. __ __ __ __ (__) __ __ __   ____

3. (__) __ __ __ __ __ __ __   ____

4. __ __ __ __ (__)   ____

5. (__) __ __ __ __ __ __ __   ____

6. (__) __ __ __   ____

7. __ (__) __ __ __ __ __ __ __   ____

Unscrambled word __ __ __ __ __ __ __

1. Improper storage of _____ gas cylinders can cause injury.

2. _____ is typically used for tissue preservation.

3. When _____ exotic animals, their defenses can injure.

4. Lifting requires the use of _____, not the back.

5. Raccoons, bats, and skunks spread _____ diseases such as rabies.

6. Material Safety _____ Sheets are in a binder for all employees to view.

7. Never operate _____ without a safety guard in place.

FILL IN THE BLANK

1. OSHA stands for the Occupational Safety and Health _____.

2. If an employee is terminated for willful violation of safety rules, they will likely be denied

   _____ benefits.

3. The _____ is required to provide safety equipment and training.

4. Written safety-related policies are known as the Hospital Safety _____.

5. Some injuries are caused by _____ and/or dirty areas.

6. Chemicals on shelves should be stored at _____ level or below.

7. One of the first rules of safety is to _____ appropriately.

8. Excessive _____ may be a hazard when animals struggle during restraint.

9. One in every five workplace injuries is _____ related.

10. The best defense against ergonomic injury is good _____.

11. _____ and _____ are always stored away from biologic materials.

12. _____ from autoclave steam and cautery irons can be serious.

13. Portable dryers or electrical equipment cords must be properly _____.

14. _____ items such as gasoline and ether must be stored in an approved cabinet.

15. Newspapers, boxes, and cleaning supplies must be stored at least _____ feet away from an ignition source.

16. Always keep nonclient doors _____ to prevent unauthorized entry.

17. OSHA's "_____ to Know" law requires training for all hazardous chemicals in the facility.

18. Employees must know the location of eye _____ stations.

19. _____ is a potent chemical used to sterilize hand instruments without the use of an autoclave.

20. Since injury cannot be eliminated, the next best thing is to _____ it.

21. If you enter an animal's stall, remain on the side by the _____ for easy escape.

22. Noise levels above _____ dB are considered dangerous.

23. Use a _____ fan to keep fumes at a safe level.

24. _____ is a viral disease of humans and animals spread by contact with saliva.

25. *Borrelia burgdorferi* is the cause of _____ disease.

26. Microsporum is a fungus of the skin known as _____.

27. _____ mange can typically affect the bra line or waist band areas.

28. High-dose exposure to _____ can cause cell damage.

29. Long-term exposure to _____ agents can lead to liver and kidney damage.

30. The most serious hazard from needles and sharp objects is by a _____ or laceration.

CROSSWORD PUZZLE

Across

1. A class of drugs that are toxic to cells, and are frequently used to treat cancer
5. A type of outlet or circuit designed to prevent electrocution by detecting the leakage of current, such as what happens when an electrical current comes in contact with water
6. An agency of the U.S. Department of Health and Human Services working to protect public health and the safety of people
8. Any piece of clothing or article that is worn by the user that is designed to prevent injury
9. A viral infection of cats that is not considered contagious to humans but is highly contagious from cat to cat
13. The study of how the human body moves
14. A gaseous substance used as a sterilant for instruments and articles that would be damaged by steam sterilization (2 words)
16. The agency of the U.S. Government that is charged with making sure places of employment are safe and healthy
17. A biologic organism (fungi, bacteria, virus, etc.) that causes disease or illness
19. The device used to capture, transport, or remove waste anesthetic gases from an anesthesia machine
21. The gas used in inhalation anesthetic machines that is not metabolized by the patient and given off in respiration
22. Also known as sarcoptic mange
24. A protozoan parasite in the small intestine of mammals, which is spread from one animal to another (including humans) by ingestion of water contaminated with cysts or contact with infected feces

Down

2. Caused by a single-celled parasite, this disease is primarily a disease of concern for pregnant women and people with compromised immune systems
3. Microscopic, single-celled parasites that spread from one animal to another (including humans) by contact with infected feces
4. The aqueous solution of formaldehyde used as a disinfectant and tissue fixative in medicine
6. A device that filters or "focuses" a stream of x-rays so that only those inside the open part of the device are allowed through
7. The use of chemical substances to treat disease, primarily with drugs used to treat cancer
10. A measure of loudness
11. Also known as Lyme disease
12. A disease that is common to both animals and humans
15. A contagious fungal infection of the skin
18. A commonly used acronym for a hazardous chemical
20. A viral disease spread by the saliva of infected animals, primarily through bite wounds
23. A medical condition in which the median nerve of the hand is compressed at the wrist, leading to pain, paresthesia, and muscle weakness in the forearm and hand

Chapter **6** Occupational Health and Safety in Veterinary Hospitals

2. The ideal environment to rope a horse is:
   a. In an open field
   b. In a round pen made of wood
   c. In a round pen made of pipes
   d. In a grazing pasture

3. A single handler should approach a foal:
   a. Directly from the front
   b. From the rear
   c. From the left side only
   d. Midway between the head and tail

4. When a cow is cast, what position should it be kept in to minimize the chance of bloat?
   a. Lateral recumbency
   b. Cows should never be cast
   c. On their left side
   d. Dorsal recumbency

5. Which venipuncture site used in dogs requires that the dog be placed on its side?
   a. Cephalic
   b. Jugular
   c. Saphenous
   d. Lumbar

FILL IN THE BLANK

1. The most obvious reason for restraint of an animal is to _____.

2. _____ is necessary for the purpose of physical examination, diagnostic, or therapeutic procedures.

3. _____ are used to protect the animal from self-mutilation following procedures.

4. In the _____, the sympathetic nervous system releases the hormone epinephrine from the adrenal gland, causing an increased heart rate and a subsequent increase in blood flow to the skeletal muscles, lungs, and brain.

5. The clinical stare of veterinary personnel as they examine a dog can be taken as a _____ challenge by a dog.

6. _____ should be worn when attempting to rope any animal.

7. Lifting a horse's _____ leg is only done for examination procedures. It is not performed as a means of restraint.

8. The horse's tail may be tied during _____, _____, and

   _____.

9. _____ is the key to the restraint of a horse lying in lateral recumbency.

10. To examine a horse's mouth and dental arcades, the handler's hand nearest the horse's nose is inserted into the

   _____ space. The hand must be kept in a _____ position to protect the handler's fingers from being bitten.

11. The _____ is a stainless steel tube commonly used in cattle for passage of oral-gastric tubes.

12. When using chemical restraint on ruminants it must be remembered that they are sensitive to

_____, such as xylazine.

13. A useful technique for capturing goats is the use of a _____.

14. To administer fluid to a sheep via an oral syringe, the jaw should not be lifted above a line _____. The nozzle of the syringe should be inserted well back into the mouth so that the fluid does not dribble out. Caution

must be used to keep the animal's head under control so as not to traumatize the _____.

15. The correct position of the head during jugular venipuncture should be no more than slightly above

_____° from the neck.

16. _____ is recommended to extend a turtles or tortoises head away from the shell over the use of delivery forceps.

17. A mouse should be initially restrained _____, whereas a hamster should be initially

restrained by the _____.

TRUE OR FALSE

1. _____ The veterinarian and associated personnel are legally responsible for any injuries to the client while performing a veterinary procedure.
2. _____ A handler is less likely to be seriously injured by a kick if she stands very close to (up against) a horse's hind quarters rather than 3 feet behind the horse.
3. _____ Under any circumstances, a handler should stand on the same side of the horse as the veterinarian working on the horse.
4. _____ A cow in a narrow chute will avoid a human, so generally it is safe to move in and about chutes when driving cattle.
5. _____ While horses generally kick straight to the rear, cattle usually kick forward and to the side with a hooking action.
6. _____ Heavy tranquilization is the most foolproof method of keeping a snappy dog from biting and an agitated horse from kicking.
7. _____ The feline's first line of defense is its teeth.

SHORT ANSWER

1. List five examples of why you must assess the condition of the capture area *before* beginning to capture the animal:

   A. _____

   B. _____

   C. _____

   D. _____

   E. _____

Chapter **7** **Restraint and Handling of Animals**

2. List three reasons why proper restraint is necessary:

A. _____

B. _____

C. _____

3. Why is a female rabbit (doe) always taken to the males (buck) cage for mating?

_____

_____

4. List the four classic signs that a dog is being intimidated and may attack:

A. _____

B. _____

C. _____

D. _____

5. Describe six head restraint techniques used for cattle.

A. _____

B. _____

C. _____

D. _____

E. _____

F. _____

6. List the steps in casting an adult cow:

A. _____

B. _____

C. _____

D. _____

E. _____

F. _____

7. What steps should be used to capture a pig inside a small enclosure?

A. _____

B. _____

C. _____

D. _____

E. _____

8. A dog you are restraining suddenly breaks free and is frantically running around in the clinic. What are some techniques you should try to recapture the dog?

A. _____

B. _____

C. _____

D. _____

E. _____

F. _____

G. _____

9. Give two reasons why you should offer the back of your hand to an unknown dog instead of your palm.

A. _____

B. _____

10. Describe how you would restrain a dog or cat on an examination table for cephalic venipuncture.

_____

_____

_____

_____

_____

_____

_____

_____

_____

_____

11. Describe two techniques to prevent a turtle or tortoise from walking during an examination.

A. _____

B. _____

12. List two common errors in positioning a dog for jugular venipuncture and how they interfere in the procedure:

A. _____

B. _____

13. Why may jugular venipuncture be more appropriate for some cats?

_____

14. List things that will stress an exotic animal in a veterinary hospital:

A. _____

B. _____

C. _____

D. _____

15. List the steps to capture and restrain a small bird:

A. _____

B. _____

C. _____

D. _____

E. _____

F. _____

G. _____

H. _____

I. _____

J. _____

16. The general approach to restraint of any snake is to:

_____

17. A client brings in a rabbit complaining that it is not eating. The vet wants to view its mouth to see if the incisor teeth need to be trimmed. How would you restrain the rabbit for examination of the mouth?

_____

_____

_____

18. Describe four classic signs seen in a dog about to bite you because she is afraid of you.

    A. _____

    B. _____

    C. _____

    D. _____

19. What is the key to restraining a horse in lateral recumbency to keep it lying down?

_____

20. Briefly describe, in five steps, how you would capture a dog that has escaped from the kennel and is running loose down the street.

    A. _____

    B. _____

    C. _____

    D. _____

    E. _____

21. List the three most commonly accessed veins in the cat.

    A. _____

    B. _____

    C. _____

Restraint and Handling of Animals

```
N  H  D  D  K  O  R  P  W  U  T  T
O  A  R  E  M  T  N  E  E  R  M  W
I  W  Y  G  O  L  O  H  T  E  O  I
T  E  S  L  T  A  I  C  E  L  T  T
A  U  T  O  T  O  M  I  Z  E  A  C
D  N  D  V  W  O  R  T  C  T  E  H
O  L  C  I  E  D  I  S  R  A  E  N
M  O  I  N  L  H  A  I  N  P  S  G
M  A  E  G  I  U  C  N  G  E  K  T
O  L  F  A  C  T  I  O  N  T  C  A
C  P  I  T  L  P  D  G  H  U  O  R
C  M  A  T  E  R  N  A  L  M  T  A
A  K  C  I  K  W  O  C  P  O  S  T
```

accommodation	agonistic	autotomize
cast	cow kick	degloving
ethology	halter	maternal
near side	olfaction	pinnae
sow	stocks	tapetum
twitch		

8 History and Physical Examination

LEARNING OBJECTIVES

When you have completed this chapter, you will be able to:

1. Explain the role of the veterinary technician in obtaining the patient medical history
2. List questions commonly used to obtain a patient medical history for small and large animals
3. List the sections of information found in a medical history for small animal patients
4. Describe the types of information contained in each section of the patient medical history for small animal patients
5. List the sections of information found in a medical history for large animal patients
6. Describe the types of information contained in each section of the patient medical history for large animal patients
7. Describe the general procedures used to obtain a patient physical examination in dogs and cats
8. Describe the general procedures used to obtain a patient physical examination in horses and cattle
9. Discuss the methods for performing a comprehensive evaluation of each of the body systems
10. List and describe unique procedures used in examination of horses and cattle

MATCHING

Match the question in *Column A* with the correct answer in *Column B*

Column A

1. _____ Increased lens opacity
2. _____ Nictitating membrane
3. _____ Yellow discoloration of MM or sclera
4. _____ Absence of a palpable pulse with heart beat
5. _____ Decreased body temperature
6. _____ Limb weakness associated with abnormal gait
7. _____ Thoracic fluid accumulation
8. _____ Excessive urine production
9. _____ Pupil asymmetry
10. _____ Normal variation in heart rhythm
11. _____ Presence of a third heart sound
12. _____ Excessive water consumption
13. _____ Containing or producing pus
14. _____ High-pitched inspiratory wheeze
15. _____ Itching
16. _____ Bright red mucous membranes
17. _____ Malperfusion of blood flow
18. _____ Pus in the uterus

Column B

A. Purulent
B. Hyperemia
C. Shock
D. Gallop rhythm
E. Polydipsia
F. Stridor
G. Anisocoria
H. Pyometra
I. Sinus arrhythmia
J. Pulse deficit
K. Nuclear sclerosis
L. Ataxia
M. Hypothermia
N. Pleural effusion
O. Pruritus
P. Third eyelid
Q. Icterus
R. Polyuria

TRUE OR FALSE

1. _____ The ovaries cannot be palpated in the dog or cat.

2. _____ Masses should be described based on whether they are cutaneous or subcutaneous.

3. _____ Axillary and inguinal lymph nodes are typically palpable only when they are enlarged.

4. _____ Evaluation of muscle tone cannot be determined by anal sphincter tone.

5. _____ Aggressive pinching of the bones of the toe with hemostats is testing for deep pain or for withdrawal.

6. _____ Ejection murmurs in the horse should disappear with exercise or exertion.

7. _____ Animals with neurologic disease can still have normal gain and posture.

8. _____ The urethra can be palpated during a rectal examination.

9. _____ Penile examination of the male cat is not typically performed unless the patient is sedated.

10. _____ Horses cannot breathe through their mouth.

11. _____ Abdominal palpation should be consistently performed as part of the physical examination.

12. _____ Canine testicles typically should descend into the scrotum by 8 months of age.

13. _____ Mammary glands should be gently palpated for heat, swelling, or discharge.

14. _____ The urinary bladder is located in the cranial-dorsal aspect of the abdomen in the dog and cat.

15. _____ Abdominal auscultation should be performed on the left side of the horse.

16. _____ Cardiac sounds S-1 and S-2 are components of two heart beats.

17. _____ Ejection murmurs are the result of large volumes of blood moving at slow speeds through the heart valves.

18. _____ Skin turgor is less reliable in assessing hydration status in the geriatric animal.

19. _____ Resting heart rates are typically lower in large animals.

20. _____ Eructation is a normal finding in the ruminant.

21. _____ Questions about the severity, duration, frequency, progression, trigger situations, time of day, and character of the problem should be asked about every new problem, in addition to the reason the client brought the animal in for evaluation.

22. _____ The systems review is part of a patient's medical history.

23. _____ During the physical examination, only observations that appear significant need be recorded.

24. _____ If a scale is available, an animal should be weighed at every visit to the veterinarian.

25. _____ The oral cavity of a cat should *not* be examined when the cat is awake because of the risk of getting bitten.

MULTIPLE CHOICE

1. Heart murmurs are assessed for:
   a. Loudness, character, and timing
   b. Heart rate
   c. Pulse deficits
   d. Abnormal rhythm

2. Which aspect of the physical examination can help assess GI motility?
   a. Diet history
   b. Rectal temperature
   c. Abdominal auscultation
   d. Body condition scoring

3. What are the anatomic landmarks commonly used to auscultate a horse's heart?
   a. Level of the shoulder for heart base

   b. Intercostal space 6 on right side
   c. Cranial border of the flexor muscle
   d. Midsternum

4. Complete absence of GI sounds is termed:
   a. Borborygmi
   b. Ileus
   c. Colic
   d. Normal

5. Icteric mucous membranes suggest:
   a. Liver disease
   b. Cardiac disease
   c. Hemolysis
   d. a and c

6. Key aspects in determining hydration status include:
   a. Capillary refill time
   b. Body condition score
   c. Skin turgor
   d. a and c

7. The most common cause of increased capillary refill time in the horse:
   a. Shock and dehydration
   b. Neurologic disease
   c. Poor nutrition
   d. Fever

8. Purple-colored gums that appear along the margin of the teeth are termed:
   a. Hyperemia
   b. Icterus
   c. Toxic lines
   d. Petechiations

9. Gas accumulations can be detected in the ruminant by:
   a. Percussion and auscultation of the abdomen
   b. Presence of a "papple" shaped abdomen
   c. Radiographic analysis only
   d. a and b

10. The physical examination of the ruminant typically begins with:
    a. Abdominal auscultation
    b. Rectal palpation
    c. Temperature
    d. Visual observation of behavior and interaction with the herd

11. Conscious proprioception is tested by:
    a. Aggressive toe-pinching with hemostats
    b. Checking reflexes with a pleximeter
    c. Picking up one paw and placing the dorsal surface onto the floor
    d. Pupillary light reflex

12. Lymph node enlargement may indicate:
    a. Hypertension
    b. Hypotension
    c. Neoplasia
    d. Poor nutrition

13. A neurologic examination includes:
    a. Abdominal auscultation
    b. Evaluation of mentation
    c. Postural reactions
    d. b and c

14. Common skin abnormalities suggestive of a coagulopathy include:
    a. Papules or pustules
    b. Petechia or ecchymosis

c. Wheals or hives
d. Alopecia

15. During a routine cardiac auscultation, a murmur is detected solely on the right side. Which valve is most likely insufficient?
    a. Tricuspid
    b. Pulmonic
    c. Aortic
    d. Mitral

16. Auscultation of pulmonary crackles may indicate:
    a. Cardiac disease
    b. Neurologic insufficiency
    c. Severe allergies
    d. Hypothermia

17. Sinus arrhythmias can best be described as:
    a. Increase in heart rate during inspiration
    b. Increase in heart rate during expiration
    c. Pulse deficits
    d. a and b

18. A 12-week-old kitten, recently adopted by the local humane society, has a history of lethargy and anorexia. What is the most appropriate first response?
    a. Immediately separate the pet from its owner and take to an isolated area
    b. Obtain a thorough history from the owner
    c. Assess respiratory function
    d. Obtain a heart rate and body temperature

19. Weak pulses generally indicate:
    a. Sinus arrhythmia
    b. Hyperthermia
    c. Poor perfusion
    d. Inflammation

20. Which is typically **not** a factor in hyperthermia:
    a. Infection
    b. Neoplasia
    c. Inflammation
    d. Decreased capillary refill time

21. Assessment of a patient's perfusion may best be achieved by:
    a. Pulse strength
    b. Capillary refill time
    c. Lung sounds
    d. a and b

22. Jugular pulses may indicate:
    a. Poor perfusion
    b. Hypothermia
    c. Hypertension
    d. None of the above

23. Heart murmurs may be a result of:
    a. Hypothermia
    b. Anemia
    c. Pneumonia
    d. Severe allergies

24. The area on the chest where a murmur is the loudest is termed:
    a. Palpable thrill
    b. Point of maximum intensity
    c. Systolic peak
    d. Target point

25. Pulse deficits are determined by:
    a. ECG
    b. Blood pressure
    c. Cardiac auscultation and arterial palpation
    d. Capillary refill time

26. What is the most common cause of pulse irregularities in the horse?
    a. Stress
    b. Hypoxia
    c. Congential defects
    d. Second degree heart block

27. Equine heart sounds are best auscultated on which side of the chest?
    a. Left
    b. Right
    c. Midsternum
    d. Heart sounds can be equally heard on both sides

28. Which statement regarding the rectal examination is most accurate?
    a. Palpation and inspection of the rectal wall should be performed on every feline patient.
    b. A fecal flotation should be performed after every rectal examination.
    c. Anal gland expression should be performed on every canine patient.
    d. The prostate gland should be palpated on every male canine patient.

29. Most likely evidence of an anal gland infection includes:
    a. Thick material easily discharged
    b. Blood- or pus-filled discharge
    c. A palpably distended anal sac
    d. Diarrhea

30. Palpation of the canine ear is necessary to aid in the diagnosis of:
    a. Coagulation disorders
    b. External parasites
    c. Aural hematoma
    d. Hearing difficulty

MATCHING

Pair each of the following mucous membrane colors to their respective cause.
1. __F__ Pink
2. __D__ Pale pink
3. __A__ Blue
4. __C__ Yellow
5. __E__ Brick red
6. __B__ White

A. Cyanosis; respiratory failure
B. Severe anemia, circulatory failure
C. Liver disease, hemolysis
D. Pain, mild anemia, hypothermia
E. Hyperthermia, vasodilation, sepsis
F. Adequate perfusion and oxygenation

CIRCLE ALL THAT APPLY

1. A neurologic examination of every patient should include:
    a. Gait
    b. Visual acuity
    c. Pulse strength
    d. Mentation
    e. Menace reflex
    f. PLR
    g. Cardiac auscultation
    h. Rectal palpation

2. Hydration status can best be assessed by which of the following?
    a. Stool composition
    b. Skin turgor
    c. Body condition score
    d. Patient history
    e. Body temperature
    f. Lung sounds

3. What are the physical examination findings that may indicate a patient is experiencing respiratory difficulty?
   a. Abdominal effort
   b. Increased respiratory rate
   c. High-pitched inspiratory noises
   d. Normal auscultation
   e. Increased heart rate

4. A neurologic examination typically does *not* include which of the following (circle all that apply):
   a. Gait evaluation
   b. Visual acuity
   c. Pulse strength
   d. Mentation
   e. Lymph node palpation
   f. Menace reflex
   g. Pupillary light response

5. A 12-year-old, female-spayed outdoor Golden Retriever has been referred to your hospital for surgery to remove an abdominal mass. Which questions listed below are appropriate to ask the client in the examination room? (Circle all that apply and include a brief explanation as to the validity of the question.)
   a. Is your pet on heartworm prevention?
   b. Has your pet ever received a blood transfusion?
   c. Do you have any other pets at home?
   d. Does your pet have any known allergies?
   e. Has she had any recent vomiting?
   f. What is her normal routine?

CASE DISCUSSION

1. A 16-year-old, female-spayed Burmese domestic long-haired cat named Asia presents for vomiting of 4 days duration. The cat is current on vaccinations and is strictly an indoor cat. This is the first visit to the veterinarian's office for being sick. Give a brief explanation as to the validity of each question asked of the client.
   A. Are there any other cats in the house?
   B. Can you describe the vomitus?
   C. What time does she vomit? When do you feed her?
   D. What does she like to eat?
   E. When was the last time she was normal?
   F. Do you keep the windows open at home?
   G. Does she drink out of the toilet?
   H. Has there been a change in her appetite? Water consumption?
   I. Does she like to play with toys?

2. Asia is quiet and depressed, but purrs as you begin your physical examination. Findings are as follows:
   A. Body temperature of 97.5° F
   B. Heart rate of 235 beats per minute
   C. Poor pulse quality
   D. Pale, dry mucous membranes
   E. Normal respiratory effort
   F. No abnormal lung sounds noted
   G. Decreased capillary refill time
   H. Poor body condition score
   I. Increased skin turgor
   J. Cool extremities
   K. Severe halitosis
   L. Poor dentition
   M. Vomit stains under chin and sternum
   N. Oral ulcerations along gingiva

Chapter **8** History and Physical Examination

3. Which six findings suggest poor perfusion? Explain.

* _____

* _____

* _____

* _____

* _____

* _____

* _____

4. Which four physical examination findings suggest dehydration?

* _____

* _____

* _____

* _____

5. Should Asia be taken immediately to triage? Explain.

_____

_____

_____

6. Asia's heart rate is 235 beats per minute. Explain the most likely cause(s).

A. _____

B. _____

C. _____

D. _____

E. _____

F. _____

G. _____

7. It would be prudent to reauscult Asia's heart once she is acclimated to the hospital environment, particularly before her intravenous fluids are instituted. Explain.

_____

_____

_____

_____

8. The owner inquires about her halitosis, and tells you that it was noticed several months ago. What other physical examination findings listed above are possibly linked to the bad breath?

A. _____

B. _____

C. _____

9. What are the most likely causes for the oral ulcerations?

A. _____

B. _____

C. _____

D. _____

MATCHING

Interpretation of Respiratory Sounds

Match the auscultation finding (Column A) with correct medical term (Column B)

Column A

1. _____ Snap-crackle-pop sounds on inspiration
2. _____ A whine or high-pitched inspiratory wheeze, typically heard over upper airway
3. _____ A "musical" sound noted mainly on expiration
4. _____ Congested or fluttering upper airway noises heard mainly on inspiratory and but also on expiration; common in the Brach cephalic breed

Column B

A. Stertor

B. Wheeze

C. Crackles

D. Stridor

CASE STUDY

1. The receptionist asks you to take a phone call from an upset client. The client just discovered her puppy has climbed into a cabinet and has chewed through several cleaning detergent bottles and feels the puppy has swallowed some of the contents. What should you tell her to do?

_____

_____

_____

2. What questions are important to ask?

A. _____

B. _____

C. _____

SHORT ANSWER

1. Involuntary, rhythmic movement of the eyes is termed _____.

2. The eye blinking in response to touch at the medial canthus is termed _____.

3. Name the four most common areas to find petechia or ecchymosis in the patient with suspected coagulopathy.

A. _____

B. _____

C. _____

D. _____

4. List the most convenient anatomic locations locating a pulse rate in the dog. The horse?

A. _____

B. _____

C. _____

TRUE OR FALSE

1. _____ In viewing a normal ruminant abdomen, the left side may appear slightly fuller than the right.
2. _____ When taking a history of large animal patients, it is important to focus more on the chief clinical problem as opposed to the entire herd health and husbandry.
3. _____ The large animal signalment should include intended use of the animal (e.g., breeding, commercial use).
4. _____ In nonemergency situations, the patient history should be taken before the physical examination.
5. _____ Puppies may have resting heart rates up to 300 beats per minute.
6. _____ Shared food or water can allow transmission of infectious agents in the herd.
7. _____ Pulling back of a limb after an aggressive toe pinch does not necessarily indicate an intact withdrawal reflex.
8. _____ A feces-filled rectum may interfere with the accuracy of a rectal temperature.

MATCHING

The following four questions concern observations made or tests performed during a physical examination. Match the correct body system with which each observation or test corresponds.

1. _____ Capillary refill time
2. _____ Mammary gland palpation and expression of milk
3. _____ Ability to swallow
4. _____ Femoral or patellar reflex

    A. Eyes
    B. Gastrointestinal
    C. Respiratory
    D. Circulatory
    E. Genitourinary
    F. Neurologic
    G. Integumentary
    H. Musculoskeletal

SHORT ANSWER

1. Name the three pairs of peripheral lymph nodes palpable in the normal animal.

   A. _____

   B. _____

   C. _____

2. Name the two pairs of peripheral lymph nodes *not* generally palpable in the normal animal.

   A. _____

   B. _____

3. Briefly describe how you would perform a complete lung examination, including the best patient position in which to perform the examination.

   _____

   _____

   _____

4. A heart murmur is heard over the right, cranioventral chest wall. Which heart valve is most likely diseased?

   _____

5. Name six functions present in an animal with normal cranial nerves.

   A. _____

   B. _____

   C. _____

   D. _____

   E. _____

   F. _____

6. How would you describe a heart murmur heard over the mitral valve that occurs throughout systole, gets louder throughout the duration of the murmur, and is of low-to-moderate intensity?

_____

CROSSWORD PUZZLE

Across

6. The age, sex, and breed of a patient
9. Complete absence of borborygmus, associated with absence of intestinal motility
12. Accumulation of gas within certain portions of the GI tract that produces visible enlargement of the abdomen
13. A condition of decreased perfusion and decreased oxygen delivery to vital organs
16. A foul odor to the breath
17. Enlargement of one or both kidneys
19. Nostrils
20. Inspiratory noise similar to snoring
24. Elevation of body temperature
26. Elevation of body temperature caused by a temporary increase in the body's thermoregulatory set-point usually caused by infection, inflammation, or neoplasia
27. A type of murmur that is a normal heart sound in large animals produced by large volumes of blood moving at high speeds through the heart valves
28. Under the armpit
29. The technique of identifying abdominal gas accumulations by simultaneous percussion and auscultation of the abdominal wall
30. A behavioral problem where the animal obsessively grooms to the point of damaging the hair and skin

Down

1. Skin lesions caused by the self-trauma of scratching
2. The presence of glucose in urine
3. Decreased circulating blood volume
4. High-pitched inspiratory noise usually caused by obstruction to airflow at the pharynx or larynx
5. Yellow discoloration of the skin and mucous membranes resulting from accumulation of excess bilirubin
7. Audible intestinal motility sound produced by intestinal peristalsis
8. Uncoordinated gait usually associated with neurologic dysfunction
10. An aortic __ is a congenital cardiac anomaly resulting in resistance to the flow of blood from the left ventricle into the aorta
11. Presence of pus in the uterus, usually caused by bacterial infection
14. Inflammation of the colon
15. The type of hernia that results in herniation of abdominal contents through the pelvic diaphragm resulting in swelling on either side of the anus
16. Decreased body temperature
18. In or of the ear
21. The type of hemorrhage that results in small, visible, pinpoint hemorrhage lesions <1 mm in diameter
22. Drinking more water than normal
23. Plural __ is fluid buildup in the space surrounding the lungs within the thorax
25. The mental activity or acuity of a patient

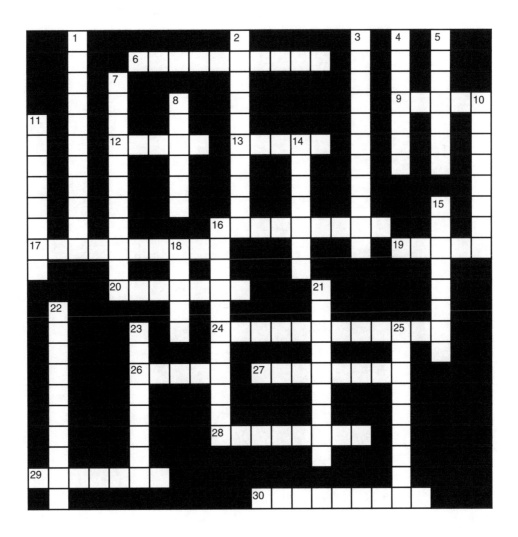

9 Preventive Health Programs

When you have completed this chapter, you will be able to:

1. Describe storage, handling, reconstitution, and routes of administration for animal vaccines
2. Differentiate between core and elective vaccines
3. Name the core vaccines for dogs and cats
4. Name the elective vaccines for dogs and cats
5. List recommended anatomic locations for each vaccine commonly administered to dogs and cats
6. List and describe potential vaccine adverse reactions in dogs and cats
7. List commonly used products to prevent parasite infection and infestation in dogs and cats
8. List and describe commonly performed diagnostic screening tests in dogs and cats
9. Provide a general outline of a routine preventive health program for horses
10. List the core and elective vaccines used in livestock

FILL IN THE BLANK

1. The effective immune periods of licensed rabies vaccines are either _____ or

   _____ years.

2. In addition to protecting against itself, the current canine adenovirus vaccine-2 (CAV-2) also protects against

   _____.

3. The intranasal vaccine for infectious tracheobronchitis should be administered to a puppy

   _____ to _____ weeks before being admitted to a
   boarding facility or before being shipped.

4. A common source of giardiasis for dogs is _____.

5. The canine parvovirus of cats is known as _____.

6. Oral ulcerations in cats may be seen due to _____ but not due to feline viral
   rhinotracheitis.

7. The _____ and feline leukemia vaccines have been associated with the development
   of soft tissue sarcomas at the vaccination site in cats.

8. _____ should always be available to administer immediately if an animal undergoes
   anaphylaxis after being vaccinated.

9. To reduce the risk of abortions, stillbirths, failure to thrive, and weak neonatal foals associated with

   rhinopneumonitis, it is recommended that pregnant mares be vaccinated against _____
   during the fifth, seventh, and ninth months of gestation.

10. Prevention of infectious bovine keratoconjunctivitis or pinkeye includes control of _____ during warm weather.

11. The preferred anatomic location for the intramuscular administration of any vaccination in food producing animals is the _____ muscles.

12. The most important aspect of successfully rearing baby calves is to ensure that they ingest _____ soon after birth.

13. Acute rhinitis and destruction of the nasal turbinates in young pigs may likely be caused by either _____ or _____, or both.

14. SMEDI stands for stillbirths, birth of weak piglets, mummified fetuses, embryonic death, and infertility and refers to porcine _____ infection.

15. _____ is the most common nutritional disease of pot-bellied pigs.

16. Urinary acidifiers may help to prevent _____ in pet pigs.

17. Fast growing young sheep and goats that receive heavy grain rations and nurse from dams with heavy milk production are at increased risk of developing _____.

18. Dehorning, castration, and tail docking of sheep and goats warrant vaccinating against _____.

19. In selenium soil-deficient areas, ewes should be supplemented with selenium to prevent weakness caused by _____.

20. A zoonotic disease of cattle for which replacement dairy heifers are vaccinated, tattooed, and ear tagged while less than 12 months of age is _____.

Find the following words:

ADENOVIRUS
BRUCELLOSIS
CALICIVIRUS
ENTEROTOXEMIA
ERYSIPELAS
LEUKEMIA
LYME DISEASE
PANLEUKOPENIA

PARAINFLUENZA
PARVOVIRUS
PSEUDO RABIES
RABIES
RHINOTRACHEITIS
SHIPPING FEVER
TETANUS

```
A P S F L E G L N G G S F R L
S Z S I B E D J Q W U W H U Y
U U N E S Z U X A R G I T A M
R M B E U O V K I L N O E I E
I E P W U D L V E O G K T M D
V B H U N L O L T M X J A E I
O W P B G N F R E N I R N X S
V V V T E B A N A C A A U O E
R U P D K C C U I B U S S T A
A H A F H J I N I A I R O O S
P L Z I J W E E A O R E B R E
N Q T E R Y S I P E L A S E N
A I N E P O K U E L N A P T T
S H I P P I N G F E V E R N F
F S U R I V I C I L A C H E G
```

ACTIVE IMMUNITY
ADJUVANT
ANAPHYLAXIS
ANTITOXIN
BIOSECURITY
COLOSTRUM
CONGENITAL

CRYPTORCHID
FOMITE
INTERFERON
NEEDLETEETH
PASSIVE IMMUNITY
TOXOID

```
L G A A W C M Y S A G L Y P Y
A O N I M U R T S O L O C A W
T S T Y M Z B I E E T Y S H
I L I R N J X N N T V N K S J
N X T B R D N U I O K A Z I C
E F O V I R D M B T W V W V R
G E X T J O O M H H G U J E Y
N F I G U F S I T D I J H I P
O I N T E R F E R O N D K M T
C X E O N D X V C Z K A H M O
N Q K N E N D I L U L B W U R
L Z W H V E U T L S R L E N C
T O X O I D Z C R J H I K I H
A N A P H Y L A X I S F T T I
H T E E T E L D E E N L G Y D
```

MATCHING

For the next four questions, match the canine vaccine or disease with its description.
  A. Canine distemper vaccine
  B. Canine parvovirus type 2 vaccine
  C. Giardiasis
  D. Canine leptospirosis vaccine

1. _____ This protects against a serious, often fatal disease affecting dogs of any age that results in severe bloody diarrhea, vomiting, dehydration, fever, and a low white blood cell count. Doberman pinschers, Rottweilers, and Labrador retrievers are at higher risk for serious infection than many breeds, so they often receive an extra booster.

2. _____ Traditionally, two serovars (*canicola* and *icterohaemorrhagiae*), which cause hepatic and renal disease, were included in this vaccine. However, new species (*grippotyphosa, pomona,* and *hardjo*) are emerging as disease-causing agents in the dog, and it is important that these serovars be included in this vaccine.

3. _____ This disease is characterized by recurrent diarrhea when dogs are continuously exposed to water contaminated with the organism.

4. _____ This vaccine can be used with a measles vaccine to increase the chance of protecting 6- to 12-week-old puppies from the respiratory, gastrointestinal, and neurologic effects of this usually fatal and extremely contagious disease.

For the next four questions, match the horse vaccine with its description.
  A. Tetanus vaccine
  B. Equine encephalomyelitis vaccine
  C. Equine rhinopneumonitis vaccine
  D. Equine influenza vaccine
  E. Strangles vaccine

5. _____ This vaccine protects against a viral neurologic disease transmitted by biting insects. A trivalent vaccine is commonly used for horses in states bordering Mexico to create a buffer zone that may prevent the spread of the Venezuelan strain into the United States. In areas where winter freezes are uncommon, semiannual vaccination may be advisable.

6. _____ The toxoid version of this vaccine is given to immunize horses against a disease characterized by muscle rigidity and spasms that may result in respiratory arrest and convulsions. Administration of an antitoxin to unvaccinated horses induces immediate protection that lasts approximately 2 weeks.

7. _____ The duration of protective immunity from this vaccine is short-lived, requiring vaccination every 2 to 3 months during periods of exposure. Disease outbreaks usually occur in horses 1 to 3 years of age after mixing with infected horses at the racetrack or show grounds. Infection is characterized by fever, depression, anorexia, muscle soreness, and coughing.

8. _____ Pregnant mares should be vaccinated with this vaccine in the fifth, seventh, and ninth months of gestation to prevent a viral disease whose strains can cause upper respiratory disease, abortions, stillbirths, and weak neonatal foals that fail to survive.

For the next three questions, match the swine vaccine with its description.
  A. *Erysipelothrix rhusiopathiae* vaccine
  B. *Escherichia coli* vaccine
  C. Mycoplasma bacterin

9. _____ This vaccine protects against an extremely common disease known as *diamond skin disease,* which causes acute septicemia, skin discoloration, arthritis, and heart-valve disease. Routine vaccination of gilts and sows before parturition and of pigs at weaning is highly recommended.

10. _____ This vaccine administered to sows or gilts protects against a common bacterial disease causing profuse and watery diarrhea, vomiting, and anorexia that can lead to death in newborn pigs.

11. _____ Vaccination at the time of weaning for this disease can reduce the incidence of pneumonia in young, growing pigs.

MATCHING

Choose the correct word from the column on the right.

1. _____ Test for equine infectious anemia		A. Wolf tooth
2. _____ Term for retained testicle(s)		B. *Clostridium*
3. _____ First milk		C. Panleukopenia
4. _____ "Diamond skin disease" of pigs		D. Lyophilized
5. _____ First upper premolar of horses		E. Cryptorchid
6. _____ Zoonotic disease of cows		F. *Dirofilaria*
7. _____ Vaccine-induced tumor in cats		G. Coggins
8. _____ Another name for distemper in cats		H. *Bordetella*
9. _____ Infectious cause of abortion in mares		I. Sarcoma
10. _____ Common name for Enterotoxemia of sheep		J. Mastitis
11. _____ Parasite that causes heartworm disease		K. Anaphylaxis
12. _____ Cause of cat scratch fever in humans		L. Attenuation
13. _____ Common endoparasite of sheep and goats		M. Colostrum
14. _____ Postvaccination immediate hypersensitivity		N. *Bartonella*
15. _____ Substance in vaccines; alerts the immune system		O. Overeating disease
16. _____ Term for freeze-dried vaccines		P. Adjuvant
17. _____ Infection of the mammary gland		Q. Erysipelas
18. _____ Tetanus causing organism		R. *Haemonchus*
19. _____ Modification of microbes for vaccine manufacture		S. Brucellosis
20. _____ Bacterium of canine kennel cough		T. Rhinopneumonitis

SHORT ANSWER

1. What do the letters in the canine DA$_2$LPP vaccine represent?

   D _____

   A2 _____

   L _____

   P _____

   P _____

2. What do the letters in the feline FVRC-P vaccine represent?

   FVR _____

   C _____

   P _____

3. Name two reasons why proper manure disposal is important to livestock health.

   A. _____

   B. _____

4. Name five procedures commonly performed with newborn pigs (not including vaccination).

A. _____

B. _____

C. _____

D. _____

E. _____

5. Suggest three strategies to control coccidiosis in sheep.

A. _____

B. _____

C. _____

6. For Equine diseases, what do the letters EEE, WEE, EIA, WNV, PHF stand for?

A. EEE _____

B. WEE _____

C. EIA _____

D. WNV _____

E. PHF _____

7. List at least five diseases that can be prevented with effective tick control.

A. _____

B. _____

C. _____

D. _____

E. _____

8. Suggest two strategies for biosecurity on a hog farm.

A. _____

B. _____

9. If a broodmare has been on a regular vaccination program and is boosted for infectious diseases 4 to 6 weeks before foaling, when should the foal start to be vaccinated for tetanus and encephalomyelitis?

_____

63

10. Suggest at least five strategies to control internal parasites in horses.

A. _____

B. _____

C. _____

D. _____

E. _____

11. List four emergency treatments that may be used for anaphylaxis.

A. _____

B. _____

C. _____

D. _____

CRITICAL THINKING QUESTIONS

1. Why is neutering or spaying earlier in life a good strategy to explain to a new cat owner?

A. Female cat

_____

_____

_____

B. Male cat

_____

_____

_____

2. Why does maternal antibody interference affect antibody production in a young puppy?

_____

_____

_____

_____

_____

3. Differentiate between core and noncore vaccines for a new kitten's owner.

_____

_____

_____

_____

_____

4. Why are screening tests such as for feline leukemia best done before vaccination?

_____

_____

_____

_____

5. What is different about the immune system reaction to intranasal versus parenterally administered vaccines?

_____

_____

_____

_____

_____

6. Explain why protection and safety are different with MLV versus killed vaccines.

_____

_____

_____

_____

_____

_____

7. List potential adverse vaccine reactions in cats or dogs.

A. _____

B. _____

C. _____

D. _____

E. _____

F. _____

8. Explain why vaccinations are not indicated when an animal is or has recently been sick with another illness.

_____

_____

_____

_____

9. Why are vaccinations never 100% effective for protection against disease?

_____

_____

_____

_____

_____

_____

10. Why is the dose of vaccine the same for a Chihuahua and a Great Dane *or* a miniature horse and a draft horse?

_____

_____

_____

_____

CASE PRESENTATION

1. A new client has just gotten a 12-week-old Rottweiler puppy during the summertime, and they live in a neighborhood with many other dogs. It is typical in this urban area that puppies are taken to puppy behavior classes. The puppy had one vaccine at 6 weeks of age, but the client does not know what the puppy was given. The client has called today to find out what they need to do to verify that their puppy is eligible for the puppy behavior class that starts next week.

A. Should this puppy come into the clinic soon?

_____

_____

B. What does the puppy need from a preventive care standpoint? Are other vaccinations needed?

_____

_____

_____

C. What other care should be discussed?

_____

_____

_____

D. Should the puppy go to the behavior class when another class starts in 8 weeks?

_____

_____

_____

_____

2. A client has just gotten her first horse and just moved the horse to a small, local boarding facility that is very conscientious about preventive care. The horse has an unknown health history and now has a puncture wound on its shoulder.

A. What advice should we give the client when she calls to inquire about the wound?

_____

_____

_____

_____

B. Other than immunizations, what other preventive care should be discussed?

_____

_____

_____

C. Should the horse be tested for equine infectious anemia? How long should the horse be segregated from the other horses at the boarding stable?

_____

_____

_____

3. A client comes in with a 16-month-old Yorkshire Terrier that they had gotten as a puppy. They are new clients and report that the dog had a "vaccine reaction" as a puppy but that it responded well to reaction treatments given at the time at their previous veterinary clinic.

   A. Should the dog be given booster vaccines at this time? Should we attempt to get the previous clinic's patient file?

_____

_____

   B. What was the most likely antigen that stimulated the previous reaction?

_____

_____

   C. Are there other precautions to take with vaccinating this dog? Are all vaccine reactions life threatening?

_____

_____

_____

4. A client has a new kitten and they know someone whose cat may have died from a tumor caused by vaccines at another veterinary clinic. They have brought the kitten in to be checked for internal parasites, but they have told the clinic's receptionist that they are reluctant to have the kitten vaccinated. Should we discuss all aspects of preventive care and insist on vaccinations for the kitten? Are there other questions that need to be asked? Do we need to review the risk versus benefits of vaccinations with the client? What vaccine may have produced the tumor on the cat that they referred to?

_____

_____

_____

_____

_____

_____

5. You have just been hired to work at a busy small animal veterinary clinic. You start your new job on a Monday morning. One of your stated responsibilities is inventory management, including vaccine inventories. You see that the clinic received a box of vaccines that arrived on Friday and has been sitting on the table waiting for you to open it today.

   A. What is your next step?

_____

_____

_____

B. How are vaccines shipped and stored?

_____

_____

_____

C. What is the difference between a MLV versus a killed vaccine?

_____

_____

_____

D. You also see that someone reconstituted a feline leukemia vaccine that they did not use on Saturday. They labeled the reconstituted vaccine and left it in the refrigerator. What should you do with this vaccine?

_____

_____

_____

6. A regular equine client at the veterinary clinic where you work has just gotten a pet pygmy goat to keep as a "buddy" for the horse. She has contacted you outside of work to ask your opinion about a goat as a buddy for a horse. She also wants to know "can I feed the goat just horse food?" Is there other preventive care that should be discussed with this client? Can she just give the goat a "small dose of the horse's worming medication?" Should you go into the details of a preventive care program with someone when you're not at work?

_____

_____

_____

_____

_____

_____

_____

_____

_____

Across

1. A substance added to a vaccine to increase inflammation and stimulation of the immune system to respond to the antigen
4. Inanimate object that transmits an infectious organism from one animal to another
6. Antiserum targeted against a specific toxin and used to provide passive immunity
7. Type of immunity made specifically by the animal's immune system after stimulation of the immune system by exposure to the antigen
10. A surgical procedure that sutures (attaches) the stomach wall to the abdominal wall so that the stomach is less likely to become twisted in a life-threatening gastric torsion
11. A condition where one or both testicles has not descended normally into the scrotum
12. A life-threatening and immediate (within 30 minutes) reaction to a foreign substance

Down

2. Nontoxic portions of a toxin used to provide active immunity
3. A test for equine infectious anemia
5. Glycoproteins in the family of cytokines made by cells of the immune system in response to foreign antigens
8. A trait an individual is born with, which could be genetic (inherited) or a result of an environmental cause during gestation
9. The type of immunity (antibodies) not made by the individual, for instance, from the mother

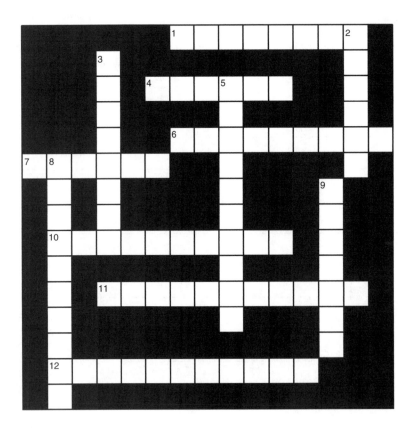

Chapter **9** **Preventive Health Programs**

Neonatal Care of the Puppy, Kitten, and Foal

LEARNING OBJECTIVES

When you have completed this chapter, you will be able to:

1. Describe special requirements for examination of neonates
2. List normal physiologic and behavioral parameters of neonatal puppies
3. Describe diagnostic sampling techniques used for neonatal puppies
4. Define hypothermia and describe problems related to hypothermia in neonatal puppies and kittens
5. Explain how neonatal isoerythrolysis occurs and is managed in kittens
6. List the symptoms, causes, and treatments of fading puppy/kitten syndrome
7. Describe considerations for care of orphan puppies and kittens
8. Describe care of the high-risk perinatal mare and list supplies needed to attend a high-risk foaling
9. Describe the events that occur in each of the stages of labor in the mare
10. Describe normal development and routine nursing care, medical care, and diagnostic procedures in the neonatal foal

MATCHING

The Fading Puppy/Kitten Syndrome
Using the following word bank, place the correct terms into each section.

Word Bank
- Anorexia
- Birth defects
- Congenital and genetic defects
- Death
- Die of starvation at time of weaning
- Emaciation
- Environmental conditions
- Frequent introduction of new animals
- Hypoglycemia
- Hypothermia
- Inappropriate temperature or humidity
- Inappropriate use of medication or exposure to chemical toxins
- Infections
- Lethargy
- Malnutrition
- Necropsies of neonates who have died
- Overcrowding
- Poor hygiene
- Poor management
- Removal of inciting causes
- Small, weak, and unable to nurse
- Stillborn
- Supportive care

Symptoms or Signs
A. _____

B. _____

C. _____

D. _____

E. _____

F. _____

G. _____

H. _____

I. _____

J. _____

Causes

A. _____

B. _____

C. _____

D. _____

E. _____

F. _____

G. _____

H. _____

I. _____

J. _____

Treatment

A. _____

B. _____

C. _____

FILL IN THE BLANK

Physical Examination of Neonates

1. For the physical examination of a neonate, a pediatric stethoscope with a _____ bell is helpful.

2. The neonate can have a body temperature lower than _____.

3. Neonates cannot regulate their body temperature for the first _____ of life.

4. Checking the oral mucous membranes assesses _____ on the neonate.

5. The neonate is born with hair that covers most of the body except the _____.

6. Lack of hair or a sparse hair coat may indicate either a _____ of the skin or premature birth.

7. Bluish or dark red discolorations are indicative of a neonate in _____.

8. Other than _____, discharge from any orifice is abnormal in the neonate.

9. The head is specifically examined for fontanelles, _____, bulging eyes from behind closed eyelids, and the formation of the nose and external ears.

10. The presence of _____ or malformations of the chest are noted.

11. Neonatal puppies are generally mildly _____.

12. Neonatal kittens are generally on the _____ side.

13. The genitals and the anus are checked for _____ by stimulating urination and defecation using a moistened cotton ball.

14. The presence of hair coat abnormalities over the dorsum may indicate the presence of _____.

15. Abnormalities in tone may be indicators for associated defects or problems such as _____ of the distal pelvis.

SHORT ANSWER

Normal Development of the Neonate

1. During the first week of life about how often do newborn puppies and kittens sleep?

   _____

2. About how often should a newborn puppy or kitten nurse?

   _____

3. Neonates will respond only to what stimuli?

   A. _____

   B. _____

   C. _____

4. How does the queen or bitch stimulate urination or defecation in the newborn?

   _____

5. What milestone should the puppy or kitten have reached at the age of 3 days and then at the age of 1 week?

   A. _____

   B. _____

6. At what age does the shiver reflex develop?

_____

7. When does the umbilical cord dry out and when could you expect to see it fall off?

_____

8. How can one determine the sex of a kitten at birth?

_____

9. At what age do puppies and kittens open their eyes and the external ear canals?

_____

10. By the end of what week are puppies and kittens able to stand and have good postural reflexes?

_____

TRUE OR FALSE

Neonatal Isoerythrolysis in Kittens and Malnutrition

Select T (true) or F (false) for each statement below.

1. _____ Overfeeding or high lactose content in the milk replacer often causes diarrhea.
2. _____ Milk replacer is better than the mother's milk.
3. _____ Neonates should be weighed weekly on a suitable scale until 3 weeks of age.
4. _____ A puppy or kitten should never be tube-fed if its body temperature is lower than normal for its age.
5. _____ Tube feeding is performed by first measuring the distance from the tip of the neonate's nose to the beginning of the chest.
6. _____ When tube feeding you may need to exert force as most neonates will not swallow the tube easily.
7. _____ Negative pressure indicates that the feeding tube is indeed in the lower esophagus and not in the lungs.
8. _____ When feeding milk replacer alone to puppies or kittens, use a 5 French feeding tube.
9. _____ As a rule of thumb, about 5 ml of milk replacer can be given to a 160 g puppy or kitten.
10. _____ Cats with blood type A have low titers of naturally occurring antibodies against blood type A red blood cells.
11. _____ All blood type B cats have high titers of naturally occurring antibodies against type A red blood cells.
12. _____ Kittens at risk for neonatal isoerythrolysis must be removed from their queens only during the first week of life.
13. _____ Kittens can be tested at birth for isoerythrolysis at birth using blood typing cards.
14. _____ It is rare for a kitten to show no signs of having neonatal isoerythrolysis.

MULTIPLE CHOICE

Diagnostics and Common Concerns and Disorders of the Puppy and Kitten

1. Blood can easily be obtained from what vein in neonates?
   a. Cephalic vein
   b. Jugular vein
   c. Saphenous vein
   d. Femoral artery

2. Radiography of neonates requires:
   a. Low-detail intensifying screens and single emulsion film
   b. High-detail intensifying screens and double emulsion film
   c. High-detail intensifying screens and single emulsion film
   d. Low-detail intensifying screens and double emulsion film

3. If possible, you should radiograph normal littermates for what reason?
   a. Comparison
   b. Size
   c. Weight
   d. Abnormalities

4. As long as neonates are close to their dams and mammary glands, they can maintain:
   a. Body weight
   b. Comfort
   c. Thermal balance
   d. A bond

5. As the neonate begins to take up food, this increases:
   a. Metabolic rate
   b. Heart rate
   c. Blood pressure
   d. Hunger

6. At what age do puppies and kittens have a temperature that is similar to an adult's temperature?
   a. 2 weeks
   b. 4 weeks
   c. 6 weeks
   d. 8 weeks

7. Name two complications of tube feeding a hypothermic neonate.
   a. Pneumonia and a full stomach
   b. Pneumonia and bloat
   c. Pneumonia and colic
   d. Colic and bloat

8. A neonate is considered hypothermic if its body temperature drops below what?
   a. 88° F
   b. 90° F
   c. 92° F
   d. 94° F

9. What range is the body temperature of a neonate that appears lethargic and uncoordinated but responsive?
   a. 90° F to 95° F
   b. 88° F to 92° F
   c. 78° F to 85° F
   d. 75° F to 78° F

10. Treatment of hypothermia consists of slowly reheating the patient at a rate of _____ ° F/hr.
    a. <1° F/hr
    b. <2° F/hr
    c. <3° F/hr
    d. <4° F/hr

11. Do not give anything orally until the patient has:
    a. Audible gut sounds and is moderately warmed.
    b. Audible gut sounds and is fully rewarmed.
    c. Inaudible gut sounds and is slightly rewarmed.
    d. Inaudible gut sounds but is not rewarmed.

12. Any disease process or imbalance of fluid or electrolytes will quickly lead to:
    a. Hypothermia
    b. Colic
    c. Lethargy
    d. Dehydration

13. Fluids can be given:
    a. Intravenously
    b. Intraosseously
    c. Intraperitoneally
    d. Intravenously, intraosseously, intraperitoneally, or subcutaneously

14. When administering fluid intraosseously, an 18- or 19-gauge needle can be placed in the:
    a. Proximal tibia or proximal femur
    b. Proximal tibia or distal femur
    c. Distal tibia or distal femur
    d. Distal tibia or proximal femur

15. Failure to suckle will result in _____ after 24 to 36 hours because of depletion of hepatic stores.
    a. Hypothermia
    b. Hyperthermia
    c. Hypoglycemia
    d. Hyperglycemia

16. Dextrose solutions should never be given _____ as they may cause tissue damage.
    a. Intravenous
    b. Subcutaneous
    c. Intraosseous
    d. Intraperitoneally

The Perinatal Period and the High-Risk Mare

1. Sometimes the mare will develop a problem in late term pregnancy, these mares are referred to as:
   a. Healthy
   b. High-risk mares
   c. Late-risk mares
   d. Problem mares

2. The average gestational length in the mare is:
   a. 200 days
   b. 240 days
   c. 300 days
   d. 340 days

3. The veterinarian will perform a rectal examination and a transrectal ultrasound at approximately:
   a. 15 days, 30 days, and then 90 days
   b. 15 days
   c. 30 days
   d. 90 days

4. If vaginal discharge is present, it may indicate:
   a. Nothing, this is normal
   b. Twins
   c. Placentitis or urine pooling
   d. Pregnancy

5. By performing a transrectal ultrasound, the veterinarian can evaluate gross fetal movement and measure the eye orbit to:
   a. Estimate fetal age
   b. Check for blindness
   c. Measure reflexes
   d. Predict labor

6. Vaginal examination in a late-term mare is not recommended unless:
   a. There are twins
   b. Delivery is imminent
   c. Ascending placentitis occurs
   d. There is urine pooling

7. _____ can be used in a noninvasive way to measure the foal and mare's heart rates during labor:
   a. Ultrasound
   b. Stethoscope
   c. Telemetry
   d. ECG

8. In late-term pregnancy, the foal will have a heart rate between:
   a. 20 to 120 bpm
   b. 40 to 80 bpm
   c. 40 to 150 bpm
   d. 150 to 250 bpm

9. A late-term pregnant mare should have a heart rate around:
   a. 40 to 50 bpm
   b. 50 to 150 bpm
   c. 80 to 160 bpm
   d. 60 to 120 bpm

10. Mares often foal:
    a. First thing in the morning
    b. In the afternoon
    c. At night
    d. At varying times with each foal

11. Agitation, pacing, nickering, lifting the tail head, turning and biting at sides, and kicking the abdomen all describe what stage of labor in the mare:
    a. Stage 1
    b. Stage 2
    c. Stage 3
    d. Stage 4

12. If you observe sweating around the shoulders of a mare in labor:
    a. This is an emergency, something is wrong
    b. This means nothing
    c. The mare will foal in the next 48 hours
    d. The mare will foal in the next ½ hour

13. What stage of labor in the mare is explosive and starts when the mare's placenta ruptures and allantoic fluid escapes?
    a. Stage 1
    b. Stage 2
    c. Stage 3
    d. Stage 4

14. If the foal is not delivered within a ½ hour of the stage described in question 13, the foal will experience:
    a. Hypoxemia
    b. Hypotension
    c. Hypocapnia
    d. Death

15. In what stage does the mare pass her placenta?
    a. Stage 1
    b. Stage 2
    c. Stage 3
    d. Stage 4

The Neonatal Foal: Normal Development, Routine Nursing Care, and Medical Care

1. At what age should the foal be doing the following:

    A. Standing: _____

    B. Nursing: _____

    C. First urination: _____

2. A normal temperature, pulse, and respiration at birth would be:

    T: _____

    P: _____

    R: _____

3. How long will a neonatal foal sleep and stand to nurse on average?

    Sleep: _____

    Stand: _____

4. An average foal will gain an average of how many pounds per day?

    _____

5. In comparison to an adult's, how does the neonatal foal's PCV range?

    _____

6. Routine care for all foals includes:

    A. _____

    B. _____

    C. _____

    D. _____

7. It is important to measure the foal's antibody levels how soon after birth?

    _____

8. Reasons for failure of passive transfer include:

    A. _____

    B. _____

    C. _____

9. Name the three main sites of entry for bacteria and viruses.

    A. _____

    B. _____

    C. _____

10. Name the five classic early clinical signs of disease in a critically ill foal.

    A. _____

    B. _____

    C. _____

    D. _____

    E. _____

11. Initial triage of a critically ill foal entering an NICU includes:

    A. _____

    B. _____

    C. _____

    D. _____

    E. _____

12. Initial treatment of the critically ill patient usually entails:

    A. _____

    B. _____

    C. _____

    D. _____

13. When providing fluid therapy what two things do you want to perform to ensure the foal is not losing glucose in the urine and the kidneys are responding appropriately.

    A. _____

    B. _____

14. When venous samples are required, what two veins are ideal for collection?

    A. _____

    B. _____

15. Complications during hospitalization include:

    A. _____

    B. _____

    C. _____

    D. _____

FILL IN THE BLANK

Orphan Care

Time consuming   Hydrated
Feeding tubes   Feeding
Hand-raised   Over
Daily   Diarrhea
84° F to 90° F   Growth factors
79° F to 84° F   Cow
73.4° F to 79° F   Metabolized
Second

1. The neonate must be kept warm and well _____ at all times.

2. Materials needed for orphan care include warm clean bedding, milk bottles, _____,
   syringes, a gram scale, and cotton balls.

3. Ambient temperature and humidity of _____ and 55% to 60%, respectively, should
   be provided during the first week of life.

4. Because of the differences in physiology, medications will not be taken up and _____
   at the same rate as in adults.

5. Homemade formulas are often deficient in _____ amino acids, and other nutrients
   essential for growth.

6. Many of the commercial milk replacers are made using _____ milk as a base and are
   therefore not always complete either.

7. Fostering neonatal puppies and kittens is _____.

8. During the second week of life, the ambient temperature may be kept at _____.

9. Shivering reflexes will set in after the _____ week of life.

10. Kittens or puppies need to be _____ because of maternal death or abandonment,
    lack of milk in the mother, maternal aggression, large litter size, malformations, or trauma.

11. Overfeeding milk replacers often results in _____.

12. Each orphan must be weighed _____ and records should be kept.

13. Ambient temperature during the third week of life should be kept at _____.

14. After _____ the orphan must be stimulated to urinate and defecate.

15. Common pitfalls of orphan care are _____ and underfeeding.

TRUE OR FALSE

Select T (true) or F (false) for each statement below.

1. _____ Overfeeding or high lactose content in the milk replacer often causes diarrhea.

2. _____ A puppy or kitten should never be tube-fed if its body temperature is lower than normal for its age.

3. _____ Negative pressure indicates that the feeding tube is indeed in the lower esophagus and not in the lungs.

4. _____ Cats with blood type A have low titers of naturally occurring antibodies against blood type A red blood cells.

5. _____ Kittens at risk for neonatal isoerythrolysis must be removed from their queens only during the first week of life.

CROSSWORD PUZZLE

Across

4. Lower than normal levels of blood glucose
6. Adult female horse
7. Insufficient body water caused by loss either through vomiting, diarrhea, lack of intake, hypothermia, overheating, or other illnesses
9. The period in puppies and kittens during the first 2 to 4 weeks of life are characterized by complete dependence on the mother
12. One-year-old horse
14. Born with a specific condition; can be genetic or environmentally induced
15. Castrated male horse; reproductive organs, the testes, have been removed
16. Inherited
17. Adult female horse used for breeding

Down

1. Female horse less than 4 years old
2. Juvenile horse nursing from its mother
3. The ability to generate heat through physiologic processes
5. The period from birth to puberty
8. Young horse not nursing from its mother
10. Abnormally low body temperature
11. Noncastrated male horse used for breeding
13. Male horse less than 4 years old, usually noncastrated

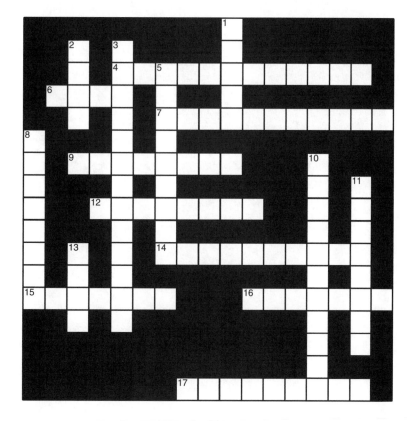

11 Animal Behavior

LEARNING OBJECTIVES

When you have completed this chapter, you will be able to:
1. Define behavior wellness and explain the importance of behavior wellness programs in pet animal practice
2. Differentiate between positive reinforcement, positive punishment, negative reinforcement, and negative punishment
3. Describe aspects of social behavior and social hierarchies in dogs and cats
4. List criteria that define behavioral health in dogs and cats
5. Define socialization and identify critical periods of social development in dogs and cats
6. List and describe the five steps in the Five-Step Positive Proaction Plan
7. List the five major areas of a behavioral assessment
8. List the most common agnostic behaviors exhibited by animals
9. Describe methods for dealing with threatening and aggressive animals
10. List and describe common products used for behavior modification in dogs and cats and handling aggressive animals

MATCHING

1. _____ Behavior wellness
2. _____ Negative reinforcement
3. _____ Socialization
4. _____ Positive reinforcement
5. _____ Sensitive period
6. _____ Closed social group
7. _____ Negative punishment
8. _____ Positive punishment
9. _____ Open social groups
10. _____ Reward
11. _____ Lure
12. _____ Intermittent reinforcement
13. _____ Continuous reinforcement
14. _____ Time-out

A. Puppy is given a treat immediately after eliminating in an appropriate area
B. Puppy is squirted with water while chewing on table leg
C. State of normal and acceptable pet conduct that enhances the human-animal bond and the pet's quality of life
D. Food is shown to an animal to elicit a behavior
E. Food is given to reinforce every occurrence of a correct behavior
F. Owner stops playing with puppy that begins to bite
G. The process by which an animal develops appropriate social behaviors toward members of its own and other species and inanimate elements of the environment
H. Dog learns to stop barking when he sees the owner get a rolled up newspaper
I. When socialization to their own species, to humans, and to other animals occurs most easily
J. Food is given for some correct behavior responses but not others
K. Between species
L. Within the species
M. Food is used after the behavior has been performed to acknowledge the behavior
N. As a consequence of unwanted behavior, the animal is immediately taken to a place where he doesn't want to be

MULTIPLE CHOICE

1. How many times should you recommend that an owner use a positive punishment before it is determined that it has not been successful?
   a. After the first time it is used
   b. After three to five applications
   c. After 10 to 15 applications
   d. Positive punishment always works if it is done correctly.

2. An animal that displays the following physical signs: crouching, lowered ears, and tail is exhibiting the following behavior:
   a. Aggressive
   b. Submissive
   c. Avoidance
   d. Threatening

3. Animals exhibiting this type of behavior tend to respond better if they are allowed to approach a person, rather than the other way around.
   a. Submissive
   b. Happy
   c. Fearful or threatening animals
   d. Dominant

4. Displacement behaviors are normal behaviors but are displaced out of their expected context and indicate an animal is stressed and unsure about how to respond. An example of a displacement behavior is:
   a. A dog barking
   b. A cat playing with a treat
   c. A cat twitching it's ears
   d. A dog yawning

5. Threats can be either offensive or defensive and may overlap with this.
   a. Acquiescence
   b. Submission
   c. Aggression
   d. Dominance

FILL IN THE BLANK

1. Ethology is the study of animal behavior. It needs to include the knowledge of _____ and _____, whereas animal learning must include principles of _____ and _____ conditioning.

2. Dogs are frequently mislabeled as _____ when in fact they are quite fearful.

3. The most common reasons for cat aggression to employees in a veterinary practice are _____ and _____.

4. In dogs, the socialization period occurs from _____ weeks of age; in cats it is from _____ weeks of age; in horses, it occurs _____.

5. Owners should actively _____ the behaviors they desire.

6. An animal should be released from its time-out after about _____ minutes.

7. Any punishment must be delivered within a _____ after the undesirable behavior occurs.

8. The first step in lowering patient stress is to understand species' _____ when an animal feels threatened or challenged.

9. Most aggressive behavior that technicians will see in the veterinary context is likely _____ rather than _____.

10. The _____ amount of physical restraint necessary for the technician's safety is the maximum that should be used.

SHORT ANSWER

1. List general health care tasks that a veterinary technician can perform to relieve the veterinarian's work load.

   A. _____

   B. _____

   C. _____

   D. _____

2. What are four things in behavior wellness care that veterinary hospitals can implement to decrease dog bites in the community and society at large?

   A. _____

   B. _____

   C. _____

   D. _____

3. Explain the behavioral consequences of operant conditioning by describing the concepts of positive, negative, reinforcement, and punishment.

   _____

   _____

   _____

   _____

   _____

4. List several of the behaviors that some dogs exhibit that are mistakenly categorized as dominance patterns.

   A. _____

   B. _____

   C. _____

   D. _____

   E. _____

   F. _____

   G. _____

   H. _____

I. _____

J. _____

5. List 10 criteria that technicians should look for to determine if a dog or cat is exhibiting normal and acceptable pet conduct and desirable behaviors.

A. _____

B. _____

C. _____

D. _____

E. _____

F. _____

G. _____

H. _____

I. _____

J. _____

6. List four submissive behaviors that owners misinterpret as guilt when an animal has done something unacceptable.

A. _____

B. _____

C. _____

D. _____

7. Why do pets seem to engage in certain unacceptable behaviors only in the owners' absence?

_____

_____

_____

_____

8. What is a good way to open a line of communication with a client concerning potential relationship problems between a new and an established pet in a household?

_____

9. Why is it important to adequately socialize animals?

   _____

10. The best time to at least introduce elements of the Five-Step Positive Proaction Plan is:

    _____

11. List the five steps in the Five-Step Positive Proaction Plan.

    A. _____

    B. _____

    C. _____

    D. _____

    E. _____

12. Why is praise alone often not adequate reinforcement when an owner is first establishing a relationship with a new pet?

    _____

    _____

13. It is recommended that owners prevent unwanted behaviors from occurring by managing the pet's environment through constant supervision in the new household. What suggestions would you make to clients to accomplish this for dogs and cats?

    _____

    _____

    _____

    _____

14. Behavior problems that can result from lack of physical activity and mental stimulation include:

    A. _____

    B. _____

    C. _____

    D. _____

    E. _____

    F. _____

15. List the five major areas of behavior assessment.

    A. _____

    B. _____

    C. _____

    D. _____

    E. _____

16. Why should technicians make note of the pet's demeanor at the veterinary hospital?

    _____

    _____

17. Once the behavior assessment is performed and the results discussed with the veterinarian an action plan should be composed. What are some things that an action plan could include?

    _____

    _____

    _____

    _____

18. List ways to manage the waiting room better to reduce stress on the animal and the clients and staff.

    A. _____

    B. _____

    C. _____

    D. _____

    E. _____

    F. _____

    G. _____

19. Why should animals that are upset or overly excited be moved out of the waiting area as quickly as possible?

    _____

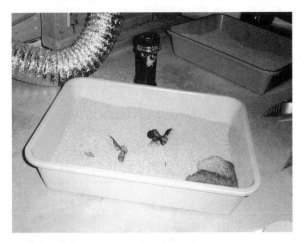

1. List at least four reasons why this litter box would be unacceptable to most cats.

   A. _____

   B. _____

   C. _____

   D. _____

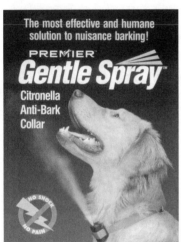

2. The use of a Citronella Anti-Bark Collar such as this is an

   example of _____ punishment.

3. What other citronella oil product on the market can be used for this type of punishment?

   _____

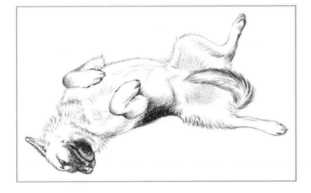

4. What type of behavior is this dog displaying?

   _____

5. What are some other behaviors besides rolling over that this dog might display for this behavior?

   A. _____

   B. _____

   C. _____

   D. _____

   E. _____

   F. _____

Chapter **11** **Animal Behavior**

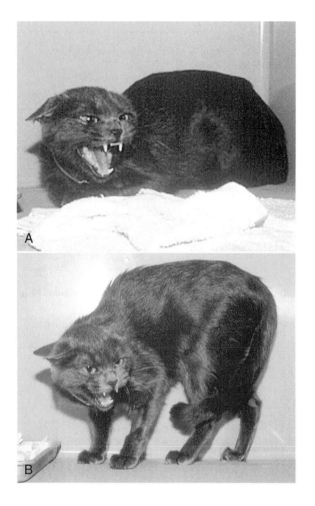

A

B

6. What behavior is this cat displaying?

   _____

7. What physical signs led you to this conclusion?

   A. _____

   B. _____

   C. _____

   D. _____

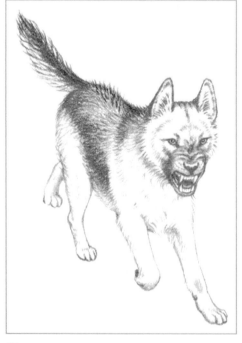

8. What behavior is the dog in this figure displaying?

   _____

9. What physical signs indicate this?

   A. _____

   B. _____

   C. _____

   D. _____

   E. _____

   F. _____

   G. _____

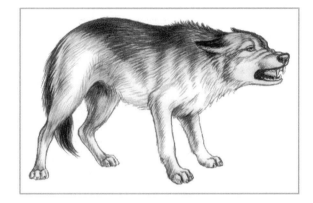

10. What behavior is the dog in this figure displaying?

    _____

11. What physical signs indicate this?

    A. _____

    B. _____

    C. _____

    D. _____

    E. _____

    F. _____

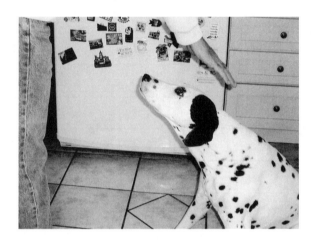

12. The person in this photo is reaching over the dog's head, facing the dog, and leaning over the dog. How may some dogs wrongly interpret these actions?

    _____

    _____

    _____

13. How should the person have approached the dog to turn this into a nonthreatening greeting?

    A. _____

    B. _____

    C. _____

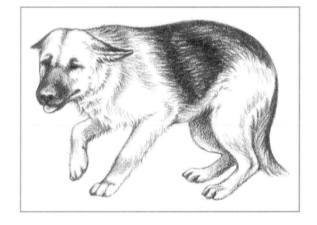

14. What behavior is the dog in this figure displaying?

    _____

15. What physical signs are often identified with this behavior?

    A. _____

    B. _____

    C. _____

DEFINE THE FOLLOWING TERMS

1. Aggression _____

    _____

    _____

2. Defensive aggression _____

    _____

    _____

3. Offensive aggression _____

    _____

    _____

4. Agonistic behaviors _____

    _____

    _____

5. Anthropomorphism _____

6. Classical conditioning _____

    _____

    _____

7. Operant conditioning _____

    _____

    _____

    _____

8. Socialization _____

    _____

    _____

    _____

9. Social hierarchies _____

_____

_____

_____

_____

10. Species typical behavior _____

_____

_____

11. Submissive behaviors _____

_____

12. Subordinate role _____

_____

TRUE OR FALSE

Select T (true) or F (false) for each statement below.

1. _____ Cats are typically undersocialized.

2. _____ The ideal time for socialization for horses begins at 8 weeks.

3. _____ The most proactive behavior wellness service one can offer is to educate clients on pet selection.

4. _____ Toys and food are tools used to elicit and reinforce appropriate behavior.

5. _____ Positive stimuli should be presented to pets with a firm, authoritative voice from the beginning of training.

6. _____ Remote punishment is more likely to be immediate and consistent even if the owner is not around at the time of the unwanted behavior.

7. _____ It is always appropriate to knee a dog in the chest when it jumps up.

8. _____ An important role of the veterinary technician in animal behavior counseling involves knowing the correct questions to ask and discussing the case with the veterinarian.

9. _____ Puppy socialization classes are designed specifically to help puppies and kittens become accustomed to the veterinary clinic under enjoyable conditions.

10. _____ Owners can be shown how to place Elizabethan collars on their pets before they enter the clinic to prevent bites to personnel.

11. _____ The appropriate time to begin socialization in horses is approximately 4 to 12 weeks of age.

12. _____ Positive and negative punishment refer to adding something and taking something away, in learning theory terminology.

13. _____ While interviewing clients about their pet's behavior, asking open-ended questions is discouraged because this does not lead to informative answers.

Across

3. Behaviors that result in harm to the opponent
6. A social structure that allows for division of resources, rights, and privileges
8. A _____ role is a superior position in a rank order or social hierarchy
10. _____ aggression is behaviors that result in harm done to another individual when the aggressor initiates the conflict
14. Negative _____ increases the frequency of behavior because something unpleasant is taken away or avoided (subtracted) following a behavior
15. The process by which an animal develops appropriate social behaviors
16. Behaviors that occur when other behaviors are thwarted or interrupted and when an animal is in conflict about choosing between two incompatible behaviors
17. A _____ role is a lower position in a rank order or social hierarchy

Down

1. The attribution of human characteristics to animals
2. Negative _____ decreases the frequency of behavior because something pleasant is taken away (subtracted) following a behavior
4. Also known as instrumental conditioning, based on the principle that the consequences of a behavior will influence its frequency
5. _____ aggression is behaviors that result in harm to another individual as a result of defending oneself
7. Behaviors that function as signals to "turn off" threatening and aggressive behaviors from other individuals
9. Behaviors which signal an intent or willingness to attack or become aggressive
11. For a period of time, the animal is prevented from receiving any reinforcement for any behavior (2 words)
12. Behaviors having to do with social conflict, which typically include avoidance, appeasement, threats, and aggression
13. Also known as classical conditioning; the animal learns the association between events

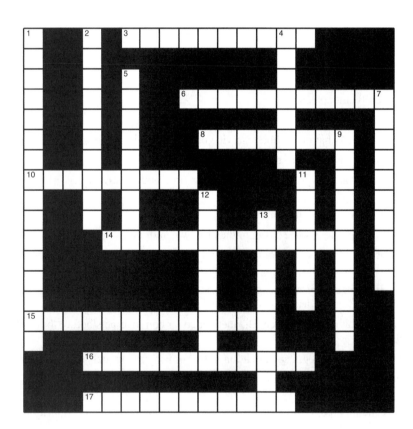

Chapter **11** Animal Behavior

Copyright © 2010 by Saunders, an imprint of Elsevier Inc.

12 Small Animal Nutrition

LEARNING OBJECTIVES

When you have completed this chapter, you will be able to:
1. List the energy-producing and nonenergy producing components of food
2. List the classes of carbohydrates and describe the catabolism of carbohydrates
3. Differentiate between lipids and fats and describe the general structure of triglycerides
4. Describe the structure and functions of proteins
5. Differentiate between essential and nonessential amino acids
6. Explain the importance of water in metabolic reactions
7. Differentiate between microminerals and macrominerals and give examples of each
8. List the fat-soluble and water-soluble vitamins and explain the importance of vitamins in metabolism
9. Define the following terms: nutrient, ingredient, formula, nutrient profile, calorie, and kilocalorie
10. Differentiate between dry, semi-moist, and moist foods and describe the characteristics of each
11. Describe considerations in evaluating home-prepared diets
12. List the legal requirements of pet food labels and considerations in evaluating pet food label information
13. Describe components of a nutritional assessment for dogs and cats
14. List special considerations in feeding adult, pediatric, geriatric, pregnant, lactating, injured, and ill dogs and cats
15. List and describe routes and procedures for providing nutritional support to hospitalized patients

MATCHING

Match the term to its correct definition listed in the table below.

1. _____ Anorexia
2. _____ Body condition scoring system
3. _____ Calorie
4. _____ Carbohydrates
5. _____ Energy
6. _____ Enteral tube feeding
7. _____ Phosphorous
8. _____ Selenium
9. _____ Sodium
10. _____ Clinical sign of hepatic lipidosis
11. _____ Refeeding syndrome
12. _____ A potential complication
13. _____ Minerals
14. _____ Fats
15. _____ Nutrients
16. _____ Obesity
17. _____ Parenteral feeding
18. _____ Protein

A. Typically limited in patients with renal insufficiency
B. A common nutritional deficiency in birds
C. Aspiration
D. Provide essential fatty acids
E. Intravenous nutritional delivery
F. An estimate of an animal's body composition
G. A safe, relatively inexpensive alternative to force feeding
H. Essential component of food necessary to sustain all life forms
I. A consequence of poor diet choice and physical inactivity
J. The body's main source of energy
K. Energy released from nutrients in the form of heat
L. A period of decreased nutritional intake to tube feeding
M. Metabolic derangements associated with feeding after prolonged starvation
N. Provides amino acids to support metabolism
O. Components of food that do not produce energy
P. Typically limited in patients with cardiovascular disease
Q. Inorganic chemicals that are an important part of a balanced diet
R. Icterus

95

FILL IN THE BLANK

Choose the correct answer from the list provided.

Humectants
Glycogen
Preservatives
Triglycerides
Antioxidants
Monosaturated
Metabolic rate
Fat
Polysaturated

Vitamins C and E
Additives
Essential fatty acids
Saturated
Monosaturated
Polysaturated
Proteins
Essential amino acids

1. Stores of _____ provide a rapid supply of glucose to tissues when sugar is urgently needed.

2. Nonenergy-producing, nonnutrient substances purposely added to food to enhance color, flavor, texture, and stability

   are termed _____.

3. Substances capable of inhibiting food-deteriorating microbes are identified as _____.

4. Preservative additives that bind to water to inhibit mold and fungal growth are called _____.

5. _____ can inhibit oxidation of fatty acids and fat-soluble vitamins, which protects
   them from becoming rancid and losing potency.

6. Dietary fats are primarily made up of units called _____.

7. There are several families of fatty acids, named according to the position of the first double bond. Fatty acids with no

   double bonds in the primary hydrocarbon chain are referred to as _____. Subsequently,

   the fatty acid with one double bond is called _____, and the one with more than

   one double bond is called _____.

8. The principal source of energy which also provides palatability, texture to food, supplies essential fatty acids, and

   acts as a carrier for the fat-soluble vitamins is called _____.

9. Deficiencies of _____ include alopecia, dull hair coat, anemia, and hepatic lipidosis.

10. The principle structural component of all body organs and tissues, which serve as enzymes, hormones, and

    antibodies are called _____.

11. Protein substances that cannot be synthesized in the body in adequate quantities, and therefore must be supplemented

    in the diet are called _____.

12. Prolonged starvation or food deprivation in normal animals results in a reduction in _____,
    to slow fat and muscle catabolism in an effort to survive long-term starvation.

TRUE OR FALSE

Select T (true) or F (false) for each statement below.

1. _____ A balanced diet should supply all the key nutrients and energy needed to meet the daily requirements of the animal at its particular stage of life.

2. _____ Fiber plays an important role in maintaining normal colonic function by decreasing pathogenic intestinal bacteria.

3. _____ Feeding a food with higher digestibility may lead animals to consume more of a particular food.

4. _____ Foods higher in fiber will be lower in digestibility.

5. _____ Dogs and cats lack certain salivary enzymes; consequently, digestion of starchy substances is not initiated in the mouth.

6. _____ Iron deficiency can be seen in animals with chronic blood loss such as those with hookworm or other parasitic infestations.

7. _____ Fiber differs from starch in that fiber is digestible by the monogastric stomach and small intestines.

8. _____ Amino acids are classified as either monosaturated or polysaturated.

9. _____ Fiber is an important part of the diet for dogs with diabetes mellitus because it helps to stabilize blood sugar levels by extending the time that nutrients are absorbed.

10. _____ Continuous protein catabolism limits the cat's ability to conserve protein, leading to higher requirements than found in the dog.

11. _____ Special-purpose foods provide specialized nutrition for individual need.

12. _____ Horses, cattle, and other grass-eaters house microbes and protozoa in their GI tracts (rumen, cecum, and large intestine) that break fiber down via fermentation.

13. _____ The ingredients listed on pet food labels are listed by weight, with the heaviest ingredients first and the lightest ones last.

14. _____ Guinea pigs lack an enzyme in the glucose to the vitamin C pathway, thus requiring a daily dietary ascorbic acid supplement.

15. _____ Proteins are the principle structural component of all body organs and tissues.

16. _____ Mammals cannot synthesize essential fatty acids; therefore, they must be obtained by the food.

17. _____ Food higher in fiber will be higher in digestibility.

18. _____ High-quality protein is especially needed during periods of growth, physical exertion, pregnancy, lactation, and for the repair of damaged tissues.

19. _____ A deficiency of a single essential amino acid can be detrimental.

20. _____ Small birds have high metabolic rates and high-energy requirements; therefore a continuous supply of food should be available.

21. _____ Cats are specifically adapted to low protein, high-carbohydrate diets.

22. _____ Most vitamins cannot be synthesized in the body and therefore must be present in the diet.

23. _____ Nutritional antioxidants in canine foods help protect immune function and improve cognitive dysfunction in senior dogs.

24. _____ Low birth weight is correlated with an increase in mortality.

25. _____ Percentages listed in the guaranteed analyses food label state only maximal and minimal levels and do not reflect the exact amounts of each nutrient.

26. _____ Dentition patterns of the cat demonstrate herbivorous eating behaviors.

27. _____ Amino acids are not stored to the same degree that excess fat and carbohydrates are stored.

28. _____ Dogs and cats lack certain salivary enzymes; consequently, digestion of starchy substances is not initiated in the mouth.

29. _____ Developmental skeletal diseases, such as wobbler syndrome, hip dysplasia, and osteochondrosis are thought to be associated with low-protein diets.

30. _____ Nursing pediatric patients are particularly susceptible to anemia because milk is low in iron.

31. _____ Dietary excesses of trace elements can be toxic.

32. _____ By AAFCO regulations, the nutritional adequacy of a food only requires recommended levels of essential nutrients at two different life stages: pediatric and geriatric.

33. _____ The AAFCO Animal Feeding Test statement is required on pet food labels, and lets the consumer know that the product was used in animal feeding tests and that it performed at acceptable levels.

34. _____ Daily energy requirements are the number of calories needed to maintain an animal's weight and are roughly equivalent for both the dog and cat.

35. _____ There are no human daily supplements that can be added to make a complete and balanced homemade pet diet.

36. _____ Proteins serve as enzymes, hormones, and antibodies.

37. _____ Certain feline diets are formulated to induce acidic urine because struvite crystal formation is not possible at a urine pH below 8.0.

38. _____ Guinea pigs should not be fed rabbit or any other diet designed for another species.

MULTIPLE CHOICE

1. In the critical patient, essential fatty acid deficiency will increase susceptibility to:
   a. Infection
   b. Poor wound healing
   c. Hypertension
   d. A and b

2. Simple sugars and complex sugars are broken down to provide energy, which are stored in the form of:
   a. ATP
   b. Linoleic acid
   c. Amino acids
   d. Protein

3. Clinical signs of taurine deficiency includes:
   a. Bradycardia
   b. Tachypnea
   c. Vision changes
   d. Obesity

4. The breakdown of circulating and structural protein into glucose is called:
   a. Gluconeogenesis
   b. Lactation
   c. Hepatic lipidosis
   d. Hyperglycemia

5. There are three known essential fatty acids; linoleic acid, α-linoleic acid, and:
   a. Taurine
   b. Arachidonic acid
   c. Lysine
   d. Glargine

6. The feline liver has limited capacity to synthesize which of the following amino acids?
   a. Taurine
   b. Lysine
   c. Arginine
   d. Tryptophan

7. A central component of hemoglobin and myoglobin molecules, which carry oxygen in blood and muscle respectively, is the macromineral:
   a. Selenium
   b. Vitamin k
   c. Iron
   d. Methionine

8. A physiologic process wherein electrolyte shifts occur from extracellular to intracellular compartments as amino acids are reintroduced is termed:
   a. Refeeding syndrome
   b. Gluconeogenesis
   c. Fatty acid synthesis
   d. Anaerobic catabolism

9. Metabolism of excess amino acids:
   a. Increases liver and kidney workload
   b. May decrease gastrointestinal motility
   c. May cause excessive weight gain
   d. May stimulate pancreatitis

10. Pets with trauma, infection, severe sepsis or burns will:
    a. Increase protein turnover
    b. Have decreased metabolism
    c. Have increased protein requirements
    d. Both a and c

11. Signs of protein deficiency include:
    a. Weight gain
    b. Immunodeficiency
    c. Urinary retention
    d. Poor GI motility

12. Calcium and phosphorous:
    a. Sustain the structural rigidity of bones and teeth
    b. Sustain visual acuity
    c. Are responsible for hair growth
    d. Are necessary for lung function

13. A calcium deficiency can result in:
    a. Secondary hypoparathyroidism
    b. Increased bone resorption to restore circulating calcium levels
    c. Refeeding syndrome
    d. Renal insufficiency

14. Proteins are essential to all living cells. One of the many functions include:
    a. ATP synthesis muscle breakdown
    b. Tissue growth and repair
    c. Sustaining normal digestive function

15. Calcium is a necessary ingredient in:
    a. Gastrointestinal motility
    b. Digestion
    c. Normal blood clotting
    d. Liver function

16. One of the many clinical signs of refeeding syndrome includes which of the following?
    a. Hyperthermia
    b. Anisocoria
    c. Hypertension
    d. Hemolytic anemia

17. Large meals should be avoided before exercise, particularly in large breed dogs, to minimize the potential of:
    a. Diarrhea
    b. Vomiting
    c. Gastric dilation and torsion
    d. Long bone injury

18. Colostrum provides:
    a. Protective maternal antibodies
    b. Antibiotics
    c. Amino acids needed for respiration
    d. Essential fatty acids

19. The onset of bone developmental disorders is usually associated with rapid growth of the long bones in large breed dogs. The most common of these disorders are:
    a. Canine hip dysplasia
    b. Osteoarthritis
    c. Hypertrophic osteodystrophy
    d. A and c

20. Technicians should advise pet owners to feed small meals several times a day and not allow the puppies continuous access to food because:
    a. Puppies may develop gastric torsion
    b. Many puppies will overeat when fed ad lib
    c. Puppies will develop diarrhea
    d. Puppies will lose interest in food

21. During lactation, proper dam nutrient intake is directly linked to successful milk production; technicians should recommend:
    a. Feeding larger amounts of a maintenance food
    b. Feeding a canned maintenance food
    c. Feeding a growth or lactation formula to meet the increased requirements
    d. Feeding a homemade diet supplemented with vitamins

22. Key nutritional factors in the lactating bitch include:
    a. Highly digestible starches
    b. Decreased concentrations of fat
    c. Approximately two to five times more calcium than during the maintenance life stage
    d. Vitamins C and E

23. For weaning purposes, food intake of the dam should be:
    a. Terminated for 24 hours to help the bitch slow and stop her milk production
    b. Terminated for 48 to 72 hours to help the bitch slow and stop milk production
    c. No termination—restrict water only to reduce nutrients needed for milk production
    d. No food or water restriction, simply remove the puppies from the dam

24. Obesity is a predisposing factor for:
    a. Hepatic lipidosis in cats
    b. Anesthetic complications
    c. Laryngeal paralysis
    d. A and b

25. Common nutritional factors to take into consideration when recommending a balanced senior diet in the healthy pet include:
    a. Reduced protein
    b. Increased phosphorous and sodium
    c. Decreased fiber concentrations
    d. Increased protein for hepatic function

26. The two most common calculi that can lead to lower urinary tract diseases in cats are:
    a. Struvite and calcium oxalate calculi
    b. Sodium urates
    c. Calcium sulfates
    d. Cystine

27. Factors in urinary calculi formation include:
    a. Low dietary magnesium
    b. Urine production
    c. Urinary pH
    d. Low dietary protein

28. Acidifying diets are recommended to safely prevent and manage struvite-related LUTD. These diets are not recommended for:
    a. Kittens
    b. Tomcats
    c. Obese cats
    d. Underweight cats

29. What is the preferred method of feeding the hospitalized patient (when possible)?
    a. Intravenous nutritional delivery
    b. Enteral nutritional delivery
    c. Tube feeding
    d. Force feeding

30. After placement of an esophagostomy or gastronomy tube, how long before the tube can be safely used to deliver nutrition?
    a. Immediately
    b. 48 to 72 hours
    c. 24 hours
    d. 4 to 6 hours

31. On the first day of tube feeding, it is generally recommended to feed:
    a. ⅓ of daily caloric requirement divided into six feedings
    b. ½ of the daily caloric requirement divided into 12 feedings
    c. ½ of the daily caloric requirement divided into two feedings
    d. 100% if the daily caloric requirement divided into 12 feedings.

32. Before tube feeding, food substances should be aspirated to ensure:
    a. Adequate gastric motility
    b. Adverse reactions such as stomach bleeding is not occurring
    c. Correct tube placement
    d. A and c

33. To prevent a feeding tube from clogging, the technician should:
    a. Flush with warm water after each feeding
    b. Flush with Coca-Cola products after each feeding
    c. Clean the entry site of the tube daily
    d. Pass a small wire gently down the tube to remove debris

34. Common complications to tube feedings include:
    a. Excessive weight gain
    b. Vomiting and diarrhea
    c. Decreased albumin
    d. Pain

35. Patient response to feedings is important during administration as it may suggest improper tube position. Common signs of discomfort include:
    a. Head pressing
    b. Seizures
    c. Abdominal bleeding
    d. Hypersalivation

36. Parenteral nutrition refers to the delivery of nutrients:
    a. Through a feeding tube
    b. Intravenously
    c. By mouth
    d. Through a specialized filter

37. Candidates for parenteral nutrition include:
    a. Patients who are unable to digest or absorb nutrients via the GI tract
    b. Recumbent patients
    c. Most postoperative patients needing nutritional support
    d. Patients with severe dehydration

38. The addition of lipids to partial parenteral nutrition (PPN) may be associated with:
    a. Pancreatitis
    b. Inflammatory bowel disease
    c. Immunosuppression
    d. Anemia

39. In general, slow "trickle" tube feedings through a fluid or enteral feeding pump:
    a. Is indicated when time does not allow for intermittent bolusing
    b. Is not recommended because of digestive complications
    c. Has less incidences of gastric bloating or vomiting than intermittent-bolus feedings
    d. Is less tolerated by the patient than intermittent feedings.

40. Nursing management of parental nutrition catheters includes:
    a. Strict sterile technique, including sterile bandage changes and avoiding disconnection of IV line from the catheter
    b. Changing administration sets every 6 to 8 hours
    c. Frequent heparin saline flushing to avoid thrombus formations
    d. A and c

41. All birds have similar nutritional requirements; the mineral required in the largest quantity is:
    a. Phosphorous
    b. Magnesium
    c. Iron
    d. Calcium

42. Commercially prepared seeds are rarely, if ever, an appropriate sole nutritional source for the bird because:
    a. They provide inadequate levels of protein, vitamins, and minerals
    b. Commercially available seed mixtures can cause inappetence
    c. Uninformed owners create a mixture based primarily on the price and physical appearance
    d. A and c

43. Insoluble and soluble mineral grit are often given to birds to:
    a. Facilitate mechanical digestion
    b. Prevent gizzard impaction
    c. Provide glucose
    d. Promote beak and feather growth

44. The best pet rabbit diet is:
    a. An alfalfa-based pellet with a hay supplement given on a daily basis
    b. An alfalfa-based pellet with an occasional hay supplement
    c. A primarily hay diet with commercial pellet supplement
    d. Fresh dark leafy greens only

45. Regular feeding schedules are important to the rabbit; when do they consume most of their feed?
    a. During the night as they are nocturnal in nature
    b. During early morning hours
    c. They generally eat all throughout the day
    d. They generally do not have specific eating habits in captivity

46. Rabbit pellets high in calcium or excessive vitamin D can occasionally produce:
    a. Chalky-white or cream colored urine
    b. Polyuria
    c. Seizures
    d. Vomiting

47. Guinea pigs are notoriously fastidious eaters and are primarily:
    a. Carnivores with normal caprophagic behavior
    b. Herbivores with normal caprophagic behavior
    c. Omnivores with abnormal caprophagic behavior in captivity
    d. Omnivorous with normal caprophagic behavior

48. Recommended diets for guinea pigs include food types with:
    a. Increased fiber to avoid cecal impaction and fur chewing
    b. Decreased fiber to avoid cecal impaction and fur chewing
    c. Decreased fiber to avoid GI upset
    d. Decreased fiber to avoid caprophagic behavior

49. The most common nutritional deficiency in captive turtles is:
    a. Vitamin A deficiency
    b. Vitamin C deficiency
    c. Calcium deficiency
    d. Phosphorous deficiency

50. Frequency of feeding snakes varies on the size of prey and on both the time of year and the signalment of the snake. However, most species of snake are fed:
    a. Once every month
    b. Once every other day
    c. Once every 1 to 2 weeks
    d. Once a month

51. As snakes eat infrequently, inappetence or weight loss may go undetected. How can a nutritional deficiency possibly be avoided?
    a. Periodic weighing
    b. Ensure water is always available
    c. Monitor urine production
    d. A and b

CIRCLE ALL THAT APPLY

1. The veterinary technician should help evaluate the patient on a homemade diet by noting:
    a. Body weight
    b. Body condition score
    c. Activity level
    d. Abnormalities on a thorough physical exam

2. Specific instructions as to feeding and storing of homemade food are of utmost importance. Pet owners should be advised to:
    a. Refrigerate or freeze homemade food
    b. See a veterinarian monthly for nutritional reviews and a thorough physical examination
    c. Never store food; use immediately
    d. Monitor food for color and odor changes

Chapter **12 Small Animal Nutrition**

3. Cooking techniques of homemade diets need to be discussed with the client. Longer periods of cooking may:
   a. Depreciate vitamin concentration
   b. Cause protein denaturation of meat sources
   c. Decrease digestibility of starch
   d. Add caloric density

4. Factors contributing to clinical obesity of the dog and cat include:
   a. Genetic background
   b. High protein diets
   c. Owner compliance to suggested diets
   d. Physical inactivity
   e. Presence of endocrine or neuroendocrine disorders
   f. Gonadectomy
   g. Dentition

5. The health risks of obesity are numerous. Among the most common include:
   a. Coronary heart disease
   b. Type 2 diabetes and insulin resistance
   c. Pulmonary thromboembolism
   d. Hypotension
   e. Intervertebral disk disease
   f. Liver, kidney, and gall bladder disease
   g. Lymphoma
   h. Joint stress, hip dysplasia, and osteoarthritis
   i. Muscular injuries, including cranial cruciate ligament rupture

6. Many tube feeding complications can be prevented by:
   a. Radiographic confirmation of correct tube position
   b. Force feeding and avoiding tube placement overall, especially in the critically ill
   c. Measuring gastric residue before each feeding
   d. Prophylactic administration of antibiotics to avoid tube infection
   e. Monitoring gastric tubes for migration during daily bandage changes
   f. Discontinuing concurrent medications during feedings
   g. Flushing tube with warm water before and after use

7. Land tortoises are predominantly herbivores, but will occasionally eat insects and small rodents. In captivity, diets should vary in proper amounts to ensure good health. List the following food substances from highest amount required, to least amount required.
   a. High-protein foods such as dry maintenance dog food, parrot chow, cereals, mice, scrambled eggs
   b. Vegetables such as collards, radish and turnip greens, dandelions, kale, cabbage, bok-choy, broccoli, cauliflower, summer and winter squash
   c. Fruit, such as grapes, apples, oranges, pears, peaches, plums, dates, melons, strawberries, raspberries, mangos, and tomatoes

FILL IN THE BLANK AND SHORT ANSWER

1. Normal growth rate for puppies is _____ of the anticipated adult weight. What are some of the clinical signs that a puppy is not receiving adequate amounts of milk?

   A. _____

   B. _____

   C. _____

2. Neonatal puppies that are unable to nurse should be fed what type of food? _____
Because canine milk is higher in protein and lower in lactose than bovine milk, what should be used to mix the replacement formula?

_____

3. The orphan formula dose is initially _____ of the puppy's weight per day

divided into several doses. If the animal has a strong _____, a small

animal nursing bottle or doll's baby bottle may be used. Why may a syringe or eyedropper be contraindicated?

_____

4. If a feeding tube is used, care must be taken not to place it in the trachea. The stomach capacity of the neonate

is approximately _____. Initially, puppies are fed _____ ml q4-6h, and kittens are

fed _____ ml q4-6h. The amount is gradually increased by _____ ml/feeding (dog)
or 1 ml/day (cat) until the recommended guidelines are reached.

5. Typically, the stomach is full from feeding when the belly is _____
or the animal turns its head away from the nursing bottle and squirms.

   a. How often should new formula be made? _____

   b. How is the reconstituted formula stored? _____

   c. At what temperature should food substances be fed? _____

6. When the puppy reaches 2 to 3 weeks of age, the food dose should approximate _____
of the body weight divided into four to six daily feedings. Monitoring weight gain by the use of a

_____ is a good way to evaluate food intake.

7. If the puppies or kittens are unable to consume formula through bottle feedings or syringe, and are too weak to obtain dam's milk on their own, are there any options to provide nutrition?

_____

8. What are the proper placement techniques for tube feeding?

_____

_____

9. Easy tube passage to the premeasured distance usually indicates _____.
After delivery of the fluid, are there special precautions to prevent aspiration?

_____

10. The animal should be burped after feeding by _____

_____.

11. Assist elimination every 2 to 4 hours or _____ for up to 4 weeks using cotton balls soaked in warm water to wipe the caudal abdomen and anogenital region.

12. In general, the stomach volume of the dog is approximately _____ ml/kg.

    However, the amount fed typically should not exceed _____ ml/kg.

    In the cat, general stomach capacity should never exceed _____ ml.

13. The most common cause of dietary-induced diseases in companion birds is the practice of adding fruits and vegetables sold for human consumption to commercially prepared food or supplemented seed mixtures. Explain.

    _____

    _____

    _____

FILL IN THE BLANK

Choose the correct answer from list provided below (one answer per question, answers may be used only once)

Semisolid gruel   Gastrointestinal paralysis
Hypothermia   External warming
Diarrhea   Gag reflex
Hypoglycemia

1. Puppies with low body weights prone to _____.

2. _____ should always be provided if the neonate is separated from its mother.

3. Hypothermia is common in neonates and is associated with _____.

4. Feeding is contraindicated if the animal is _____.

5. What is a common complication to formula feeding? _____

6. During administration of food substrates, patient response may not be typical, as the

   _____ does not develop until 10 days of age.

7. Three weeks of age is a suitable time to introduce _____, except for toy breeds and weak animals, which need more time before being offered solid food.

CASE DISCUSSION

A 16-year old, 6 lb male domestic shorthair cat was taken to surgery for an exploratory laparotomy for chronic vomiting. A gastronomy tube was placed at the time of surgery.

  1. How soon can you start feeding? Are there any side effects to feeding soon after anesthesia?

     _____

     _____

     _____

2. How do you calculate his estimated caloric intake? What type of food should be used initially?

_____

_____

_____

3. The cat has been anorectic for 2 weeks. How quickly should you achieve full caloric intake after such a long period of anorexia? Are there any special considerations due to his age in terms of food type? Are there special considerations to the rate of administration of food if concurrently on intravenous fluids?

_____

_____

_____

_____

_____

_____

4. The cat is on pain medication and is generally sedate. How can you tell if the amount being fed is being tolerated?

_____

5. Is refeeding syndrome a concern? Why or why not? What are some typical clinical and laboratory markers to monitor?

_____

_____

_____

_____

_____

_____

6. What are the nursing responsibilities in terms of tube care?

_____

_____

_____

7. How should the food be prepared before tube feeding? When should the cat be reintroduced to food by mouth?

_____

_____

_____

_____

_____

_____

_____

Across

3. The amount of heat (energy) needed to raise the temperature of 1 g of water 1° C
5. A type of feeding that delivers nutrients intravenously
6. Organic compounds necessary for normal physiologic function
9. A type of feeding that uses the upper alimentary tract for assisted feeding
11. Nourishing substances, food, or components of food
12. A body composition with a ratio of too much fat to lean tissue, or body weight 15% to 20% greater than optimal
14. A flexible tube with a rounded end that is passed through the nasal cavity to the stomach.
16. Can be broken down into triglycerides
17. The type of feeding tube that is inserted directly into the stomach
18. They are a quick source of energy and may be stored in the body as glycogen; sugars

Down

1. The type of feeding tube that is surgically positioned beyond the stomach to bypass the upper GI tract
2. A group of minerals called the trace elements
4. Long chains of amino acids held together by peptide bonds
7. A condition caused by a diet that contains all of the essential nutrients but in suboptimal amounts
8. Lack or loss of appetite for food
9. The type of tube that is placed into an artificial opening in the esophagus when oral feeding is impossible
10. The amount of heat (energy) needed to raise the temperature of 1 kg of water 1° C
13. Derived from food, it is essential for every body process, including the building up of cells, motion of the muscles, and maintenance of body temperature
15. The association that establishes standards for label information and the description of ingredients on pet food sold in the United States

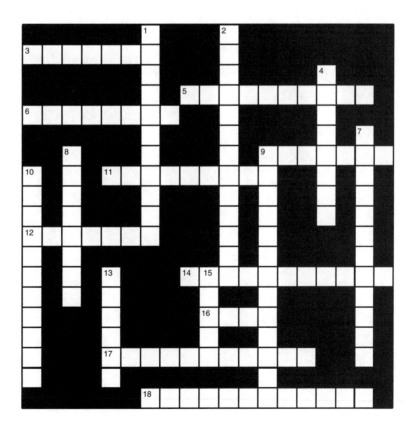

13 Large Animal Nutrition

LEARNING OBJECTIVES

When you have completed this chapter, you will be able to:

1. Explain the relationship between productivity and profitability in livestock production
2. List the energy-producing and nonenergy producing components of food
3. Define the following terms: digestion, maintenance nutrient requirements, biologic value, protein efficiency ratio, total digestible nutrients, gross energy, digestible energy, metabolizable energy, and net energy
4. List the variables affecting energy requirements of livestock and factors affecting water intake of livestock
5. Differentiate between essential and nonessential amino acids
6. Explain the importance of water in metabolic reactions
7. Differentiate between microminerals and macrominerals and give examples of each
8. Describe the two commonly used feeding systems for dairy cattle
9. Describe special considerations for feeding of beef cattle, sheep, and swine for specific productive purposes (maintenance, growth, finishing, lactation, work, wool, or eggs)
10. List advantages and disadvantages of pasture feeding of livestock

SHORT ANSWER

1. List the two methods by which digestion occurs within the body.

   A. _____

   B. _____

2. List two of the four items that are a part of amino acids.

   A. _____

   B. _____

3. Name the two categories in which carbohydrates are commonly categorized in animal feeds.

   A. _____

   B. _____

4. Name two ways to measure feed energy value.

   A. _____

   B. _____

5. Explain why total digestible nutrients (TDN) are not as useful as other measurements when looking at the nutritional value of a feed.

   _____

6. Name two values used when evaluating horse feeds.

    A. _____

    B. _____

7. Define total mixed ration.

    _____

8. Name the two feeding programs that are used predominantly in dairy production systems.

    A. _____

    B. _____

9. What is the main annual goal of the profitable cow-calf producer?

    _____

10. Explain the goal of the beef finishing feeding program.

    _____

11. In the ewe, energy requirements increase during the _____ trimester, making

    supplementation of forages with grain necessary _____.

12. Name two common problems attributed to poor nutrition in ewes.

    A. _____

    B. _____

13. How many times per day should the lactating sow be fed to ensure fresh feed and improved energy intakes?

    _____

14. What mineral is lacking in the sow's milk and therefore anemia may occur in young pigs if not properly

    supplemented? _____

15. List the 10 elements that influence nutrient requirements of livestock.

    A. _____

    B. _____

    C. _____

    D. _____

    E. _____

    F. _____

G. _____

H. _____

I. _____

J. _____

16. List the five variables affecting energy requirements.

A. _____

B. _____

C. _____

D. _____

E. _____

17. List the eight factors that affect water intake in the dairy cow.

A. _____

B. _____

C. _____

D. _____

E. _____

F. _____

G. _____

H. _____

18. Explain why water is important for the dairy cow.

_____

_____

19. List the two methods that can be used when watering livestock.

A. _____

B. _____

20. What can be done to keep water available in the winter?

_____

_____

21. List the eight factors that can affect the dry-matter intake in the dairy cow.

A. _____

B. _____

C. _____

D. _____

E. _____

F. _____

G. _____

H. _____

22. List five signs of undernutrition that may occur before death.

A. _____

B. _____

C. _____

D. _____

E. _____

23. List the energy intake variables in the sheep.

A. _____

B. _____

C. _____

D. _____

E. _____

F. _____

G. _____

H. _____

I. _____

J. _____

24. List the advantages of pasture feeding livestock.

    A. _____

    B. _____

    C. _____

    D. _____

    E. _____

25. List the disadvantages of pasture feeding livestock.

    A. _____

    B. _____

    C. _____

26. List the variables in protein requirements of sheep.

    A. _____

    B. _____

    C. _____

    D. _____

    E. _____

    F. _____

27. List the optimal requirements for lamb milk replacement.

    A. _____

    B. _____

    C. _____

28. What steps can be taken to prevent iron-deficiency anemia in baby pigs?

    A. _____

    B. _____

    C. _____

    D. _____

    E. _____

FILL IN THE BLANK

1. Minerals are divided into two categories: _____ and _____.

2. _____ is the cheapest and most abundant resource.

3. The major energy source for the lactating cow is _____.

4. The use of animal protein sources derived from ruminant species is not allowed in any rations to prevent the possible transmission of _____.

5. In beef cattle production is usually divided into two primary areas: _____ and _____.

6. _____ supplementation will be necessary and is usually offered on a free-choice basis when beef animals are on pasture.

7. Creep-fed calves can weigh _____ to _____ more pounds by weaning.

8. Sheep production is divided into two principal areas: _____ and _____.

9. Large fast-growing lambs are susceptible to overeating disease, which is also called _____.

10. Pig production is divided into three distinct areas: _____, _____, and _____.

11. Horse production is divided into three areas: _____, _____, and _____.

TRUE OR FALSE

Select T (true) or F (false) for each statement below.

1. _____ Proteins of plant origin have a greater biologic value than do proteins of animal origin.
2. _____ The crude protein measurement shows the quality or use potential of the protein in the feed.
3. _____ Carbohydrates are the primary energy source in livestock rations.
4. _____ A feed can possess high protein content, yet the biologic value of that protein is low.
5. _____ In the pig, overfeeding energy during gestation has a direct negative impact on lactation feed intake, which can impair lactation performance.
6. _____ Peak lactation in the mare occurs 3 to 4 weeks after foaling.
7. _____ In the maintenance phase of a horses life, they need constant supplement feeds to survive.
8. _____ Cows milk is the best milk replacement for lambs.
9. _____ Essential amino acids must be supplied in the diet because the animal body cannot synthesize them fast enough to meet its requirement.
10. _____ Colostrum can be successfully frozen and used at a later date.
11. _____ Lambs do *not* require colostrum immediately after birth to achieve adequate immunity.
12. _____ Many pigs in the swine industry are raised in confinement.

Chapter **13** **Large Animal Nutrition**   Copyright © 2010 by Saunders, an imprint of Elsevier Inc.

MATCHING 1

Match the following definition to the correct term.

1. _____ Digestion
2. _____ Maintenance nutrient requirements
3. _____ Biologic value
4. _____ Protein efficiency ratios
5. _____ Total digestible nutrients

A. General measurement of the nutritive value of a feed
B. Number of grams of body weight gain per unit of protein consumed
C. Process of protein, carbohydrate, and fat breakdown in absorbable nutrients
D. True amount available for productive body functions
E. Level of nutrients needed to sustain body weight without gain or loss

MATCHING 2

Match the following definition to the correct term.

1. _____ Gross energy
2. _____ Digestible energy
3. _____ Metabolizable energy
4. _____ Net energy

A. Energy that was digested or absorbed
B. The actual portion of energy available to the animal for use in maintaining body tissues or during pregnancy or lactation
C. Total energy potentially available in a feed consumed by an animal
D. Used to account for energy losses and is a step beyond DE or TDN

MATCHING 3

Match the following substance with the correct category.

1. _____ Stored carbohydrates
2. _____ Structural carbohydrates
3. _____ Glucose
4. _____ Sucrose
5. _____ Cellulose
6. _____ Grains
7. _____ Hemicellulose
8. _____ Fructose

A. Fiber-forages
B. Sugars
C. Starches

MATCHING 4

Match the following substance with the correct category.

1. _____ Salt
2. _____ Potassium
3. _____ Zinc
4. _____ Cobalt
5. _____ Chromium
6. _____ Phosphorus
7. _____ Zinc
8. _____ Selenium
9. _____ Molybdenum
10. _____ Magnesium
11. _____ Calcium
12. _____ Manganese
13. _____ Iodine
14. _____ Fluorine
15. _____ Silicon

A. Macrominerals
B. Microminerals

Chapter **13** **Large Animal Nutrition**

16. _____ Iron

17. _____ Copper

18. _____ Sulfur

MATCHING 5

Match the breed usage with the correct breed.

1. _____ Polypay

2. _____ Leicester

3. _____ Rambouillet

4. _____ Suffolk

5. _____ Dorset

6. _____ Merino

7. _____ Hampshire

8. _____ Tunis

9. _____ Shropshire

10. _____ Texel

11. _____ Debouillet

12. _____ Oxford

13. _____ Columbia

14. _____ Cheviot

15. _____ Southdown

16. _____ Targhee

A. Wool breed

B. Meat breed

C. Combination breed

MATCHING 6

Match the statements with the correct animal.

1. _____ Ensure calf nurses within 2 hours of birth

2. _____ Can sometimes be grafted to another cow

3. _____ Days 5 to 84: starter and free-choice water through weaning

4. _____ Days 1 to 3: obtain colostrum from dam

5. _____ Days 4 to 7: begin offering starter and free-choice water

6. _____ Ensure that calf continues to thrive and that cow does not show signs of mastitis or decreased milk production

7. _____ Days 5 to 84: begin offering forage

8. _____ Ensure that colostrum has been administered

9. _____ Days 4 to 7: transition to milk replacer or other liquid feed

10. _____ Feed like dairy calves

A. Dairy calves

B. Beef calves

C. Orphans

MATCHING 7

Match the statements with the correct rule.

1. _____ Continue to rotate salt

2. _____ 3 to 5 lb in each spring and summer month

3. _____ Make salt available at all times

4. _____ Manger throughout pasture

5. _____ 1 to 1.5 lb in each fall and winter month

A. Rule 1: Supply

B. Rule 2: Availability

C. Rule 3: Rotation

Match the terms to the definitions.

1. _____ Amino acids
2. _____ Forages
3. _____ Gross Energy
4. _____ Digestible Energy
5. _____ Metabolizable Energy
6. _____ Protein efficiency ratio
7. _____ Biologic value
8. _____ Net Energy
9. _____ Concentrates
10. _____ MNR
11. _____ TDN
12. _____ Digestion

A. A term which indicates the energy value of a feedstuff.

B. The percentage of the protein of a feed which is usable as a protein by the animal. A protein which has a high biologic value is said to be of good quality.

C. Nitrogen-containing compounds that constitute the "building blocks" or units from which more complex proteins are formed.

D. Energy available to the animal after energy from feces, urine, and combustible gases has been subtracted from gross energy.

E. The number of grams of body weight gain per unit of protein consumer.

F. A broad classification of feedstuffs which are high in energy and low in fiber.

G. The levels of nutrients needed to sustain body weight without gain or loss.

H. The vegetative portion of plants in a fresh, dried, or ensiled state, which is fed to livestock (as pasture, hay, or silage).

I. The energy remaining after the energy lost in feces is subtracted from gross energy.

J. The process of protein, carbohydrate, and fat breakdown into absorbable nutrients.

K. Energy available to the animal after energy from feces, urine, combustible gases, and body heat loss has been subtracted from gross energy.

L. The total potential energy of a foodstuff determined by measuring the total heat produced when the food is burned in a bomb calorimeter.

MULTIPLE CHOICE

1. Which animals may develop copper toxicity because of their ability to store copper in various organs and tissues?
   a. Cattle
   b. Horses
   c. Pigs
   d. Sheep
   e. Goats

2. Lambs must receive colostrum within:
   a. The first day
   b. The first month
   c. The first hour
   d. The first minute
   e. The first week

3. At what age are pigs given supplemental iron, either orally or by injection?
   a. 3 hours
   b. 3 days
   c. 3 weeks
   d. 3 months
   e. 3 years

MATCHING 9

Match the vitamin(s) with the correct description.

1. _____ This is the only fat-soluble vitamin readily synthesized by rumen microorganisms; supplementation is normally not required.

2. _____ This vitamin is synthesized through ultraviolet radiation by the skin or added to a dairy ration as sun-cured forage or a vitamin supplement; supplementation is not necessary in beef cattle.

3. _____ Forages of good quality that are properly harvested normally contain adequate levels of the precursor for this vitamin, carotene.

4. _____ Although these water-soluble vitamins are synthesized by the rumen microflora, some evidence indicates that supplementation may be beneficial in cows undergoing heavy stress or in various disease states.

A. Vitamin K

B. Vitamin A

C. Vitamin D

D. Thiamine, choline, and niacin

CROSSWORD PUZZLE

Across

6. The vegetative portion of plants in a fresh, dried, or ensiled state, which is fed to livestock
7. Energy available to the animal after energy from feces, urine, combustible gases, and body heat loss has been subtracted from gross energy
8. Nitrogen-containing compounds that constitute the "building blocks" or units from which more complex proteins are formed. (2 words)
9. A term that indicates the energy value of a foodstuff
10. The process of protein, carbohydrate, and fat breakdown into absorbable nutrients
11. The levels of nutrients needed to sustain body weight without gain or loss

Down

1. The percentage of the protein of a feed which is usable as a protein by the animal (2 words)
2. The total potential energy of a foodstuff
3. Energy available to the animal after energy from feces, urine, and combustible gases has been subtracted from gross energy
4. The energy remaining after the energy lost in feces is subtracted from gross energy
5. Feedstuffs that are high in energy and low in fiber

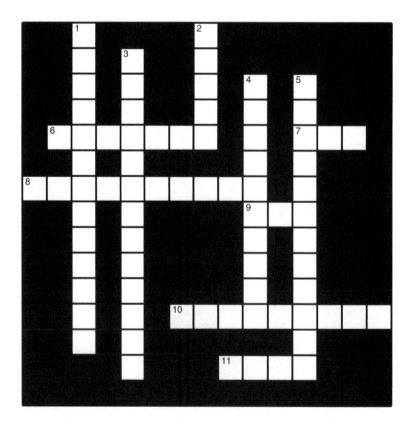

14 Animal Reproduction

LEARNING OBJECTIVES

When you have completed this chapter, you will be able to:
1. List the stages of the canine estrous cycle and describe the events that occur in each stage
2. List the female reproductive hormones and describe their roles in the process of reproduction
3. Describe the formation and structure of the placenta in domestic animals
4. List and describe methods used to confirm pregnancy
5. Describe the events that occur in each of the stages of whelping in the canine
6. List clinical signs of pyometra, eclampsia, metritis, mastitis, and brucellosis in canines
7. List the stages of the feline estrous cycle and describe unique features of the feline reproductive process
8. Differentiate between polyestrous, seasonally polyestrous, induced ovulator reproductive cycles
9. Describe the procedures and tests used for performing a breeding soundness examination in the mare
10. Describe methods for synchronization of estrous in herd animals

TRUE OR FALSE

Select T (true) or F (false) for each statement below.

1. _____ The brain is the initiator of the reproductive cycle.
2. _____ The fetus has two fluid-filled sacs surrounding it.
3. _____ During proestrus the bitch is attractive to male dogs and will allow mating.
4. _____ A vaginal cytology shows 100% cornified cells during estrus in the bitch.
5. _____ The bitch ovulates mature oocytes that require 2 to 3 more days for maturation.
6. _____ The fertile period is best identified using hormone assays for LH or progesterone.
7. _____ Although false negatives are common with in-house *Brucella canis* screening, false positives are rare.
8. _____ The queen is not an induced ovulator.
9. _____ The normal postpartum discharge is a red-black, nonodorous fluid that can be seen for as long as 3 weeks after queening.
10. _____ Queens with pyometra tend to be older, whereas bitches can be any age.
11. _____ Estrus, or the period of receptivity, is shown by teasing "in."
12. _____ All vaginal procedures in mares should be performed aseptically.
13. _____ Endometrial cytology should always be performed in conjunction with an endometrial culture to aid in interpretation of results.
14. _____ Pregnancy examination in the mare is usually performed 21 days after ovulation with the aid of ultrasonography.
15. _____ Parturition is a slow process in the mare.
16. _____ A retained placenta for more than 6 hours in duration requires veterinary attention.
17. _____ The most common reason for failure of a cow to show estrus is pregnancy.
18. _____ Dystocia is much more common in mares than in cattle.
19. _____ Artificial insemination with fresh or cooled semen is commonly performed in the swine industry.
20. _____ Metritis and mastitis are the main diseases of the postpartum period in cows, and consequently lead to a disturbance in milk production.

MATCHING

Correctly match each statement about whelping, with:

1. _____ Averages 6 to 12 hours but can be as long as 36 hours.
2. _____ A blackish-green discharge is normal.
3. _____ Lasts a total of 3 to 6 hours but may be as long as 24 hours.
4. _____ Bitch is usually restless and may show nesting behavior.
5. _____ Bitch often appears nervous, pants, and may tremble and shiver.
6. _____ When the bitch pushes the puppies out.
7. _____ Lasts approximately 20 to 60 minutes per puppy.
8. _____ Body temperature drops to 99° F.
9. _____ Presentation of the puppies is 60% anterior in the bitch.
10. _____ Abrupt decline in progesterone.

A. Stage 1
B. Stage 2

WORD SEARCH—TERMINOLOGY

Fill in the blanks and then find these words in the word search on the following page.

1. A synthetic progestin mainly indicated to suppress estrus in mares. _____

2. Portion of the uterine tube (oviduct) that connects to the uterus. _____

3. The expanded "bulb" of the proximal canine penis. _____

4. Cellular change indicative of cell proliferation and death. _____

5. The blood-filled remnant of the ovarian follicle immediately after ovulation. _____

6. A specific antiinflammatory steroid secreted by the adrenals. _____

7. Luminal cell layer in the follicle that converts testosterone to estradiol. _____

8. Fingerlike portion of the uterine tube (oviduct) that captures the ova upon ovulation _____

9. Portion of the uterine tube (oviduct) that connects the infundibulum and the ampulla. _____

10. Characteristic sign of estrus in the queen. _____

11. The female gamete that has half the number of chromosomes. _____

12. Absorption of protective antibodies from colostrum by the newborn. _____

13. Portion of the brain that secretes melatonin via light stimulation through the eyes. _____

14. Twenty-carbon fatty acid produced in the uterus and involved in luteolysis. _____

15. Condition in which the cervix does not dilate at parturition. _____

16. A group of hormones having a common ring structure and a similar synthetic pathway. _____

17. Inner cell layer in a follicle that converts cholesterol into testosterone. _____

18. Embryologic precursor of the male tubular reproductive tract. _____

```
L H K E K J K T S E G O N E R T L A V X
O M F N A U P A U U T V U D B X E Z H R
S U K I H M A L Q G C E X U U D N E I E
I C S V C E S L O B U H V O L U O C C Y
T I P R C H S U K L D B N G B D M N E A
R G V I O R I P G Q N U T H U Y R I L L
O A M N A E V M G B A H D M S L O D O L
C H U G Q Y E A K C I O O K G M H N R L
W R L W P A T L I L F P E O L H D A D E
L R U O Q L R J D N F I V P A S I L O C
S O B M Y L A I T S L N R E N Q O G S A
Y M I B F L N P E U O E J T D C R A I S
V E D P I E S H P M W A G Y I A E T S O
P H N O N C F A A H P L E C S K T S N L
C S U A R L E P L T F G D O E F S O W U
F U F C O A R T C S S L V O R F O R J N
W P N Y C C J M L I B A I G B E K P O A
L R I S X E W Q J U N N P H E R O M E R
B O N A A H V C X N B D S X Z W Y D I G
Q C Y J X T G O T E L W B E E L C J W A
```

FILL IN THE BLANK

Use the following key terms to fill in the blanks.

Teasing in
Queen
Estrus
Flaccid paralysis
21
Bitch
Radiology
Twinning

2
Goats
14
Heterospermic insemination
Placenta
Hormone assays
Mare

1. During Stage 3 of parturition, the _____ is expelled.

2. During _____, vaginal epithelial cells are cornified.

3. No more than _____ hours should elapse between the delivery of each puppy.

4. To best estimate the day of ovulation, _____ should be used.

5. Palpation to determine pregnancy in the bitch can be performed around day _____ after D1.

6. _____ is the only reliable method to accurately determine the number of pups in utero.

7. The _____ has the longest postpartum uterine involution of domestic species.

8. The _____ is a seasonal breeder.

9. Pregnancy can be diagnosed in the queen _____ days postcoitus to term by ultrasound.

10. The natural breeding season of the _____ centers around long day length.

11. Estrus in the mare is shown by _____.

12. Milk fever is characterized by _____.

13. In a commercial swine unit, _____ is sometimes used and reportedly increases pregnancy rate.

14. In goats and sheep, _____ is common.

15. Pseudopregnancy is a common condition in _____.

MULTIPLE CHOICE

Canine Estrus Cycle and Reproduction

1. The normal stages of reproduction are:
   a. Proestrus, metestrus, anestrus
   b. Proestrus, estrus, diestrus
   c. Estrus, diestrus, anestrus
   d. Diestrus, metestrus, proestrus

2. The time of progesterone domination is called:
   a. Diestrus
   b. Proestrus
   c. Estrus
   d. Anestrus

3. The time of first ovulation is called:
   a. Estrous
   b. Anestrous
   c. Pregnancy
   d. Puberty

4. After ovulation, the follicle transforms into the:
   a. Oviduct
   b. Uterine tube
   c. Corpus luteum
   d. Ampulla

5. The uterine tube is often called the:
   a. Oviduct
   b. Follicle
   c. Infundibulum
   d. Oocyte

6. The oviduct consists of what three segments?
   a. Infundibulum, ampulla, isthmus
   b. Infundibulum, ampulla, follicle
   c. Corpus luteum, uterine tube, follicle
   d. Corpus luteum, infundibulum, oocyte

7. The time of growing follicles after the death of the corpus luteum is called:
   a. Diestrus
   b. Proestrus
   c. Estrus
   d. Anestrus

8. The fetus has _____ fluid filled sacs surrounding it.
   a. One
   b. Two
   c. Three
   d. Four

9. Parturition is normally divided into how many stages?
   a. 1
   b. 2
   c. 3
   d. 4

10. What stage of parturition is expulsion of the fetus?
    a. 1
    b. 2
    c. 3
    d. 4

11. Name the four stages of the estrous cycle.
    a. Proestrus, estrus, diestrus, anestrus
    b. Proestrus, estrous, diestrus, malestrus
    c. Preestrus, estrous, diestrus, anestrus
    d. Proestrus, metestrus, diestrus, anestrus

12. Noncornified cells:
    a. Have a more angular shaped nucleus
    b. Have a nucleus that is either pyknotic or not apparent
    c. Increase approximately 10% a day
    d. Have a round cytoplasm and a large stippled nucleus

13. During estrous the vaginal cytology is:
    a. Fully noncornified
    b. Fully cornified
    c. Half cornified and half noncornified
    d. Slightly cornified

14. The end of estrus is typified by an abrupt decline in the:
    a. Percentage of WBCs
    b. Percentage of noncornified cells
    c. Percentage of bacteria
    d. Percentage of cornified cells

15. Ovulation occurs approximately _____ day(s) after the LH surge.
    a. 1
    b. 2
    c. 3
    d. 4

16. Serum progesterone _____ before ovulation in the bitch.
    a. Slightly drops
    b. Dramatically decreases
    c. Rises
    d. Stays the same

17. Insemination of the bitch with frozen semen is performed _____.
    a. Never
    b. Surgically or by a transcervical endoscopic method
    c. Only surgically
    d. Only by a transcervical endoscopic method

18. In-house tests for progesterone analysis are:
    a. Easy to perform and yield results in 20 minutes
    b. Easy to perform but take a long time
    c. Are very difficult to perform but yield results in 5 minutes
    d. Are very difficult and take a long time

SHORT ANSWER

Breeding Soundness Examination in the Mare

1. Name four things that a breeding soundness examination typically consists of.

   A. _____

   B. _____

   C. _____

   D. _____

2. In the breeding soundness examination, which of the procedures are performed aseptically?

A. _____

B. _____

C. _____

3. During an ultrasound examination what two things can be observed?

A. _____

B. _____

4. Describe the "clean hand-dirty hand" technique that is used when cleansing the perineal area.

_____

_____

_____

5. This item should be used when obtaining a culture and/or cytology specimen.

_____

6. When performing an ultrasound, what color will fluid-filled structures such as follicles appear?

_____

7. Name the structure whose appearance is important in determining the stage of the estrus cycle in the mare.

_____

8. Why should endometrial cytology always be performed in conjunction with an endometrial culture?

_____

9. Name four things a vaginal speculum examination can detect.

A. _____

B. _____

C. _____

D. _____

10. When cleansing the vulva, why is it better to place the soap on the cotton itself rather than placing disinfectant in the bucket?

_____

_____

CROSSWORD PUZZLE

Across

1. Embryonic malformation which has developed both male and female gender organs
6. Placental membrane formed from the hindgut
8. Portion of the uterine tube (oviduct) that connects to the uterus
9. A steroid hormone produced in the female's follicle
10. The placental membrane that directly surrounds the fetus
11. The act of giving birth
12. Cellular change indicative of cell proliferation and death
13. A condition in which the cervix does not dilate at parturition
16. A specific anti-inflammatory steroid secreted by the adrenals
18. Embryologic precursor of the male tubular reproductive tract (2 words)
20. The organ arising from the embryo that provides nutrient to the fetus via its interaction with the uterus
21. Portion of the uterine tube (oviduct) that connects the infundibulum and ampulla
23. The female gamete that has half the normal number of chromosomes
24. The first milk that contains the antibodies
25. A sexual signal that is secreted by an animal and is detected by the olfactory system of another animal
26. The corpus _____ is the structure on the ovary that produces progesterone

Down

2. The hormone produced in the pineal gland that is involved with seasonality of estrus in many species
3. A uterus full of pus
4. Stage of development when the species is recognizable
5. A specific area of placental attachment in ruminants
7. The fused chorionic and allantoic membranes
12. The outermost placental membrane that directly contacts the endometrium
14. Finger like portion of the uterine tube (oviduct) that captures the ova upon ovulation
15. A female pig that has not yet produced a litter
17. Fluid filled structure on the ovary that contains the oocyte
19. The hormone produced by the posterior pituitary that cause uterine contractions and milk letdown
22. A bovine female that has not yet had a calf

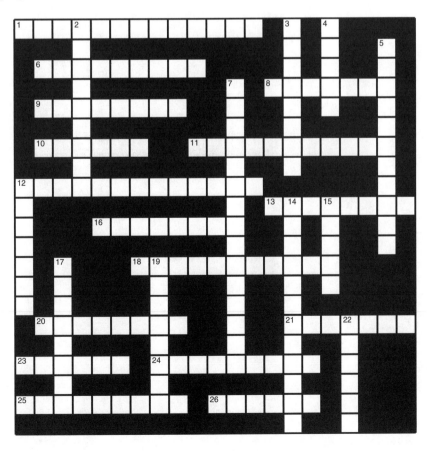

15 Care of Birds, Reptiles, and Small Mammals

LEARNING OBJECTIVES

When you have completed this chapter, you will be able to:

1. List and describe the components of the clinical history for avian and reptile patients
2. Describe physical examination considerations and sample collection procedures for avian and reptile patients
3. Describe the indications for and procedures used to perform a cloacal swab, oral examination, and crop wash in avian patients
4. Describe methods for administration of medications, trimming of nails, and clipping of wing feathers in avian patients
5. List and describe basic feeding guidelines for common pet bird and reptile species
6. List unique equipment required for care and treatment of reptiles
7. Describe the indications for and procedures used to perform a colonic wash, bone marrow and urine sample collection, and stomach lavage in reptile patients
8. Describe common diseases of ferrets and diagnostic procedures used for diagnosis and treatment of ferrets, rabbits, and rodents
9. Describe unique considerations related to administration of anesthesia in small animals
10. List and describe common zoonotic diseases of birds, reptiles, and small mammals

MULTIPLE CHOICE

Select the best answer to the question.

1. Where is the basilic vein found on the bird?
   a. Ventral surface of the wing
   b. At the back of the head
   c. On the lower leg
   d. In the roof of the mouth

2. Which of the following is a protozoan parasite that may be found on a crop wash?
   a. *Candida*
   b. *Capillaria*
   c. *Giardia*
   d. *Trichomonas*

3. Which site is most commonly used for blood collection in turtles?
   a. Caudal tail vein
   b. Jugular vein
   c. Cranial vena cava
   d. Saphenous vein

4. Which is the most common site used for IM injections in snakes?
   a. Cranial epaxial muscles
   b. Gluteal muscles
   c. Caudal epaxial muscles
   d. IM injections cannot be administered to snakes

5. Metabolic bone disease is least likely to occur in which of the following?
   a. Iguana
   b. Bearded dragon
   c. Burmese python
   d. Box turtle

6. An adult female ferret with a swollen vulva and hair loss most likely has which disorder?
   a. Hyperadrenocorticism
   b. Hypothyroidism
   c. Ovarian neoplasia
   d. Hyperthyroidism

7. Ferrets should be vaccinated against which disease?
   a. Feline panleukopenia
   b. Canine distemper
   c. Measles
   d. Leptospirosis

8. Which mite most commonly affects the fur of rabbits?
   a. *Sarcoptes*
   b. *Microsporum*
   c. *Demodex*
   d. *Cheyletiella*

9. Which of the following reduces the incidence of hairballs in rabbits?
   a. High-fiber diet
   b. High-carbohydrate diet
   c. High-protein diet
   d. High-fat diet

10. Which animal produces precocious young?
   a. Ferret
   b. Rabbit
   c. Guinea pig
   d. Sugar glider

11. Which animal requires vitamin C in its diet?
   a. Rabbit
   b. Sugar glider
   c. Hedgehog
   d. Guinea pig

12. Seizures are an inherited disorder seen in which of the following?
   a. Gerbils
   b. Hamsters
   c. Rabbits
   d. Ferrets

13. Which of the following should be fed an insectivore diet?
   a. Hedgehog
   b. Prairie dog
   c. Sugar glider
   d. Iguana

14. Which of the following is a social animal and needs special attention if housed singly?
   a. Guinea pig
   b. Sugar glider
   c. Hamster
   d. Rabbit

15. Which radiographic view is used routinely in turtles, but not in snakes, lizards, or birds?
   a. Lateral
   b. Hanging VD
   c. AP (or frontal)
   d. Lateral oblique

MATCHING

Write the name of one of these animals in the space next to the description that fits it. You can use each animal only one time.

1. _____ Smallest of the rodents
2. _____ Has the longest gestation period
3. _____ Is not a rodent
4. _____ Has the shortest gestation
5. _____ Comes from Mongolia
6. _____ Commonly develop mammary tumors

A. Mouse
B. Rat
C. Gerbil
D. Hamster
E. Guinea pig
F. Rabbit

MATCHING

Name a pet discussed in this chapter that has been shown to transmit each of the following zoonotic diseases. You may use a pet only one time.

1. _____ Monkey pox
2. _____ Chlamydiosis
3. _____ Salmonellosis
4. _____ Plague

A. Birds
B. Prairie dogs
C. Reptiles

DEFINE

Define each of the following terms as they relate to the animals covered in this chapter.

1. Cloaca _____

2. Ecdysis _____

_____

3. Renal portal system _____

_____

4. Chelonian _____

_____

5. Heterophil _____

_____

MATCHING

Match the name of the animal most commonly affected by each condition.

1. _____ Vitamin C deficiency   A. Bird
2. _____ Mycoplasmosis   B. Ferret
3. _____ Insulinoma   C. Guinea Pig
4. _____ Pasteurellosis   D. Iguana
5. _____ Metabolic bone disease   E. Rabbit
6. _____ Candidiasis   F. Rat

SHORT ANSWER

1. List four different clinical signs seen in rabbits with pasteurellosis:

A. _____

B. _____

C. _____

D. _____

2. List four questions that you would ask a bird owner that are different from questions you would ask a dog or cat owner.

A. _____

B. _____

C. _____

D. _____

3. List five questions that you would ask a snake owner that are different from questions you would ask a dog or cat owner.

   A. _____

   B. _____

   C. _____

   D. _____

   E. _____

4. Which feathers are cut on a parrot to prevent flight?

   _____

5. Why should birds and reptiles not be housed in the same room?

   _____

6. List three signs of heat stress in an avian patient.

   A. _____

   B. _____

   C. _____

7. Ferrets should be vaccinated against which two diseases?

   A. _____

   B. _____

8. List three causes of metabolic bone disease in lizards.

   A. _____

   B. _____

   C. _____

9. Estrogen toxicity causes which clinical problem in ferrets, but why is it not commonly seen in the United States today?

   _____

10. List three ways that inhalation anesthesia in rodents and rabbits differs from that in dogs.

    A. _____

    B. _____

    C. _____

11. Name three vessels that can be used for blood collection in birds.

    A. _____

    B. _____

    C. _____

12. Which vein is commonly used for blood collection in the iguana?

    _____

13. What is the principal purpose (what is the DVM looking for) of each of the following procedures?

    A. Colonic wash in snakes _____

    B. Stomach wash in snakes _____

    C. Crop wash in birds _____

PHOTO QUIZ _____

Label the diagram

A. _____

B. _____

C. _____

D. _____

E. _____

CROSSWORD PUZZLE

Across

2. A roundworm parasite lays double operculated eggs and is located in the intestinal tract of infected birds

7. A turtle

8. Inflammation of the tissue under the lid margins and surrounding the visible globe

9. A flagellated protozoan parasite that is located in the intestinal tract of infected animals and causes watery diarrhea

10. A fluid lavage of the reptile's distal intestinal tract in an attempt to collect a sample for parasite examination (2 words)

12. The genus name of an intracellular bacterium that is a zoonotic disease (psittacosis)

Down

1. In birds and reptiles the single terminus of the urinary, intestinal, and reproductive tracts

3. An area of tissue that marks externally the approximate boundary of the outlet of the pelvis and gives passage to the urogenital ducts and rectum

4. A granular leukocyte in birds and reptiles, which is the analog to the neutrophil in mammalian species.

5. The opening of the trachea within the oral cavity of birds

6. The large vein on the ventral surface of a bird's wing that courses over the humeral-ulna joint

11. A dilation of the esophagus of birds at the base of the neck, where food is stored, softened with fluids, and passed to the stomach in small amounts

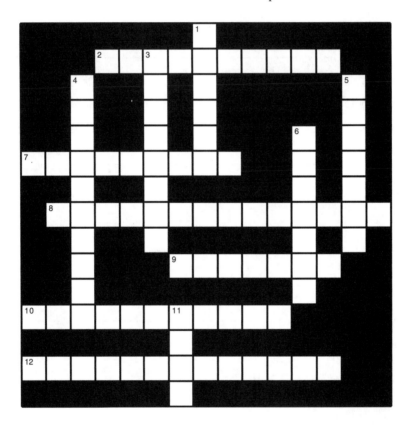

16 Clinical Pathology

LEARNING OBJECTIVES

When you have completed this chapter, you will be able to:

1. Describe proper handling of blood samples for hematology, coagulation, and clinical chemistry testing
2. List the tests included in the complete blood count and the equipment needed to perform those tests
3. Describe the procedure for counting of white blood cells and platelets with the Unopette system
4. Explain the procedures for determination of packed cell volume and plasma protein concentration
5. State the calculations for determination of erythrocyte indices
6. Describe the procedure for preparing and evaluating a differential blood cell film
7. Describe normal blood cell morphology, and list and describe common morphologic abnormalities of blood cells in a variety of species
8. State the calculations for determination of absolute values
9. State advantages, disadvantages, and limitations of automated cell counters and clinical chemistry analyzers
10. List the indications for and types of tests used in clinical chemistry testing
11. Describe methods of collection and handling of urine samples
12. List the test performed and describe the methods used for evaluation of physical properties and chemical composition of urine samples
13. Describe methods for preparing urine samples for microscopic examination of urine sediment
14. List and describe the formed elements commonly found in urine sediment
15. Describe the procedure for collection of cytology samples by fine needle aspiration and list the cytology tests performed on body fluids

DEFINE

Define the following terms:

1. Agglutination _____

   _____

2. Anisocytosis _____

   _____

3. Cystocentesis _____

   _____

4. Döhle bodies _____

   _____

5. Echinocytes _____

_____

6. Hematuria _____

_____

7. Hemacytometer _____

_____

8. Hyperchromasia _____

_____

9. Isosthenuria _____

_____

10. Left shift _____

_____

11. nRBC _____

_____

12. Poikilocytosis _____

_____

13. Refractometer _____

_____

14. Reticulocyte _____

_____

15. Rouleaux formation _____

_____

16. Spherocyte _____

_____

Find the following words:

HEMATOLOGY

AGGLUTINATION   ANISOCYTOSIS   BASOPHIL   ECHINOCYTES
EOSINOPHIL   ERYTHROCYTE   HEMACYTOMETER   HEMATOCRIT
HETEROPHIL   HYPERSEGMENTATION   HYPOCHROMIA   LEFTSHIFT
LEPTOCYTES   LEUKOCYTE   LYMPHOBLAST   LYMPHOCYTE
MACROCYTIC   MONOCYTE   NEUTROPHIL
NRBC   POLYCHROMASIA   RETICULOCYTE
ROULEAUX   SCHISTOCYTE   SPHEROCYTE

```
B O H D D R J A T K A L E B S E H E X N U T K Q S Y M V Z
C T C L Y E X V D Z I E K Q Z T I E T B K U E X T F N A N
T F I H S T F E L X M P O Y Y Y A Q U M R N E Q A M J D A
A C B R N E E T Y C O T S I H C S G M G V I K W I E Y J Z
A O C H C M A R H H R O Q Y W O W E A V C I V F M U R R L
G L I H P O R E T E H C Q L Q R J F M F Z E E W J K L J F
A A W Z N T T P D I C Y X F J E K U X K K G H F L U Q K H
P D M F E Y T A O D O T Q Q D H L Z U N C F Z A U S T P Q
W E G Q U C E L M L P E Q W Q P B H P K X N U Q Y H Y I Q
E E X A T A Z E A E Y S I R E S J T Z K O E H H L Z B S E
O E K G R M S U N N H C G S T R Q B O H X X G I W I Q Q W
S C A G O E E K I B Q W H F Y L D O L I C Z C M Q V G J X
I H A L P H T O S H S A B R C W P N Z H T Q E W U I J Q N
N I D U H Q Y C O Y Y M O F O N V S N R Z X D A G M Y F T
O N C T I R C Y C P I U C G L M P W H O Q X E A A G X M X
P O Y I L B O T Y E Z D U F U F A G N U L J Q H G Z W C U
H C G N G S R E T R V J K C C T O S Q L M U P B M A T F F
I Y F A L I H P O S A B K P I X W J I E N D S N C U Z T C
L T Y T F W T A S E P W I G T W U S L A V T J U P Z K P O
Y E M I P L Y K I G O U G K E P V E S U F T G Z D K S P P
M S A O N N R Z S M M S Q M R V O B C X Z J X Z F U T R C
P C C N F S E P Y E Q P L N O V H F O W F Z I Q W P G Q Q
H M R Q W C T N U N V G E S W Z M R O A N U O K X D Q C J
O N O L R N Y A E T O V F W O G X W D N K C D X X H T I O
B B C F M A C Z G A H A D H Q H G Z R K X R C U F A Z Q Q
L L Y M P H O C Y T E I Q N C V U V E H R D O E Y L A V L
A I T G Q O N K P I Q J G E D Y U G V W X W I N N J S Q W
S Z I U J L O O D O F H G W V Z A Z F X P Q Y V I Z S Z L
T L C M F P M S N N U U I U S O Q U C D O Y G R X J M I K
```

URINALYSIS

ACIDEMIC
ALKALEMIC
BACTERIA
BILIRUBINURIA
CASTS
CRYSTALS
CYSTOCENTESIS
EPITHELIAL
ERYTHROCYTE
GLUCOSURIA
HEMATURIA
HEMOGLOBINURIA
HYALINE
HYPOSTHENURIC
ISOSTHENURIC
KETONES
LEUKOCYTE
MYOGLOBINURIA
PROTEINURIA
REFRACTOMETER
RENAL
SEDIMENT
SQUAMOUS
TRANSITIONAL
TURBIDITY

```
A P V D P Y L A N O I T I S N A R T N O U
I R E F R A C T O M E T E R I A Y H M N I
R E T F O S C L X A K L E T U H Q O C C Z
U N J Y T I D I B R U T U I K J Q J O W M
N A E F E K P P A X G H X L Z S O Z Z W F
I L M R I F K U X G X C D Z F H K I U W J
B V H I N S S U O M A U Q S K S S D B F U
O Q U Y U D E R K R U N I S B Y Z W D B X
L J C B R B D S S D Q X P C W V O N W A P
G A I C I S I S E T N E C O T S Y C U F J
O O C R A P M G L U C O S U R I A H S I P
Y E P I T H E L I A L H Y A L I N E O J Q
M X K H D W N V R U H E M A T U R I A O X
B V C W O E T Y C O R H T Y R E G O L O I
A L K A L E M I C A S T S B U T W S E D M
C N T A L E M I C A S T S B U T W S E D M
T S L A T S Y R C K B L A B O A W F B D Y
E F H E M O G L O B I N U R I A H T J X J
R E W Y H Y P O S T H E N U R I C A O U W
I G T A D D A I S O S T H E N U R I C C V
A K E T O N E S N V E T Y C O K U E L Y O
```

MULTIPLE CHOICE

1. EDTA is the anticoagulant of choice for hematology because it:
   a. Preserves blood cell morphology
   b. Simultaneously stains and preserves WBC
   c. Destroys RBC while preserving WBC
   d. Destroys WBC while preserving RBC

2. Which measure determines the average size of an erythrocyte?
   a. Packed cell volume
   b. Mean corpuscular volume
   c. Mean corpuscular hemoglobin concentration
   d. Mean corpuscular hemoglobin

3. Drawing a blood sample from an animal that has recently eaten may result in a sample that is:
   a. Hemolyzed
   b. Icteric
   c. Lipemic
   d. Anemia

4. All of the following may cause hemolysis of a sample **except:**
   a. Excessive pressure on the syringe plunger when obtaining a sample
   b. Freezing whole blood from an EDTA tube
   c. Removing a needle from a syringe to place blood in a collection tube
   d. Centrifuging a blood sample at an overly high speed for 30 minutes

5. When mailing glass slides a technician **should not:**
   a. Send several unstained slides
   b. Send slides along with histopathology samples packed in formalin
   c. Send slides in a cardboard mailer for protection
   d. Label each slide

6. Given the following data for a dog:
   Hemoglobin = 5 gm/dl
   PCV = 20%
   RBC count = 4.7 million/μl
   A. Calculate the MCV:
      a. 25.5 femtoliters
      b. 42.5 femtoliters
      c. 60.5 femtoliters
      d. 80.0 femtoliters

   B. Calculate the MCHC:
      a. 25 g/dl
      b. 106 g/dl
      c. 45 g/dl
      d. 60 g/dl

7. Which stain is used to provide the best visualization of reticulocytes?
   a. Diff-Quik stain
   b. Giemsa stain
   c. New methylene blue stain

8. With significant dehydration in a patient (otherwise healthy), the following would likely be seen on a urinalysis and CBC?
   a. Increased urine SG and increased PCV
   b. Increased urine SG and decreased PCV
   c. Decreased urine SG and decreased PCV
   d. Decreased urine SG and increased PCV

9. In the above patient with significant dehydration, the plasma TP reading from the _____ would likely be _____.
   a. Reagent test strip, increased
   b. Reagent test strip, decreased
   c. Refractometer, increased
   d. Refractometer, decreased

10. If you count 70 reticulocytes out of 1000 erythrocytes, what is the observed reticulocyte percentage?
    a. 7%
    b. 70%
    c. 13%
    d. 4%

11. In cats, which form of reticulocytes should be counted when enumerating reticulocytes?
    a. Punctate only
    b. Punctate and aggregate
    c. Aggregate only

12. Which bovine erythrocyte parasite closely resembles a Howell-Jolly body?
    a. *Anaplasma*
    b. *Babesia*
    c. *Dirofilaria*
    d. *Ehrlichia*

13. Which sample condition *cannot* be minimized by preparing the animal or by proper sample collection and handling?
    a. Hemolysis
    b. Lipemia
    c. Icterus
    d. Evaporation

14. What is the most numerous and second most numerous leukocyte seen in canine and feline blood, respectively?
    a. Lymphocyte, neutrophil
    b. Neutrophil, monocyte
    c. Lymphocyte, monocyte
    d. Neutrophil, lymphocyte

15. A circulating neutrophil in which the cytoplasm is more basophilic than normal and contains vacuoles and Döhle bodies is known as a:
    a. Band cell
    b. Metamyelocyte
    c. Hypersegmented neutrophil
    d. Toxic neutrophil

16. What is the name of the specialized instrument on which diluted blood is placed for cell counting?
    a. Refractometer
    b. Fibrinometer
    c. Hemocytometer
    d. Leukometer

17. Where is the buffy coat found in the centrifuged microhematocrit tube?
    a. Beneath the packed red cells
    b. Above the plasma
    c. Above the packed cells and beneath the plasma
    d. Buffy coats are not seen in microhematocrit tubes

18. What is indicated by a neutrophil with a nucleus that has seven lobes?
    a. Toxic neutrophil in response to toxemia
    b. Toxic neutrophil in response to stress
    c. Hypersegmentation characteristics of an aging cell
    d. Normal finding

19. Eosinophilia is commonly seen with:
    a. Bacterial infections
    b. Parasitic infections
    c. Viral infections
    d. Hormonal disorders

20. The abbreviation "Seg" refers to which blood cell?
    a. Lymphocyte
    b. Monocyte
    c. Band
    d. Neutrophil

21. What is normally the largest blood cell in domestic animals?
    a. Monocyte
    b. Neutrophil
    c. Eosinophil
    d. Basophil

22. In the bird, what is the most common WBC seen on a smear?
    a. Neutrophil
    b. Heterophil
    c. Basophil
    d. Monocyte

23. Which cells on a blood smear are most frequently associated with DIC (disseminated intravascular coagulation)?
    a. Spherocytes
    b. Acanthocytes
    c. Basophils
    d. Schistocytes

24. An increase number of bands (>500/μl) in the peripheral blood indicates:
    a. Leukemia
    b. Leukemoid response
    c. A left shift
    d. Neutropenia

25. Under what circumstances would one need to obtain a corrected WBC count?
    a. High number of bands
    b. Decrease number of WBC
    c. High number of nRBC
    d. Decreased number of bands

26. Which cell becomes a macrophage once it enters the tissues?
    a. Plasma cell
    b. Lymphocyte
    c. Neutrophil
    d. Monocyte

27. Which equine WBC normally has large, round, red-orange staining cytoplasmic granules?
    a. Basophil
    b. Eosinophil
    c. Monocyte
    d. Neutrophil

28. Although serum is usually used for biochemical profiles, if plasma is desired, the **best** anticoagulant to use is:
    a. Heparin
    b. EDTA
    c. Citrate

29. A blood chemistry profile with an increase in BUN and creatinine indicates disease in which of the following organ systems?
    a. Pancreas
    b. Liver
    c. Kidneys
    d. Heart

30. A positive "blood" finding is determined on a reagent strip for a canine urine sample. Also included is the following data:
Plasma: clear; no RBC in the sediment; urine is dark brown in color; urine pH = 7.0
The most likely source of the positive finding is:
   a. Hemoglobin
   b. Myoglobin
   c. Blood
   d. Ketones

31. Casts are only seen in _____ urine. _____ casts almost always are indicative of severe degeneration of renal tubules.
   a. Alkaline, waxy
   b. Alkaline, hyaline
   c. Acidic, waxy
   d. Acidic, hyaline

32. Two concerns with using a reagent test strip for measuring protein in the urine are:
   a. Test strips are more sensitive to albumin and one can get false positive results with acidic urine
   b. Test strips are more sensitive to globulin and one can get false positive results with alkaline urine
   c. Test strips are more sensitive to albumin and one can get false positive results with alkaline urine

33. When evaluating canine urinary sediment, which choice best represents the relative size of elements from largest to smallest?
   a. WBC > squamous epithelial cells > RBC > transitional epithelial cells
   b. Transitional epithelial cells > squamous epithelial cells > WBC > RBC
   c. Squamous epithelial cells > transitional epithelial cells > WBC > RBC
   d. Transitional epithelial cells > RBC > WBC > renal epithelial cells

34. The ideal urine sample is:
   a. Preprandial and first morning sample
   b. Postprandial and first morning sample
   c. Postprandial and afternoon sample
   d. Preprandial and afternoon sample

35. In cases of ethylene glycol toxicity (antifreeze), which of the following crystals is most likely to be found in the urine?
   a. Ammonium biurate crystals
   b. Tyrosine crystals
   c. Calcium oxalate crystals
   d. Triple phosphate crystals

36. A urine SG of 1.010 may be described as:
   a. Concentrated
   b. Within the isosthenuric range
   c. Only reliable when a reagent test strip is used
   d. Hyposthenuric

TRUE OR FALSE

Select T (true) or F (false) for each statement below.

1. _____ When evaluating a blood film, first scan the smear on low power (10×).

2. _____ Slides prepared for cytologic analysis from a bodily fluid, tissue impression, or fine needle aspiration of a mass should always be stained before submission to a reference laboratory.

3. _____ The veterinary technician need not concern himself or herself with the routine care and maintenance of in-house laboratory equipment because a manufacturer-provided technician usually performs this service.

4. _____ Excess anticoagulant resulting from a small amount of blood in a too large tube can erroneously decrease the PCV and increase TP values determined with a refractometer.

5. _____ When collection tubes have an inadequate volume of blood, the excess anticoagulant causes the RBC to swell, erroneously increasing the PCV.

6. _____ Stains should be replaced on a regular basis to prevent bacterial contamination and accumulation of debris with repeated usage.

7. _____ Before a urinalysis is performed on refrigerated urine, the specimen should be allowed to come to room temperature.

8. _____ Good mucin clot formation usually is associated with inflammation and/or effusion, whereas a poor or absent mucin clot accompanies normal or noninflamed joints.

9. _____ Birds and reptiles have nucleated RBCs.

10. _____ Ketones are primarily one of the end products of fat metabolism and are commonly seen in the urine when carbohydrate metabolism is impaired in an animal.

11. _____ A Coombs test may be requested to further confirm the presence of immune mediated hemolytic anemia.

12. _____ The veterinary technician need not concern himself or herself with the routine care and maintenance of in-house laboratory equipment because a manufacturer-provided technician usually performs this service.

13. _____ In hematologic testing, the size of the collection tube used is not important as long as an adequate amount of blood is drawn for the test being run.

14. _____ A feline urine sample with a specific gravity of 1.010 is relatively concentrated.

15. _____ When evaluating a blood film, first scan the smear on low power (10×).

16. _____ Slides prepared for cytologic analysis from a bodily fluid, tissue impression, or fine needle aspiration of a mass should always be stained before submission to a reference laboratory.

17. _____ Blood films should always be made from fresh blood, before refrigeration, regardless of whether the CBC will be performed in the practice or sent to a reference laboratory.

MATCHING

Match the items in Column B with the appropriate one in Column A. This section focuses on the differences in species. Find the species that best characterizes the situation on the left.

Column A	Column B
1. _____ Anisocytosis of RBC	A. Normal in the cat
2. _____ Multiple forms of reticulocytes	B. Normal in the cow
3. _____ Mature RBC that are nucleated	C. Normal in the horse
4. _____ Calcium carbonate crystals in large numbers	D. Normal in the bird

Match the definition in Column B with the appropriate term in Column A.

Column A	Column B
5. _____ Pyuria	A. Increased frequency of urination
6. _____ Hematuria	B. Pus (WBC) in the urine
7. _____ Pollakiuria	C. Blood in the urine
8. _____ Oliguria	D. Decreased volume of urine produced

Match the lab finding in Column B to the appropriate description in Column A.

Column A	Column B
9. _____ Abnormal RBC morphology associated with liver disease	A. Basophilic stippling
10. _____ Nuclear remnant seen in RBCs associated with splenectomized animals	B. Heinz bodies
	C. Howell-Jolly bodies
11. _____ Lead poisoning in dogs may cause this RBC pattern	D. Poikilocytosis
12. _____ Variation in shape of a RBC indicating improper production or premature destruction of RBC's	E. Acanthocytes
	F. Spherocytes
13. _____ This abnormal RBC morphology can be associated with autoimmune disease	G. Hemobartonella
14. _____ Denatured hemoglobin seen in RBCs associated with oxidative injury	
15. _____ Feline infectious anemia associated with this RBC parasite	

Match the anticoagulant in Column B with the appropriate test in Column A.

Column A	Column B
16. _____ CBC, differential and blood smear	A. Sodium Citrate
17. _____ Plasma sample for general biochemical analysis	B. Heparin and electrolytes
18. _____ Clotting profile	C. EDTA

140

To avoid the following condition/problem in Column A, match Column B with the appropriate intervention.

Column A

19. _____ Hemolysis
20. _____ Lipemia
21. _____ Iatrogenic bacterial overgrowth in urine sample
22. _____ Artificial/iatrogenic decrease in blood glucose

Column B

A. Fast the animal before drawing blood

B. Avoid centrifugation for a prolonged period of time

C. Do not let sample sit out on counter for a prolonged period of time

D. Separate serum from RBC as soon as possible

FILL IN THE BLANKS

Use the following key terms to fill in the blanks.

Hemoglobin
Hemoglobinuria
Ketonuria
Myoglobinuria
Red blood cells

Specific gravity
Total protein
Urine protein/creatinine ratio
White blood cells

1. _____ indicates excessive fat metabolism, a deficiency in carbohydrate metabolism, or both but is most commonly seen in conjunction with glucosuria as a complication of diabetes mellitus.

2. _____ results in red to brown urine with a positive urine blood reaction and no RBC in the sediment.

3. _____ will result in red to brown urine with no RBC in the sediment, a positive blood reaction, a positive urine protein test result and the serum or plasma generally remains clear.

4. _____ is a good index of protein loss in the urine and are normally done at a reference laboratory because it requires a sensitive protein determination.

5. _____ in fresh unstained urine sediment appear colorless or yellowish and are round, slightly refractile with no internal structures.

6. _____ in fresh unstained urine sediment appear round, granular, and smaller than an epithelial cell.

7. A refractometer is used to determine the _____ of plasma and the _____ of urine.

8. _____ is the protein in RBCs that is responsible for carrying oxygen from the lungs to the tissues.

SHORT ANSWER

1. List the tests that are included in a CBC (complete blood count).

_____

_____

2. Briefly describe the procedure for performing a PCV (packed cell volume).

_____

_____

3. A cat has a total leukocyte count of 15,000. On the differential count, 50% of the cells are neutrophils. What is the absolute neutrophil count?

_____

4. Describe three methods of urine collection and describe the technique of each one.

   A. _____

   B. _____

   C. _____

5. List the physical properties evaluated in a routine urinalysis.

_____

6. Why is equine urine normally cloudy?

_____

7. Why should a fresh urine sample always be used to perform a complete urinalysis?

_____

8. Briefly describe the preparation for urinary sediment examination.

_____

_____

_____

_____

_____

_____

9. List the five main types of casts and a brief description of each.

   A. _____

   B. _____

   C. _____

   D. _____

   E. _____

10. List four potential parasites that can occur in urine.

   A. _____

   B. _____

   C. _____

   D. _____

11. Describe the procedure for making a quality blood smear and the procedure for evaluating a differential blood smear.

   _____

   _____

   _____

   _____

   _____

   _____

   _____

   _____

   _____

   _____

   _____

12. Describe the procedure for making a smear after a cytologic sample was obtained through a fine needle aspiration.

   _____

   _____

   _____

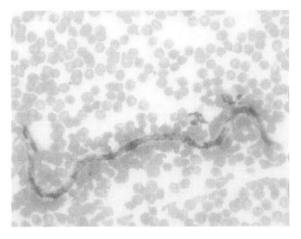

1. Identify this parasite in a canine blood smear.

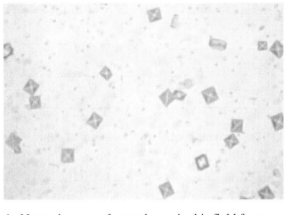

4. Name the type of crystal seen in this field from a canine urine sediment.

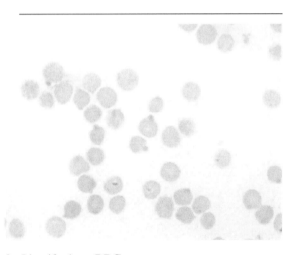

2. Identify these RBCs.

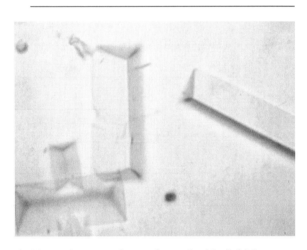

5. Name the type of crystal seen in this field from a urine sediment.

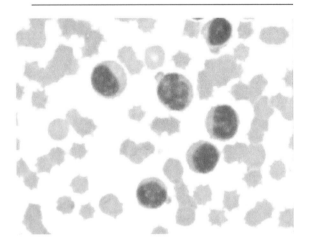

3. What type of WBCs are seen in this field?

CROSSWORD PUZZLE: CHEMISTRIES AND URINE

Across

4. Urine SG 1.008 to 1.012
7. Urine SG <1.008
8. Urine obtained when the animal voids spontaneously as the animal urinates (two words)
11. pH is the inverse logarithm of the _____ ion concentration of a fluid
13. Urinary casts that contain globules from degenerating tubular epithelial cells
14. Type of urinary casts that contain recognizable cells embedded in the protein matrix
15. Serum pH above the reference range

Down

1. Wide and homogeneous urinary casts, usually with distinct blunt or squared ends
2. Quality control solution that contains the analyte of interest at a validated true concentration as determined by the manufacturer
3. Instrument used to determine the plasma protein concentration and urine specific gravity by measuring the refractive index
5. Ratio used to quantitate protein loss in the urine
6. Urine obtained by placing a needle (with a syringe attached) through the ventral abdominal wall into the lumen of the bladder and aspirating urine
9. Serum pH above the reference range
10. A sample, possibly pooled, from representative animal(s) that has had its concentration repeatedly determined by the chemistry analyzer itself
11. RBCs in the urine
12. Homogeneous and semitransparent urinary casts

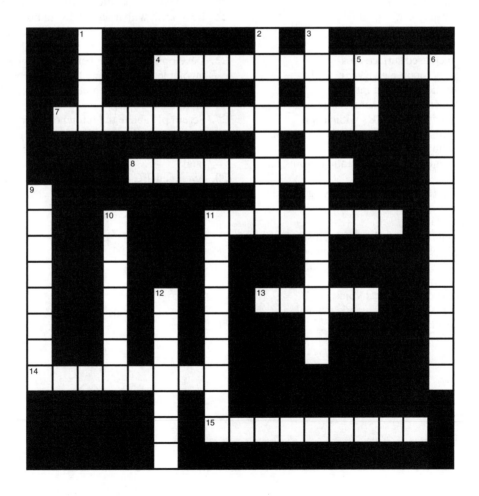

Chapter **16 Clinical Pathology**

CROSSWORD PUZZLE: CLINICAL PATHOLOGY

Across

1. A small drumstick appearing nuclear appendage representative of an inactivated X chromosome that may be present in neutrophils from females (2 words)
5. Neutrophils with increased amounts of cytoplasmic RNA
8. RBCs in the urine
9. Direct measure of red cell mass by centrifugation expressed as a percentage of blood composed of RBCs
11. Nuclei with five or more lobes
13. Type of cast that is wide and homogeneous usually with a distinct blunt or squared end
14. Neutrophil equivalent with reddish granules found in species such as avians, reptilians, amphibians, and nonhuman primates
16. Species-specific test to detect RBC surface bound antibodies and/or complement most frequently used to support the diagnosis of immune-mediated hemolytic anemia
17. A measure of anisocytosis
19. Crenated RBCs that have multiple spicule appearing projections
23. RBCs with an increased surface area
25. Solutions that may report a given expected concentration of the analyte of interest
26. Colorless, homogeneous, and semitransparent casts
29. Large immature anucleate RBCs with deeply basophilic dots or strands in the cytoplasm seen on new methylene blue (NMB) stain
30. Average RBC hemoglobin concentration expressed in g/dl
31. Immature RBC prior in developmental stage to the reticulocyte
32. Larger than normal cell
33. Solution that contains the analyte of interest at a validated "true" concentration as determined by the manufacturer using gold standard methodologies
34. A segmenter is a mature _____.
35. Urine obtained when the animal voids spontaneously or is assisted by gentle manual expression (2 words)

Down

1. Multiple tiny, lightly basophilic RBC inclusions due to staining of small amounts of cytoplasmic RNA in RBCs (2 words)
2. Leukocyte with a segmented nucleus and blue granules
3. Variation in cell size
4. A white blood cell
6. Increased MCHC
7. A measure of red cell mass expressed as a percentage of blood composed of RBCs
10. Urine with a specific gravity of 1.008 to 1.012
12. Mononuclear cell with gray-blue cytoplasm, which may contain a few clear vacuoles and a variable-shaped nucleus
15. Small, often singular, deeply basophilic nuclear remnants that are occasionally seen in RBCs on normal blood films (3 words)
18. Type of cast characterized by a nonspecific grainy matrix and designated as either coarse or fine
20. Urine with a specific gravity of less than 1.008
21. Leukocyte with a segmented to bilobed nucleus, colorless to pale blue cytoplasm, and distinct reddish orange staining cytoplasmic granules
22. Developmental stage before the segmenter with an incompletely segmented band-shaped nucleus
24. Type of left shift seen in the absence of increased mature neutrophils
27. Serum pH above the reference interval
28. A coagulopathy resulting from the uncontrolled consumption of coagulation factors that may be fatal
30. Average RBC volume expressed in femtoliters

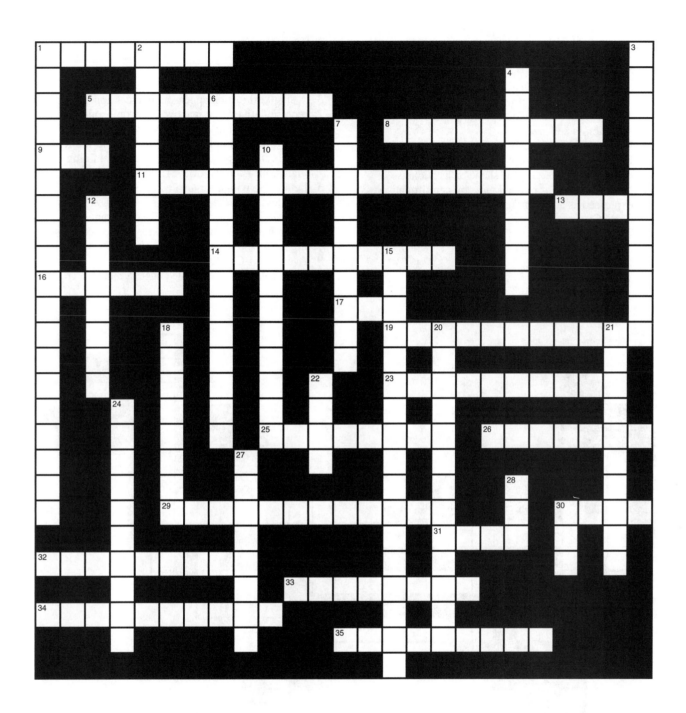

CROSSWORD PUZZLE: HEMATOLOGY

Across

2. RBCs that resemble stacked coins

6. Calculated measure of red cell mass expressed as a percentage of blood composed of RBCs

8. Variation in cell size

9. Larger than normal cells

10. Developmental neutrophil stage before the mature neutrophil; named for the shape of its nucleus

11. Direct measure of red cell mass by centrifugation expressed as a percentage of whole blood composed of RBCs

12. RBCs with an increased surface area; e.g., target cells

Down

1. White blood cells

3. A small drumstick appearing nuclear appendage representative of an inactive X chromosome that may be present in neutrophils from females

4. Denatured hemoglobin that has fused to the RBC membrane; appear as distinct, darkly staining inclusions (bodies) on NMB stain

5. Leukocyte with a segmented to bilobed nucleus, colorless to pale blue cytoplasm, and distinct reddish orange staining cytoplasmic granules

7. Average RBC hemoglobin concentration expressed in grams per deciliter

9. Average RBC volume expressed in fl

10. Leukocyte with a segmented nucleus and blue granules

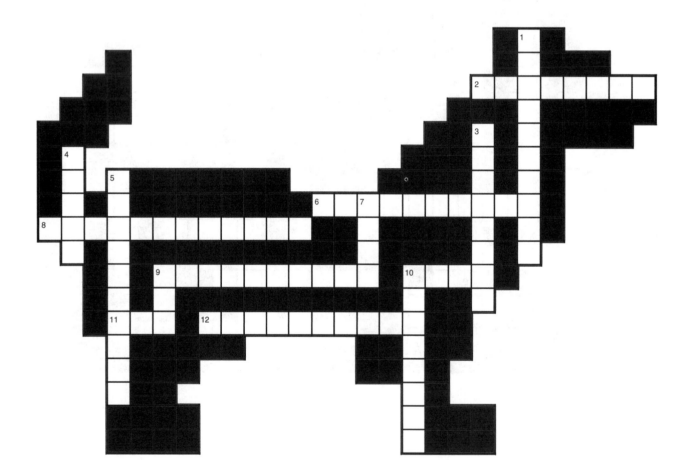

CROSSWORD PUZZLE: HEMATOLOGY

Across

2. RBCs with multiple, irregularly spaced, club-shaped projections from the cell surface
7. Large immature anucleate RBCs with deeply basophilic dots or strands in the cytoplasm seen on new methylene blue (NMB) stain
9. RBC fragment
11. Average RBC volume expressed in fl
14. A counting chamber used for microscopic determination of cell concentration in fluids
17. Developmental neutrophil stage before the mature neutrophil named for the shape of its nucleus
18. RBCs with an increased surface area; e.g., target cells
21. Smaller than normal cells
22. Leukocyte with a segmented nucleus and blue granules
23. White blood cells

Down

1. Increased numbers of bands seen on a blood smear (2 words)
3. Neutrophil nuclei with five or more lobes
4. Average RBC hemoglobin concentration expressed in grams per deciliter
5. Larger than normal cells
6. Leukocyte with a segmented to bilobed nucleus, colorless to pale blue cytoplasm, and distinct reddish orange staining cytoplasmic granules
8. Crenated RBCs that have multiple spicule appearing projections
10. Direct measure of red cell mass by centrifugation expressed as a percentage of whole blood composed of RBCs
12. Calculated measure of red cell mass expressed as a percentage of blood composed of RBCs
13. Variation in cell size
15. RBCs that resemble stacked coins
16. Neutrophil equivalent with reddish granules found in species such as elephants, rodents, avians, reptilians, amphibians, and nonhuman primates
17. A small drumstick appearing nuclear appendage representative of an inactivated X chromosome that may be present in neutrophils from females
19. Denatured hemoglobin that has fused to the RBC membrane; appear as distinct, darkly staining inclusions (bodies) on NMB stain
20. Pale bluish-gray irregular cytoplasmic inclusions (bodies) of RNA containing rough endoplasmic reticulum seen in neutrophils

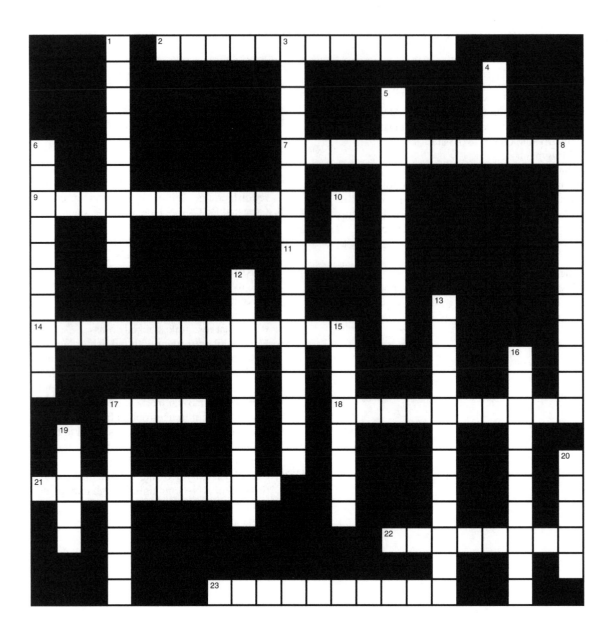

17 Parasitology

LEARNING OBJECTIVES

When you have completed this chapter, you will be able to:

1. Define the following terms: intermediate host, definitive host, reservoir host
2. State the scientific and common names for the nematode, cestode, trematode, and protozoal parasites commonly encountered in small and large animal practice
3. List the definitive and intermediate hosts for the nematode, cestode, trematode and protozoal parasites commonly encountered in small and large animal practice
4. Describe collection and handling of fecal samples from small and large animals
5. Describe the procedures for gross examination and direct examination of fecal samples and state the advantages and limitations of the procedure
6. List the methods commonly used to concentrate parasitic material in fecal samples
7. Describe the procedure for performing standard fecal flotation and centrifugal flotation
8. List and describe the procedures for identification of blood parasites
9. List the scientific and common names for ectoparasites commonly encountered in small and large animal practice
10. List and describe the procedures for collection of samples and identification of ectoparasites

PHOTO QUIZ

Match the parasites in the following figures with the names listed below.

a. Skin scraping showing *Demodex canis*
b. Life cycle stages of *Ctenocephalides felis*
c. Ovum of *Trichuris vulpis*
d. Trophozoite of *Giardia* spp.
e. Final larval stage of *Gasterophilus species*
f. Microfilariae of *Dirofilaria immitis* on a Knotts test
g. Strongyle type of ovum of horses
h. Oocyst of *Isospora* spp.
i. Adult *Otodectes cynotis* mite
j. Oocysts of *Isospora* spp. and ovum of *Ancylostoma caninum*
k. Assorted chewing lice *Mallophaga*
l. Examples of commercial fecal flotation kits
m. Ovum of *Toxocara* spp.

n. Egg packet of *Dipylidium caninum*
o. Characteristic hookworm ovum
p. Ovum of *Toxascaris leonine*
q. Proglottids of *Dipylidium caninum*
r. Ovum of *Oxyuris equi*
s. Adult *Sarcoptes scabiei* mite
t. Bovine trichostrongyle type of ova
u. *Taenia* spp. and *Dipylidium caninum* segments
v. Assorted *Anoplura* lice
w. Microfilariae of *Dirofilaria immitis* on DiFil test filter
x. Scheme of movement of the microscope field to thoroughly view entire coverslip
y. Adult *Psoroptes cuniculi* mites

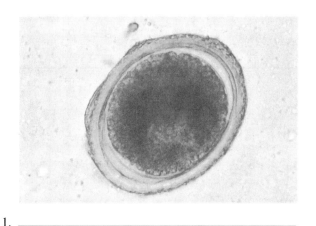

1. _____

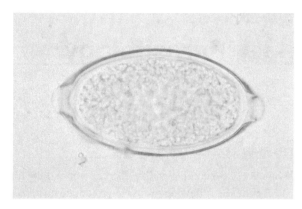

4. _____

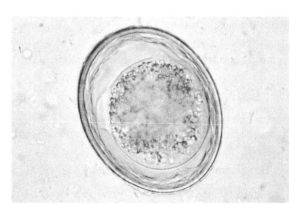

2. _____

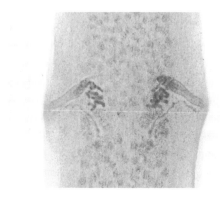

5. _____

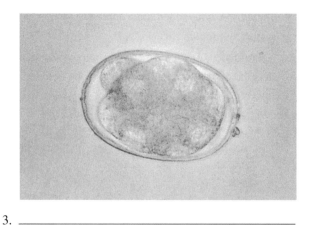

3. _____

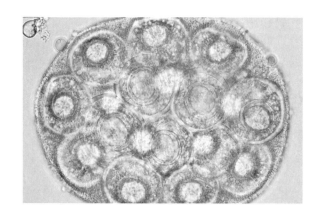

6. _____

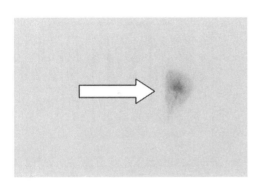

7. _____

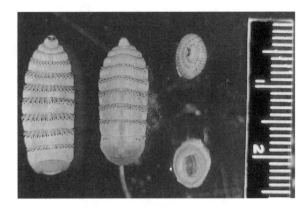

10. _____

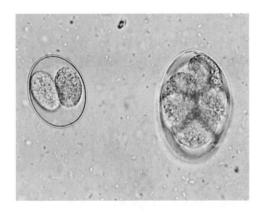

8. _____

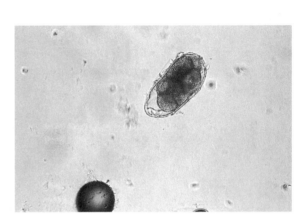

11. _____

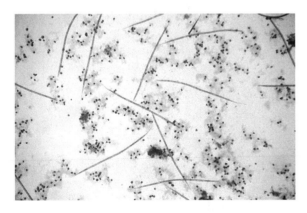

9. _____

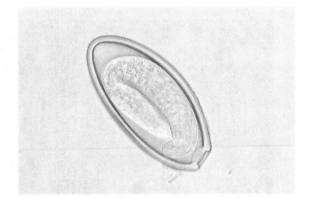

12. _____

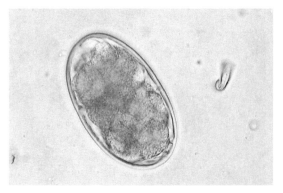

13. _____

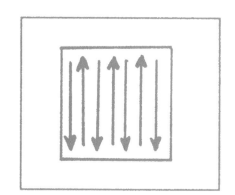

16. _____

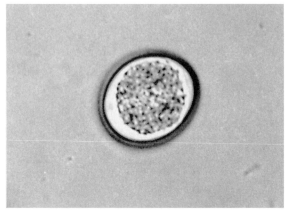

14. _____

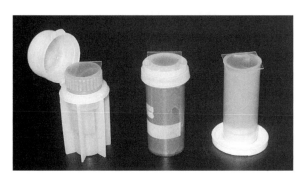

17. _____

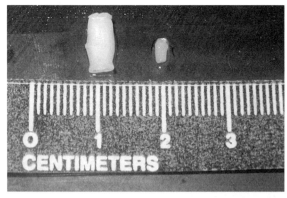

15. _____

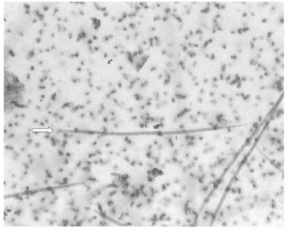

18. _____

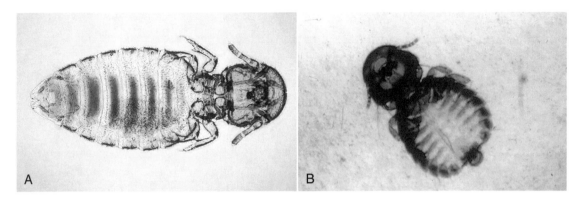

19. _____

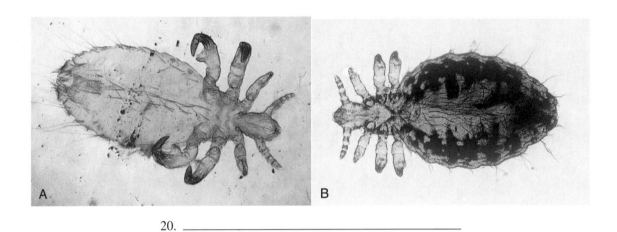

20. _____

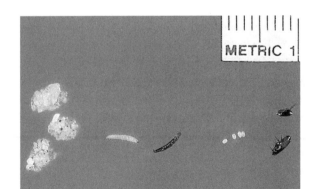

21. _____

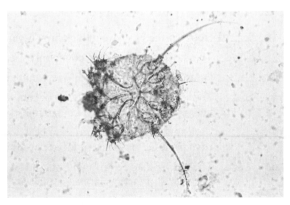

22. _____

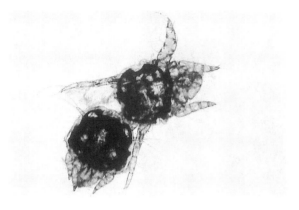

23. _____

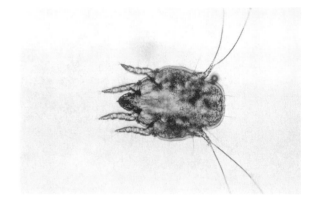

24. _____

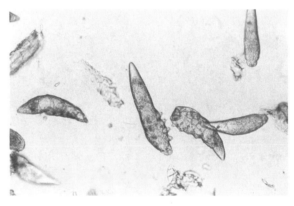

25. _____

TRUE OR FALSE

Select T (true) or F (false) for each statement below.

1. _____ Hookworm eggs have a thick brown-yellow shell with a clear polar plug at each end.

2. _____ The direct fecal smear is commonly used to identify eggs of tapeworms, nematodes, and coccidia.

3. _____ Parascaris equorum is highly resistant to environmental conditions making control difficult in horses.

4. _____ Zoonotic diseases should be a concern to veterinary personnel and requires strict attention to personal hygiene and avoidance of contaminated materials.

5. _____ Cattle and sheep lungworms are best diagnosed by using the Baermann funnel technique, which detects eggs from feces, soil, or minced tissues of animals.

6. _____ The zinc sulfate centrifugal flotation technique uses Lugol solution to stain certain eggs, larvae and cysts. The plural of larva is larvae, not larvas.

7. _____ Organophosphates should never be used on puppies younger than 16 weeks of age or on kittens younger than 6 months of age.

8. _____ The Stoll centrifugation technique provides a direct correlation between the severity of parasitism and the number of eggs.

9. _____ The roundworm's normal mode of infection is skin penetration.

10. _____ The complete life cycle of the flea occurs on the dog's or cat's body.

11. _____ The best control for *Giardia* spp. is to prevent consumption of raw flesh and contact with feces of infected cats.

12. _____ The Willis technique is a reliable test for the identification of *Giardia* spp. and lungworms.

13. _____ Diagnosis of *Oxyuris equi* is effectively performed only by the adhesive tape method.

14. _____ All tapeworms use an intermediate host in which a larval stage develops.

15. _____ Mites are usually diagnosed by the Baermann funnel technique.

16. _____ *Dirofilaria immitis* adults reside in the left ventricle and pulmonary arteries of the host.

17. _____ The filter and Knott's techniques are simple tests commonly used to detect microfilariasis.

18. _____ The most common endoparasite in pigs is *Ascaris suum*.

19. _____ *Strongyloides stercoralis* is unique because it is one of the only common intestinal nematodes of dogs and cats that is passed in the feces in a larval form *not* encased in an egg.

MULTIPLE CHOICE

1. The common name for trematodes is:
   a. Whipworms
   b. Flukes
   c. Tapeworms
   d. Pinworms

2. _____, _____, and _____ pass their eggs in dog feces and are commonly diagnosed by fecal-flotation techniques.
   a. Tapeworms; heartworms; hookworms
   b. *Dirofilaria* spp.; *Dipetalonema* spp.; *Dipylidium* spp.
   c. Ascarids; hookworms; whipworms
   d. Intestinal threadworms; coccidia; *Giardia* spp.

3. "Marty" is an adult, indoor-only Siamese cat who experiences recurrent tapeworm infections. After his most recent treatment for this infection, about what did you counsel his owner to prevent another infection with this parasite?
   a. Litter-box sanitation
   b. Flea control
   c. Diet
   d. Preventing the cat from interacting with the family's pet parrot

4. Which equine parasite has larval stages that migrate through the cranial mesenteric artery and its branches?
   a. *Strongyloides westeri*
   b. *Strongylus equines*
   c. *Strongylus vulgaris*
   d. *Anoplocephala magna*

5. The most important gastrointestinal parasites of cattle and sheep in the United States are the _____, which are diagnosed by seeing _____ in the feces.
   a. Trematodes; leaf-shaped larvae
   b. Cestodes; blood
   c. Strongyle nematodes; strongyle type of eggs
   d. Trematodes; strongyle type of eggs

6. Sulfonamide antibiotics are indicated in the treatment of:
   a. Tapeworms
   b. Coccidia
   c. Large and small strongyles
   d. Intestinal threadworms

7. Of the common domestic animal species, only _____ are infected by pinworms.
   a. Sheep
   b. Goats
   c. Cattle
   d. Horses

8. Which insecticide is considered the most toxic, especially to puppies and kittens younger than 6 months of age?
   a. Pyrethrins
   b. Lufenuron
   c. Fipronyl
   d. Organophosphates

9. Which flea-control agent is safe for judicious use in nursing animals?
   a. Lufenuron
   b. Fipronyl
   c. Imidacloprid
   d. Pyrethrins

10. Mites are diagnosed by the morphologic appearance of the adults, which most often requires:
    a. Thorough skin scrapings
    b. Close examination of the skin and hair with the unaided eye
    c. The adhesive-tape test
    d. That cut hair samples be sent to a parasitologist for species identification

11. The larvae of blowflies and screwworm flies are known collectively as:
    a. Bots
    b. Maggots
    c. Grubs
    d. Cercariae

12. For which parasite is a direct fecal-saline smear the best diagnostic test?
    a. *Trichomonas* spp.
    b. *Toxocara* spp.
    c. *Toxoplasma gondii*
    d. *Amblyomma* spp.

13. What technique is used to quantify the number of parasitic eggs and larvae per gram of feces?
    a. Willis technique
    b. Stoll dilution or Stoll centrifugation technique
    c. Baermann funnel technique
    d. Formalin-ethyl acetate sedimentation technique

14. The two most effective techniques for detecting blood microfilarial infections are:
    a. The direct blood smear and the saline-blood preparation
    b. The saline-blood preparation and the microhematocrit technique
    c. The Knott's and filter techniques
    d. The direct blood smear and the Knott's technique

15. If neither the motile trophozoites nor the cysts of *Giardia* are seen on a direct fecal-saline smear, and giardiasis is suspected, which test should you next perform on the feces?
    a. $ZnSO_4$ centrifugal flotation
    b. Maceration technique
    c. Stoll dilution technique
    d. Direct fecal smear made with distilled water rather than saline

16. A *schizont* is:
    a. Part of the life cycle of *Isospora* spp.
    b. Part of the life cycle of the cestode parasites
    c. Part of the life cycle of the trematode parasites
    d. A newborn German-breed puppy

17. "Warbles" are:
    a. Flies that lay their eggs in feces
    b. Flies that lay their eggs in a row just above the claws of cattle
    c. Seen as lumps on the backs of infested cattle
    d. The sounds a hungry cat makes when it wants to be fed

SHORT ANSWER

1. What is the common and full scientific name of the most frequently encountered parasite in pigs?

   _____

2. For each of the four stages of the flea life cycle, name and describe the stage where organisms in that stage live or are usually located, and what, if anything, they feed on.

   A. _____

   B. _____

   C. _____

   D. _____

3. Describe the premise on which fecal-egg flotation techniques are based. In other words, how do they work?

   _____

   _____

   _____

4. Why are fecal-flotation techniques unsuitable for trematode eggs (with the exception of *Troglotrema* and *Paragonimus* spp.)?

   _____

5. How is it possible for an animal to be severely parasitized yet the diagnostic test for that parasite, properly performed, is negative?

   _____

MATCHING

Match the parasite with the species and the organ it invades.

Parasite	Species	Organ
1. _____ *Ancylostoma caninum*	a. Horse	I. Large intestine
2. _____ *Trichuris vulpis*	b. Rabbit	II. Surface of skin
3. _____ *Ancylostoma tubaeforme*	c. Cat	III. Small intestine
4. _____ *Cheyletiella spp.*	d. Rabbit, cat, dog	IV. Ear canal
5. _____ *Psoroptes cuniculi*	e. Dog	V. Stomach

159

Copyright © 2010 by Saunders, an imprint of Elsevier Inc.

Chapter **17 Parasitology**

CROSSWORD PUZZLE

Across

1. Infection by a nematode using the milk of a lactating female dog to her nursing puppies
6. The "door" on one end of a trematode egg or the egg of a pseudotapeworm
7. The host that harbors the larval, asexual, or immature stages of the parasite
9. A worm
10. An organism that must live a parasitic existence
12. Infestation with either Anoplura (sucking) or Mallophaga (chewing) lice
15. An association between two organisms of different species in which one member (the parasite) lives on or in the other member (the host), and may cause harm
18. A parasite that lives within the body of the host
19. An intermediate host in which the parasite does not undergo any further development
21. The motile prelarval stage of filarial parasites
23. A parasite in a host in which it does not usually live
24. The holdfast organelle of an adult true tapeworm
26. A parasite that makes short visits to its host to obtain nourishment or some other benefit
27. The period of time between the time the infective stage of a parasite is ingested by a host to the time that the infective stage develops to the adult stage of the parasite, becomes sexually mature, breeds, and begins to produce offspring (either eggs or larvae)
28. A vertebrate host in which a parasite (or disease) occurs naturally and which is a source of infection for human beings and their domestic animals
29. Nematodes that bear live larvae
30. A tapeworm

Down

2. The entire body of the tapeworm
3. A single living organism that contains complete, functioning sets of both male and female reproductive organs
4. A parasite that has wandered into an organ or tissue in which it does not ordinarily live
5. A fluke
8. Host that harbors the adult, sexual, or mature stages of the parasite
11. Parasitism by an external parasite
12. An object that is mistaken for a parasite
13. A parasite that lives on the outside of the body of the host
14. Parasitism by an internal parasite
16. Infestation by either mites or ticks
17. The infection/infestation of Diptera larvae (maggots) into the organs or tissues of human beings, domesticated animals, or wild animals
20. An organism that is capable of living either free or as a parasite
22. Any disease that is transmissible from lower animals to human beings
23. A life cycle that uses an intermediate host
25. An arthropod that mechanically transmits bacteria, viruses, Chlamydia, and spirochetes from one host to another

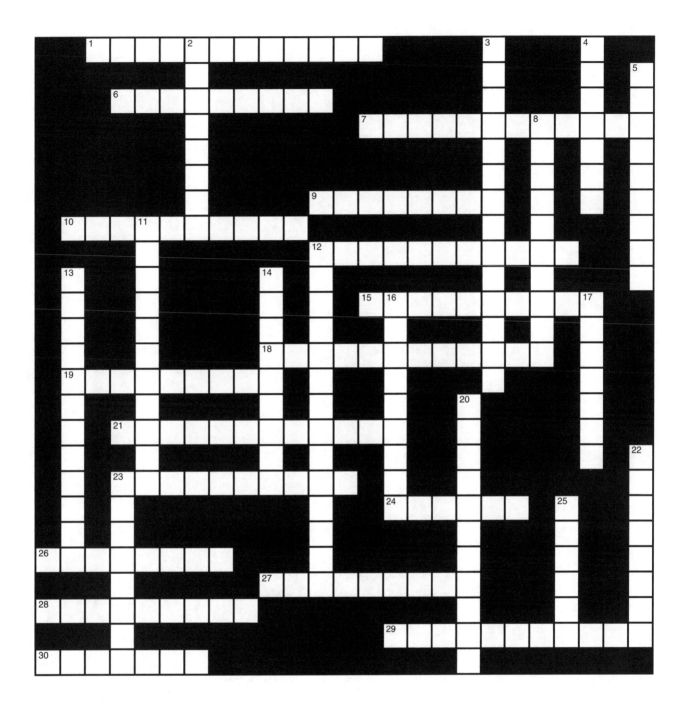

18 Clinical Microbiology

LEARNING OBJECTIVES

When you have completed this chapter, you will be able to:

1. Describe methods for collection and handling of samples for microbiology testing
2. List the steps of the Gram stain procedure
3. Describe the procedure for inoculation of agar plates, broth, and slant tube media and explain proper incubation methods for bacterial cultures
4. List types of culture media commonly used for primary isolation of microorganisms and explain the specific use of each
5. List and describe the characteristics of bacterial colonies that are evaluated on primary isolates
6. Describe common staining procedures and biochemical tests used for identification of bacteria
7. Describe the procedures for performing blood and urine cultures
8. List common bacterial species encountered in small and large animal practices
9. Describe the procedure for performing antimicrobial susceptibility testing
10. List the common fungal organisms encountered in veterinary practice and describe the procedures for sample collection and identification of these organisms
11. Describe the general principles of serologic analysis for bacterial and viral antigens
12. Define nosocomial infection and explain methods for control of nosocomial infections

DEFINE

Define the following terms.

1. MIC _____

_____

2. Selective medium _____

_____

3. Differential medium _____

_____

4. Enrichment medium _____

_____

5. Transport medium _____

_____

6. Hemolysis _____

_____

7. Nosocomial infections _____

_____

8. Gram stain _____

_____

9. Pathogen _____

_____

10. Abscess _____

_____

11. Acid-fast stain _____

_____

12. Aerobe _____

_____

13. Anaerobe _____

_____

14. Antibiogram _____

_____

15. Antibiotic _____

_____

16. Antigen _____

_____

17. Microflora _____

_____

18. Microbiology _____

_____

19. Antimicrobial testing _____

_____

20. Immunoglobulins _____

_____

21. Immunohistochemical stain _____

_____

22. Serology _____

_____

23. Catalase _____

_____

24. Oxidase _____

_____

25. Coagulase _____

_____

26. Mycosis _____

_____

27. Dermatophyte _____

_____

28. Yeast _____

_____

29. Disinfectant _____

_____

30. Antiseptic _____

_____

31. Sanitizer _____

_____

32. Fastidious _____

_____

Chapter **18** **Clinical Microbiology**

33. Infection _____

_____

34. Zoonosis _____

_____

MULTIPLE CHOICE

1. Which bacterium is *not* gram-positive?
   a. *Streptococcus*
   b. *Enterobacteriaceae*
   c. *Staphylococcus*
   d. *Erysipelothrix*

2. Which bacterium is *not* a gram-negative rod?
   a. *Enterobacteriaceae*
   b. *Pasteurella*
   c. *Pseudomonas*
   d. *Bacillus*

TRUE OR FALSE

Select T (true) or F (false) for each statement below.

1. _____ Some microorganisms present unique morphologic characteristics, host inflammatory responses, and lesions, such that a preliminary diagnosis may be made without further laboratory testing.

2. _____ For best results, the administration of antimicrobials will have little or no effect on obtaining the best culture specimens.

3. _____ Swabs are the best transport media to isolate fungi and mycobacteria.

4. _____ The same swab can be used to inoculate several media as long as the least inhibitory media is inoculated first, and the most inhibitory media is inoculated last.

5. _____ Specimens should never be cultured solely in a broth medium for primary isolation.

6. _____ Blood samples in anticoagulants (heparin and EDTA) are acceptable for culture.

7. _____ *Staphylococcus aureus* and *Staphylococcus intermedius* are usually more pathogenic than other coagulative-positive species.

8. _____ Antimicrobial susceptibility testing is always indicated for *Streptococcus* spp. suspects.

9. _____ Culturing *Bacillus anthracis* should never be attempted in a veterinary laboratory.

10. _____ Antimicrobial susceptibility testing is a necessary clinical evaluation tool.

11. _____ *Pseudomonas* spp. are usually not resistant to antimicrobials so do not need to be tested for susceptibility.

12. _____ Most veterinarians will begin antimicrobial therapy before lab results are final.

13. _____ Humans tend to be less resistant to yeast infections than animals.

14. _____ Often, IgG antibodies are less specific than IgM and may cross-react, resulting in false-positive test results.

SHORT ANSWER/FILL IN THE BLANK

1. The sophistication of diagnostic microbiology performed in a local practice lab depends on three things in comparison to services through a referral lab. List them.

   A. _____

   B. _____

   C. _____

2. The choice of method for examining a specimen in the microbiology lab depends on _____

   and _____.

3. When organisms are difficult to cultivate, or not viable in the specimen presented, the demonstration of specific

   microbial _____ or _____ may be quicker and more
   cost effective to the practice.

4. This type of assay includes enzyme immunoassays, latex particle agglutination, and protein A coagglutination
   procedures. Name this type of test.

   _____

5. Botulism and mycotoxicoses require the presence of a _____ instead of identifying
   the organism that produces it.

6. A patient showing a specific _____ to an infectious agent can establish the diagnosis
   itself.

7. Exudates and tissue biopsy specimens can be used in _____ as a diagnostic method.

8. Direct protocols using _____ and _____ have tremen-
   dous potential for detecting microbial pathogens, which are very sensitive and highly specific.

9. Nucleic acid amplification assays use primers and _____ (PCR) to provide specific-
   ity and sensitivity to detect as few as one organism or 1-10 copies of the specific gene sequence.

10. False-positive results from _____ of samples can be carried on gloves, bench tops,
    or aerosolized droplets.

11. This test method, _____, is used to discern whether DNA or RNA from an organism
    is present within a specimen.

12. What is the goal of specimen collection?

    _____

    _____

13. The best culture specimen should be from the _____.

14. Taking a swab from mucous membranes or skin will yield this result:

    _____

    _____

15. Describe the best and most useful specimen collection site.

    _____

    _____

16. Obtaining an adequate amount of material to be tested should be collected in aliquots of body fluids of this amount

    _____, and exudates or pieces of tissue of this amount _____.
    These are more useful than a sample collected on a swab.

17. In most cases, these are acceptable for transferring samples from the patient to culture media.

    _____

18. What is the function of transport media?

    _____

    _____

19. Ames Transport Medium with charcoal is best suited for this type of bacteria:

    _____

20. The Port-A-Cul Transport System is intended for this type of bacteria:

    _____

    _____

21. A culture swab placed in nutritive broth before inoculation of isolation media is not a benefit producing a good
    specimen for evaluation. Why is this true?

    _____

    _____

22. List at least six types of information that must accompany a specimen submitted for culture.

    A. _____

    B. _____

    C. _____

    D. _____

    E. _____

    F. _____

23. This is frequently the best collection device for aspirating exudate from an infected site:

    _____

24. How should a sample in a syringe be transported to the lab?

    _____

25. How are selective transport media different from anaerobic transport systems?

_____

_____

26. In processing of specimens, the laboratory worker must be very careful not to cause this.

_____

27. List one bacterial species that would cause gastroenteritis in each of the following species.

    A. Dog: _____

    B. Cat: _____

    C. Horse: _____

28. List two bacterial species that would cause abscesses in skin wounds in the following species.

    A. Dog: _____

    _____

    B. Horse: _____

    _____

    C. Ruminant: _____

    _____

29. Name two bacterial species that would cause a urinary tract infection in the following species.

    A. Dog: _____

    _____

    B. Cat: _____

    _____

30. List three reasons why you would recommend a second sample be submitted for processing.

    A. _____

    B. _____

    C. _____

31. List the two most important laboratory procedures that can be used for microbiologic diagnosis.

   A. _____

   B. _____

32. When examining urine for bacteria, which type is more easily detected without staining, cocci or rods?

   _____

33. List all the steps, in order, for preparing a gram-stained slide.

   A. _____

   B. _____

   C. _____

   D. _____

   E. _____

   F. _____

   G. _____

   H. _____

34. Gram-positive organisms stain what color?

   _____

35. Gram-negative organisms stain what color?

   _____

36. For what reasons might a gram-negative organism stain as if it were gram-positive?

   _____

   _____

37. What substances often stain gram-negative and may mask detection of gram-negative bacteria?

   A. _____

   B. _____

   C. _____

38. List at least six commonly used supplies and equipment required to perform basic diagnostic bacteriology tests.

   A. _____

   B. _____

C. _____

D. _____

E. _____

F. _____

39. Characteristics of a good quality incubator include:

A. _____

B. _____

C. _____

D. _____

E. _____

40. A solid media is designed to allow for a specimen to grow in such a way that _____ develop; each representing a single type of bacteria.

41. A selective media contains _____ for specific groups of bacteria. Name a selective type of media.

_____

42. The type of bacteria that can grow on MacConkey agar can grow in the presence of _____, which is similar to the environment found in the intestines. MacConkey agar is also a differential type of media

because it allows the _____ ability of some bacteria.

43. While there are several different streaking technique modifications, what is the goal of all these techniques?

_____

44. When a semisolid media for motility testing is inoculated, how is the inoculating wire to be used?

_____

45. How should an inoculated plate be inoculated and why?

_____

_____

46. Inoculated screw-top media tubes that are being incubated should be _____.

47. Most cultures for isolation of pathogenic bacteria are incubated at what temperature?

_____

48. While most pathogenic bacteria will grow well in room air, oxygen is toxic to _____.

49. Name two types of anaerobic systems used in small laboratories.

A. _____

B. _____

50. Most inoculated agar plates should be examined after _____ hours.

51. Slow-growing bacteria may need to be incubated for up to _____ before a negative report is issued.

52. A private veterinary practice should use a routine culture system that is designed to be _____ when used for routine aerobic cultures.

53. The most widely used primary isolation medium is _____ because of its ability to support growth of most pathogenic bacteria.

54. Blood agar is a standard medium used for describing _____ and _____.

55. The most common enrichment broth media used as part of a primary isolation media is

_____.

56. Enrichment media is formulated to facilitate cultivation of microorganisms that may be present in the specimen in

_____ or have _____.

57. The characteristics of primary cultures to be noted include:

A. _____

B. _____

C. _____

D. _____

58. In general, if there is very little aerobic growth of three or more bacteria, the result most likely reflects

_____.

59. In evaluating a colony's morphologic characteristics, these four characteristics are most likely to be significant:

A. _____

B. _____

C. _____

D. _____

60. Define the following types of hemolysis observed on blood agar plates and give the name of each one.

Complete: _____

Incomplete: _____

Nonhemolytic: _____

61. Hemolysis of blood agar is a good indication of a _____.

62. Coagulase-positive isolates of Staphylococcus spp. produces _____ hemolysis.

63. This easy-to-follow type of work chart works well for recording all observations of illustration of culture processing and observation.

_____

64. A good system of recording the relative abundance of growth of each type of colony is:

_____

65. Bacterial cultures should not be evaluated as positive or negative because of the small number recovered on the plate due to the following possible reasons:

A. _____

B. _____

C. _____

D. _____

66. For those who are highly experienced in identification procedures of bacteria, such characteristics as the following might be adequate for presumptive identification:

A. _____

B. _____

C. _____

D. _____

67. The primary differential characteristic at the start of identifying all bacteria is the reaction to

_____.

68. A more rapid test that can be used as an alternative to the Gram stain for isolated colonies is the use of a small drop

of _____. In this test, you are going to mix a colony of bacteria with this substance

and look for a _____ on your inoculating loop.

Chapter **18 Clinical Microbiology**

69. If you suspect a gram-negative organism and want to skip the Gram stain, you can usually assume this is correct if there is heavy growth on a _____ plate.

70. The quick test to differentiate between *Staphylococcus* and *Streptococcus* spp. is the _____ test. This test uses a colony of bacteria on a slide, mixed with a drop of _____.

71. This reaction indicates a positive catalase test: _____. However, if any blood agar is introduced into the test, it is a _____ result.

72. A positive reaction to this test is used for all gram-negative bacteria except strong lactose fermenters.

_____

73. Isolates of *Streptococcus* are usually characterized by the type of _____ they produce. Which type is usually considered a potential pathogen? _____

74. The TSI agar slant is used for differentiation between *Staphylococcus* and *Micrococcus*. In this test, you are looking for its _____.

75. Small gram-positive rods can be differentiated by inoculating these media:

_____

76. Members of the Enterobacteriaceae family are usually gram-_____ and oxidase-_____.

77. Why should you not ship inoculated agar plates?

_____

78. Commercial kit systems for identification of bacteria is most cost-effective for _____ laboratories.

79. An advantage in using commercial kit systems is that most bacteria can be identified within _____ hours.

80. The kit systems with a wide acceptance in veterinary bacteriology include the following:

A. _____

B. _____

C. _____

81. Blood cultures would be used for the following types of illnesses:

A. _____

B. _____

C. _____

D. _____

82. What is an important consideration in avoiding contamination of blood cultures?

_____

83. Positive blood cultures are recognized by one or more of the following characteristics:

A. _____

B. _____

C. _____

D. _____

84. Why is urine such a good growth medium for bacteria?

_____

85. Because bacteria can readily grow in urine and the sample can be contaminated, cultures must

_____ if the sample cannot be set up immediately.

86. What types of agar are used for identifying bacteria in urine?

A. _____

B. _____

87. For most samples the amount of inoculum is not important, but for urine, you must use a calibrated loop that

delivers _____ ml.

88. Describe the Gram stain characteristics and catalase test results of *Staphylococcus* spp.

_____

89. *Staphylococcus* spp. are often isolated from pyogenic lesions, such as:

A. _____

B. _____

C. _____

D. _____

E. _____

F. _____

90. *Staphylococcus* spp. are classified as _____ and _____ groups.

91. The most characteristic differentiation of the hemolytic staph organisms is the development of

_____.

92. Describe the Gram stain characteristics and catalase test results of *Streptococcus* spp.

_____

93. *Streptococcus* bacteria are the most common source of _____ and

_____ in all species of animals.

94. *Streptococcus equi* is the cause of _____ in horses.

95. *Streptococcus agalactiae* is an important cause of _____ which can be identified using

the _____ test.

96. _____ hemolysis is indicative of pathogenicity whereas _____

or _____ hemolysis usually indicates normal flora of skin and mucous membranes.

97. What site would you suspect is most commonly infected by the *Enterococcus* spp.?

_____

98. *Enterococcus* spp. are significant nosocomial agents, which are becoming more of a problem because:

_____

99. These gram-positive rod bacteria are common contaminants in the laboratory because they are ubiquitous in soil, water, air, and dust.

_____

100. Which species of *Bacillus* is the most important and pathogenic species because of its virulence in humans?

_____

101. This large, spore-forming anaerobic rod is a potent toxin and causes massive destruction of tissues.

_____

102. From where is *Clostridium perfringens* occasionally isolated?

_____

103. Which small gram-positive rod is motile at room temperature?

_____

104. What type of disease does *Listeria monocytogenes* cause in ruminants?

_____

105. A definitive characteristic that differentiates *Erysipelothrix rhusiopathiae* from other gram-positive rods

is the production of _____. This bacteria is a common cause of

_____ in pigs.

106. This family includes some clinically important bacteria that are distinguished by forming branching, filamentous gram-positive rods.

_____

107. *Nocardia* spp. may be serious pathogens in some dairy herds, causing _____.

108. *Streptomyces* spp. are aerobic, filamentous bacteria found in _____ and can be

isolated as _____.

109. Acid-fast stained impression smears can be a useful diagnostic procedure for a presumptive diagnosis

of _____ infection.

110. This family of gram-negative bacteria is the largest group of potential pathogens and most often isolated

bacteria: _____. Its normal habitat is in the _____.

111. Enteric organisms usually grow well on _____ agar.

112. Three common identifying characteristics of enteric gram-negative rods include the following:

A. _____

B. _____

C. _____

113. Most non-Enterobacteriaceae, gram-negative bacteria are oxidase-_____.

114. *Escherichia coli* is frequently identified by the strong _____ reaction it produces on MacConkey agar.

115. *E. coli* is often associated with _____ in neonates, especially pigs, calves, and lambs.

116. *E. coli* organisms are important in veterinary medicine as _____ agents after the use of antimicrobial therapy.

117. When culturing feces, it is important to use _____ and _____ media to increase the chances of isolating *Salmonella*.

118. The selective media used to isolate *Salmonella* are _____ and

_____ agar.

119. These bacteria have a unique characteristic of swarming on agar plates:

_____

120. *Actinobacillus* spp. are oxidase-positive rods and produce characteristic _____.

121. *Pasteurella* spp. are usually associated with _____ infections in animals.

122. The normal flora of mucous membranes may contain these bacteria:

_____

123. These bacteria are commonly found in water and soil and are often opportunistic pathogens of wounds and otitis:

_____

124. This small coccobacillus is frequently found in respiratory tract infections in dogs and is becoming an important respiratory pathogen of dogs:

_____

125. Due to its capability of producing abortion and infertility, this small coccobacillus isolate should be sent to a reference lab because of its regulatory and zoonotic importance:

_____

126. Species identification is rarely important when working with these gram-negative anaerobes. They are frequently involved in mixed infections in abscesses and necrotic tissue. Name two.

    A. _____

    B. _____

127. Arthritis and pneumonia are common diseases caused by this small bacterium that lacks cell walls:

_____

128. The most common mechanism for acquired resistance of an antimicrobial is _____.

129. When is susceptibility testing indicated?

    A. _____

    B. _____

    C. _____

130. Gram-_____ bacteria have unpredictable resistance patterns to require susceptibility testing.

131. The simplest type of susceptibility test is one that determines the presence of _____ that can inactivate an antimicrobial.

132. The most precise method of susceptibility testing systems is the _____.

133. What represents the degree of susceptibility of an isolate to a drug?

_____

134. The standard culture medium for the diffusion test for susceptibility is _____ agar.

135. For fastidious pathogens *(Streptococcus, Listeria, Corynebacterium, Erysipelothrix),* _____

    or _____ enrichment is necessary.

136. For best results, susceptibility tests should always be performed using a _____ of bacteria.

137. Describe the Diffusion Test Procedure.

    A. _____

    _____

    B. _____

    _____

    _____

    C. _____

    _____

    _____

    D. _____

    _____

    _____

    _____

    E. _____

    F. _____

    _____

138. Disks impregnated with different antimicrobials should be evenly distributed on the inoculated agar plate so that

    there is at least _____ mm space from the center of one disk to the center of another.

139. The antimicrobial susceptibility test should be repeated if this happens:

_____

140. How are results of the antimicrobial susceptibility test reported?

A. _____

B. _____

C. _____

141. The most common fungal agents you will expect to identify in a lab are _____ and

_____.

142. Which type of fungal agent requires specialized lab facilities and procedures for identification, but is seen infrequently?

_____

143. Dermatophytes are keratinophilic fungi. Where would they typically be found?

_____

144. Dermatophytes cause a disease, commonly referred to as _____.

145. Describe the procedure for collection of a suspected dermatophyte sample.

A. _____

_____

B. _____

C. _____

D. _____

_____

E. _____

_____

F. _____

G. _____

_____

H. _____

146. How would you prepare a direct mount of a fungal culture?

    A. _____

    _____

    B. _____

    _____

147. What is the standard medium for isolation of fungi?

    _____

148. What color are most dermatophyte colonies on the agar?

    _____

149. Dermatophytes rapidly change the normal yellowish color of DTM agar to _____.

150. _____ of fungi serve as the basis for identification.

151. The three most important systemic mycoses are:

    A. _____

    B. _____

    C. _____

152. Which disease is a chronic infection characterized by nodular lesions of skin or subcutaneous tissues?

    _____

153. The best way to isolate yeast is to inoculate _____ agar and _____ agar.

154. Name the species of yeast found in cases of external otitis and a cause of seborrheic and hypersensitivity reactions associated with dermatitis.

    _____

155. *Cryptococcus neoformans* can be differentiated from other nonpathogenic yeasts because it grows at

    _____ ° C and is urease _____.

156. Name the species of yeast usually involved in infections of mucous membranes that is frequently an opportunistic

    pathogen. _____

157. Viruses are _____ intracellular parasites that are best recovered from living tissue.

158. To collect the best viral specimen to deliver to a lab, when is it optimal to collect the sample?

_____

159. Viral infections may be identified by microscopic examination of infected tissues for the presence of

_____ or of body fluids for the presence of viral particles.

160. Direct electron microscopic examination is solely for _____ viruses, such as those found in body fluids.

161. Diagnostic labs usually perform _____ staining for virus identification.

162. List four advantages of antigen detection compared with viral isolation.

   A. _____

   B. _____

   C. _____

   D. _____

163. What does the acronym ELISA represent?

_____

164. The most common type of enzyme immunoassay test is the _____.

165. At what time during an animal's illness will you find the greatest number of microorganisms present?

_____

166. It is best to collect two samples during a viral infection. At what times during the infection will you want to collect the samples?

   A. _____

   B. _____

167. A change in antibody titer is known as _____.

168. When an animal is exposed to an infectious agent, the first antibodies produced are usually of the

_____ class, with later antibody production being _____.

169. The timing of serum collection is very important. When should the first sample be collected?

_____

170. How should blood be collected for a serum sample?

   A. _____

   B. _____

   C. _____

171. List the four types of immunologic disorders.

    A. _____

    B. _____

    C. _____

    D. _____

172. Which types of immunologic disorders are the most frequently seen?

    _____

173. Allergies are usually diagnosed by physical examination, history, and _____.

174. Autoimmune disorders can be diagnosed efficiently by evaluating _____.

175. Common sequelae to the failure of the neonate to obtain and absorb adequate colostral immunoglobulins include:

    A. _____

    B. _____

176. What test is the reference method for quantitating serum immunoglobulins?

    _____

177. Where would you observe the highest incidence rates for nosocomial infections?

    _____

178. What factors predispose an animal to a nosocomial infection?

    A. _____

    B. _____

    C. _____

    D. _____

    E. _____

    F. _____

    G. _____

    H. _____

179. Many nosocomial infections are caused by what type of microorganisms, which otherwise would not cause an infection in a healthy animal?

    _____

180. List at least five reservoirs for microorganisms found in a hospital.

   A. _____

   B. _____

   C. _____

   D. _____

   E. _____

181. What is the most important way to prevent the spread of nosocomial infections in a hospital?

   _____

182. What types of microorganisms are most resistant to disinfectants and sterilization?

   _____

183. What is the first, and most important, step in disinfection of physical structures in a hospital?

   _____

184. Name at least three precautions that the technician and others should take when working with hazardous chemical disinfectants.

   A. _____

   B. _____

   C. _____

185. Urease-positive bacteria produce a _____ color change in the slant and sometimes throughout the butt.

186. What color will you see as a positive indole test result?

   _____

CROSSWORD PUZZLE

Across

3. An antimicrobial agent that kills or inhibits the growth of microorganisms on the external surfaces of the body
5. A useful differential staining procedure that specifically stains all members of the genus *Mycobacterium* (two words)
6. An infection acquired within a hospital or hospital-like setting, but secondary to the patient's original condition
7. A disease that may be transmitted between animals and humans
10. An antimicrobial product, often a detergent, that reduces the number of bacteria to a safe level on a treated surface, but does not completely eliminate them
12. An antimicrobial agent that is applied to nonliving objects to destroy disease-causing microorganisms and their spores by physical or chemical means
19. Fungal infection in or on a part of the body
20. Immunoglobulin formed in blood or a tissue that interacts only with antigens that induced its synthesis
21. A microorganism that can live and grow in the absence of oxygen
22. A group of large glycoproteins that are secreted into blood and tissue fluids by plasma cells and that function as antibodies in the immune response by binding with specific antigens
24. A growth medium that permits preferential emergence of certain organisms that initially may have made up a relatively minute proportion of a mixed inoculum
25. Localized collection of pus in part of the body formed by tissue disintegration usually resulting from bacterial infection and surrounded by an inflamed area
26. A growth medium that contains microbial inhibitors that allow the preferential growth of desired types of microorganisms in preference to others
27. Unicellular fungi that reproduce by budding

Down

1. A fungus that causes infections of the skin, hair, and nails because of its ability to obtain nutrients from keratinized material
2. Destruction of the RBC membrane
4. Molecule or substance that is recognized by the immune system as foreign (nonself) and that elicits an immune response or specific antibody response
8. Microorganisms (mostly bacteria) with intimate and permanent associations with epithelial surfaces; also called normal flora
9. Concerned with the quantitative and qualitative detection of antibody in serum that reacts with a known antigen
11. Substance produced by a microorganism that inhibits or kills other microorganisms
13. Describes microorganisms with complex nutritional requirements, usually requiring an enriched medium for cultivation
14. A nonnutritive, buffered medium for maintaining viability without overgrowth of microorganisms while carrying specimens to the laboratory for examination
15. Catalase is an enzyme found in most living cells that catalyzes the decomposition of hydrogen peroxide into water and __
16. An enzyme that is used as an indicator of virulence and a differential identifying characteristic of some bacteria, especially *Staphylococcus*
17. An enzyme that reacts with molecular oxygen to catalyze the oxidation of a substrate
18. A growth medium that allows two or more organisms to be distinguished from one another by some characteristic
23. A differential bacteriologic stain that distinguishes bacterial cell-wall structure types, which is a common basis for bacterial classification and identification

Chapter **18** **Clinical Microbiology**

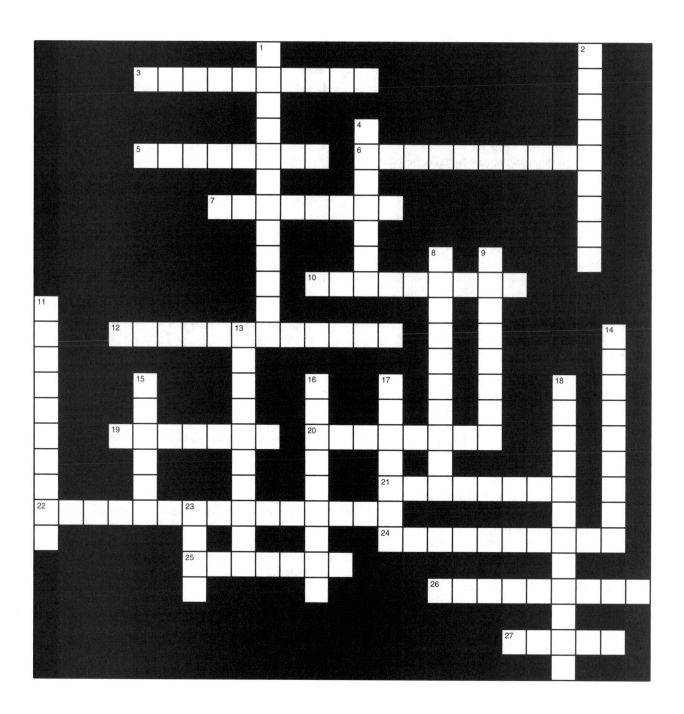

19 Diagnostic Imaging

LEARNING OBJECTIVES

When you have completed this chapter, you will be able to:

1. List and describe methods for labeling of radiographic films
2. Describe the parts of the x-ray machine and explain the production of x-rays
3. Differentiate between computed tomography, diagnostic ultrasound, nuclear medicine, magnetic resonance imaging, digital radiography, and computed radiography
4. List advantages and disadvantages of digital radiography
5. Define DICOM and explain its use in the veterinary practice
6. Explain the procedure for developing a radiographic technique chart
7. Describe the components of the x-ray intensifying screen and list the unique properties of rare earth intensifying screens
8. Differentiate between screen and nonscreen x-ray film
9. Explain the purpose and construction of the grid in radiology and differentiate between focused and nonfocused grids
10. Describe use, care, and maintenance concerns related to x-ray film processing
11. Differentiate between radiographic contrast and density and explain how kilovoltage and milliamperage affect contrast and density of the radiograph
12. List common artifacts encountered on radiographic images and methods for minimizing these problems
13. List and describe safety issues related to radiography and methods for reducing exposure to radiology hazards
14. List commonly used types of radiographic contrast agents and give examples of each
15. State general considerations in positioning of patients for radiography
16. Describe the preparation of a patient for ultrasound imaging and explain the importance of each step
17. Identify basic ultrasound artifacts and describe their cause
18. List tissues in order from most to least echogenic and identify basic anatomic structures on ultrasound images
19. Define radioactive half-life and explain its importance in veterinary medicine
20. Give the main advantages of teleradiology for the veterinary field

DEFINE

Define the following terms:

1. Anechoic _____

_____

2. A-mode _____

_____

3. Anode _____

_____

4. B-mode _____

_____

5. Cathode _____

_____

6. Computed Radiography _____

_____

7. DICOM _____

_____

8. Digital Radiography _____

_____

9. Fluoroscopy _____

_____

10. Grid _____

_____

11. Heel Effect _____

_____

12. Hyperechoic _____

_____

13. Ionizing Radiation _____

_____

14. Isoechoic _____

_____

15. Kilovoltage _____

_____

16. M-mode _____

_____

17. Milliamperage _____

_____

18. PACS _____

_____

19. Rad _____

_____

20. Rem _____
_____

21. Rotating Anode _____
_____

22. Stationary Anode _____
_____

23. Teleradiology _____
_____

24. X-rays _____
_____

25. Density _____
_____

FILL IN THE BLANKS

1. _____ is a thin sheet of lead strips with radiolucent spacers encased in an aluminum cover.

2. The presentation of a continuous image that involves the use of an image intensifier is referred to as

_____.

3. _____ is any radiation capable of displacing electrons from atoms or molecules thereby producing ions.

4. _____ are a form of electromagnetic radiation that can be used in diagnostic imaging to produce either radiographs or computed tomographic images.

5. The shorter the wavelength, the _____ the energy of the x-ray beam and the greater the penetrating power.

6. The setting that controls the amount of electrons boiled off the filament in the x-ray tube is the

_____.

7. The negatively charged side of the x-ray tube is the _____.

8. According to the Heel effect, the x-ray beam is more intense on the _____ side of the x-ray tube.

9. The practice of transmitting digital images from one hospital to the next via computer connections is

_____.

10. Portable or dental units use _____ anodes.

11. _____ is the quality factor that regulates the energy of the x-ray beam.

12. In an ultrasonic image, a structure that appears bright or white compared to adjacent structures is called

_____.

X-RAY MATCHING

1. _____ Type of anode found in dental units
2. _____ Regulates the voltage difference between the anode and the cathode
3. _____ Determines the number of electrons produced inside the x-ray tube
4. _____ Film's ability to convert absorbed x-rays into visible light
5. _____ The degree of sharpness that defines the edge of an anatomic structure
6. _____ The amount of blackness on a film
7. _____ Opacity/density difference between two areas on the x-ray
8. _____ Range of different opacities on a radiograph
9. _____ Measure of radiation exposure or x-ray machine output
10. _____ Unit of absorbed dose of ionizing radiation
11. _____ Unit equal to the absorbed radiation dose multiplied by a qualifying factor
12. _____ Usually located between the patient and the image receptor; absorbs scattered radiation
13. _____ Converts x-rays into fluorescent light allowing for a lower mA setting
14. _____ Lower-energy x-ray photons that have undergone a change in direction after interacting with structures in the patient's body
15. _____ Decrease in the energy of the x-ray photons as they pass through matter

a. Attenuation
b. Contrast
c. Density
d. Detail
e. Grid
f. Intensifying screen
g. kVp
h. Latitude
i. mAs
j. Rad
k. Rem
l. Roentgen
m. Rotating
n. Scattered radiations
o. Screen speed
p. Stationary

PHOTO QUIZ

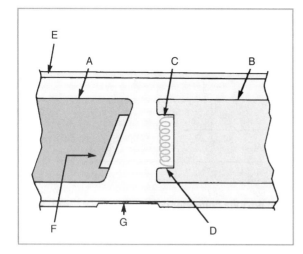

1. Identify the parts of the x-ray tube.

   A. _____

   B. _____

   C. _____

   D. _____

   E. _____

   F. _____

   G. _____

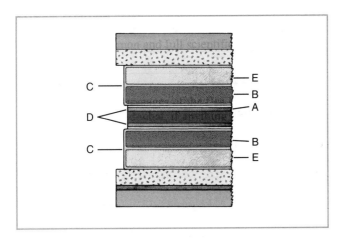

2. Identify the parts of the cassette intensifying screen system.

A. _____

B. _____

C. _____

D. _____

E. _____

SHORT ANSWER

1. What is the main disadvantage of digital radiography when compared with conventional radiography?

   _____

2. The shorter the wavelength, the _____ the energy of the x-ray beam and the greater the penetrating power.

3. List one way in which DR differs from CR. _____

4. What does the acronym DICOM stand for? _____

5. Why is it important? _____

6. Name four types of ionizing radiation.

   A. _____

   B. _____

   C. _____

   D. _____

7. List the two types of electrical circuits present in every x-ray tube.

   A. _____

   B. _____

8. List two reasons that the rotating anode is angled.

   A. _____

   B. _____

9. The actual focal spot is _____ than the effective focal spot.

10. What three primary factors must be set to produce diagnostic radiographs?

   A. _____

   B. _____

   C. _____

11. If you increase the focal-film distance, you _____ the number of x-rays reaching the film.

12. kVp controls the _____ of electron acceleration and _____ of the x-ray beam.

13. The main source of radiation exposure for veterinary personnel comes from _____.

14. List the three factors that when increased directly increase scattered radiation.

   A. _____

   B. _____

   C. _____

15. Scattered radiations are of concern because:

   A. _____

   B. _____

16. Rare earth screens have several properties that give them an advantage over other screen types. List four of the advantages.

   A. _____

   B. _____

   C. _____

   D. _____

17. What is the optimal time and temperature for hand developing?

   _____

18. List the four items that must be included as part of the identification label on a radiograph.

A. _____

B. _____

C. _____

D. _____

19. When developing a technique chart, list the factors that must remain constant.

A. _____

B. _____

C. _____

D. _____

20. A grid should be used for a thickness greater than _____ cm.

21. Unexposed film in the darkroom must be protected from:

A. _____

B. _____

C. _____

D. _____

E. _____

22. Describe the steps to take to properly hand develop a radiograph.

A. _____

B. _____

C. _____

D. _____

E. _____

23. What are the "big three" of radiation safety?

A. _____

B. _____

C. _____

24. List the protection practices that should be employed to reduce radiation exposure.

A. _____

B. _____

C. _____

D. _____

E. _____

F. _____

G. _____

H. _____

I. _____

25. Film badges are used to monitor radiation exposure; what other factors can expose them?

A. _____

B. _____

C. _____

26. List the contrast agent that would be commonly used for the following studies.

A. Esophagus _____

B. Stomach _____

C. Large bowel _____

D. Urinary tract _____

27. If an animal must be manually restrained for x-rays, list two ways to prevent unnecessary exposure to personnel.

A. _____

B. _____

28. List five advantages to using ultrasonography in veterinary medicine.

A. _____

B. _____

C. _____

D. _____

E. _____

29. As sound waves travel through the body they are attenuated by several factors:

A. _____

B. _____

C. _____

D. _____

E. _____

30. Circle the correct choice for ultrasound transducer characteristics.

High frequency
INCREASES / DECREASES resolution

INCREASES / DECREASES attenuation

INCREASES / DECREASES penetration

Low frequency
INCREASES / DECREASES resolution

INCREASES / DECREASES attenuation

INCREASES / DECREASES penetration

31. Place the following organs in order according to their echogenicity; most echogenic to least echogenic.

_____

_____

A. Liver
B. Renal cortex
C. Spleen
D. Renal sinus fat
E. Renal medulla
F. Prostate

32. Give one example of therapeutic nuclear medicine. _____

33. List four common diagnostic uses of nuclear medicine.

A. _____

B. _____

C. _____

D. _____

34. List the advantages of CT imaging when compared with standard radiography.

A. _____

B. _____

C. _____

35. List the four ways MRI is superior to CT imaging.

A. _____

B. _____

C. _____

D. _____

36. What is the most important safety consideration when using an MRI unit?

_____

CONTRAST STUDY MATCHING

1. _____ Insoluble inert radiopaque medium
2. _____ Radiolucent gases
3. _____ Soluble ionic radiopaque medium
4. _____ Soluble nonionic radiopaque medium
5. _____ Double contrast study of the bladder
6. _____ Contrast study performed to localize spinal cord lesions
7. _____ Most common contrast study of the kidneys

A. IVP
B. Myelography
C. Nitrous oxide
D. Barium
E. Diatrizoate
F. Iopamidol
G. Cystogram

ULTRASOUND MATCHING

1. _____ Brightness mode ultrasound image display
2. _____ A structure on the ultrasound image that appears bright or white compared with adjacent structures
3. _____ Attenuation of the energy of the ultrasound beam as it passes through different tissues
4. _____ Time-motion ultrasound imaging mode where the motion of the body is observed by scanning a thin slice of it over time
5. _____ The energy of the returning energy is shown as an amplitude spike at each tissue interface when the ultrasound is in this mode
6. _____ A structure on the ultrasound image that is of equal echogenicity to another structure
7. _____ A structure in the ultrasound image that does not produce echoes and appears black

A. Acoustic impedance
B. Anechoic
C. A-mode
D. B-mode
E. Hyperechoic
F. Isoechoic
G. M-mode

DEFINE

1. Computed radiography _____

_____

2. Digital radiography _____

_____

3. Computed tomography _____

_____

4. Nuclear medicine _____

_____

5. Magnetic resonance imaging _____

_____

6. Inverse square law _____

_____

7. Distortion _____

_____

8. Piezoelectric effect _____

_____

9. Reverberation artifact _____

_____

10. Acoustic enhancement artifact _____

_____

11. Radiology information system _____

_____

12. Picture archival computing systems _____

_____

_____

13. Potter-Bucky diaphragm _____

_____

14. Air gap technique _____

_____

15. Dynamic range _____

_____

CALCULATE

Calculate the mAs for the following:

1. 300 mA, $\frac{1}{120}$ s = _____

2. 100 mA, $\frac{1}{60}$ s = _____

3. 100 mA, $\frac{1}{20}$ s = _____

Calculate the mA for the following:

1. _____ mA, 0.5 s = 50 mAs

2. _____ mA, 0.3 s = 60 mAs

3. Your original exposure factors are the 100 mA and 0.5 s. If you change the mA to 400, what is the new time?

   _____

4. Your original exposure factors are 400 mA and 0.3 s. If you change the mA to 300, what is the new time?

   _____

5. The original exposure factors were the 200 mA, FFD 100 cm time 1/120. What is the mAs if the FFD is changed to

   50 cm? _____

CROSSWORD PUZZLE

Across

1. A decrease in the energy of the x-ray photons as they pass through matter
4. Screens that contain a phosphor that is highly efficient in transforming energy into light compared with calcium tungstate screens (2 words)
5. This is the maximum allowed radiation exposure a person is allowed to receive during occupational exposure over a certain time
7. The density or opacity differences between neighboring areas on the radiographic image
9. A measure of radiation exposure or x-ray machine output
13. A structure in the ultrasound image that is of equal echogenicity to another structure
16. A structure in the ultrasound image that does not produce echoes and appears black
18. Degree of sharpness that defines the edge of an anatomic structure in the radiographic image
20. Placed between the patient and the film cassette to absorb scatter radiation so it does not reach the cassette and affect image quality
21. Positively charged side of the x-ray tube
22. The unit of absorbed dose of ionizing radiation
23. Controls the quantity of electrons boiled off the filament in the x-ray tube
25. Degree of blackness of the film
26. The region on the anode that is bombarded by electrons (2 words)

Down

2. A technique that uses increasing the distance between the patient and the cassette, scatter produced by the patient does not reach the cassette as easily thereby improving image quality (2 words)
3. Negatively charged side of the x-ray tube
6. The number of shades of gray in an image (2 words)
8. Radiographic film that requires direct exposure to x-rays to create an image
10. The x-ray beam is more intense at the side of the cathode than in the center of the beam or on the anode side (2 words)
11. The distance between the target in the x-ray tube and the surface of the x-ray cassette (2 words)
12. A quality factor that regulates the energy of the x-ray beam
14. Anode block that does not move and is imbedded in copper to aid in heat dissipation
15. Partially exposed film that causes poor contrast in the resulting radiographic image
17. A structure in the ultrasound image that appears bright or white compared with adjacent structures
19. The light bulb in the darkroom that is shielded by a plastic filter that stops light that the film is sensitive to from penetrating and exposing the film (2 words)
24. Iodinated contrast medium is injected intravenously to assess the kidneys

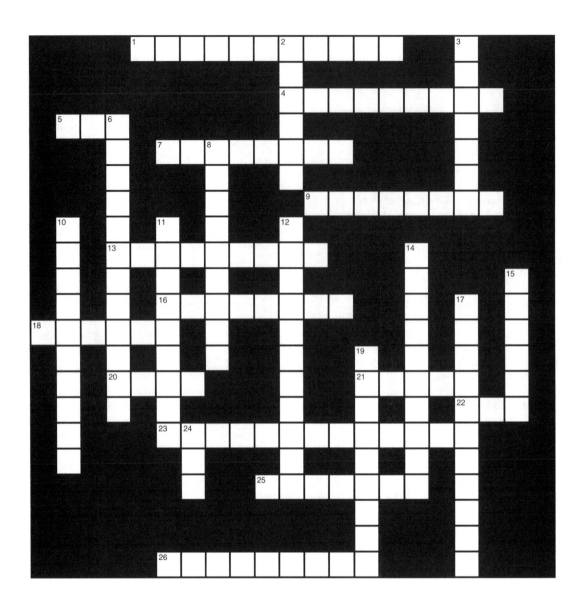

20 Diagnostic Sampling and Therapeutic Techniques

LEARNING OBJECTIVES

When you have completed this chapter, you will be able to:

1. List and describe general principles for collection of samples for laboratory testing
2. Describe patient preparation, positioning, and procedures for blood collection from peripheral veins and capillary beds in small and large animals
3. Describe indications and procedures for collection of arterial blood samples in small and large animals
4. List and describe procedures for collection of urine samples from small and large animals and give advantages and limitations of each method
5. Describe the indications and procedures for performing thoracocentesis, abdominocentesis, arthrocentesis, fine-needle aspiration, bronchoalveolar lavage, and collection of vaginal cytology samples in small and large animals
6. Describe the indications and procedures for performing diagnostic peritoneal lavage
7. Describe the two methods for performing a transtracheal wash and give advantages and disadvantages for each method
8. Describe procedures for obtaining cerebrospinal fluid and bone marrow aspirate samples and list indications, contraindications, and potential complications of the procedure
9. List the routes used for administration of medications in small and large animals and describe procedures for administration of medications by each route
10. Describe the procedure for placement and care of a peripheral intravenous catheter
11. Describe the indications and procedure for placement and care of a jugular catheter
12. List requirements for monitoring of patients with intravenous catheters
13. Describe indications and methods for administration of oral medication of enteral feeding of small and large animals
14. Describe procedures for collection and evaluation of milk samples from dairy animals
15. Describe procedures for collection of rumen fluid in large animals

SHORT ANSWER

1. Describe the appearance of thrombophlebitis at the site of catheter insertion.

   A. _____

   B. _____

   C. _____

   D. _____

2. List three tests that can be affeected by patient stress.

   A. _____

   B. _____

   C. _____

3. List the parts of the Vacutainer system used for blood collection.

A. _____

B. _____

C. _____

4. List three vessels commonly used for canine blood collection.

A. _____

B. _____

C. _____

5. List two causes of hemolysis related to blood collection.

A. _____

B. _____

6. A veterinarian hands you a patient and asks you to place an IV catheter, start IV saline at maintenance rate, administer IV antibiotics, offer food and water, and collect blood for a CBC and chemistry panel. She then leaves the room. Which procedure is best performed first and why?

_____

7. What can the person restraining a dog do to improve the visualization of the vein for blood collection?

_____

8. What are the borders of the intramuscular injection region on the neck of the horse?

A. _____

B. _____

C. _____

9. Describe the technique for administering a pill to a cat.

_____

10. List the materials needed for intravenous catheter placement.

A. _____

B. _____

C. _____

D. _____

E. _____

F. _____

G. _____

H. _____

I. _____

J. _____

K. _____

MULTIPLE CHOICE QUESTIONS

1. When collecting blood from a vein in the dog and cat, which direction should the bevel be pointed?
   a. Down
   b. Up
   c. To either side
   d. Doesn't matter

2. When collecting blood from the jugular vein, which is most important?
   a. Dog must be in lateral recumbency
   b. Rear legs must be extended
   c. Neck must be extended
   d. Forelegs must be extended

3. You are drawing blood from the medial saphenous vein of a cat using a 23-gauge needle on a 3-cc syringe. The blood begins to fill the syringe and then stops flowing. What is the most likely cause of this problem?
   a. The syringe is too large
   b. Too much suction has caused the vein to collapse
   c. The needle is too small
   d. The cat has developed an arrhythmia

4. What should be periodically infused in an IV catheter to prevent problems?
   a. Antibiotics
   b. Steroids
   c. Heparin
   d. EDTA

5. Intraosseous catheterization is most commonly placed in which bone in small animals?
   a. Humerus
   b. Femur
   c. Ulna
   d. Ilium

6. Vaginal smears are most commonly used in which animal?
   a. Bitch
   b. Queen
   c. Mare
   d. Cow

7. Due to anatomic obstacles, which male animal is rarely catheterized to obtain urine?
   a. Horse
   b. Bull
   c. Dog
   d. Goat

8. Which vaccine may be administered by the intranasal route in the dog?
   a. Leptospirosis
   b. Parvovirus
   c. Rhinotracheitis
   d. Bordetella

9. What is the term for a leukocyte count above normal?
   a. Leukemia
   b. Leucopenia
   c. Leukophilia
   d. Leukocytosis

10. Which is the vein from which you are most likely to successfully draw 10 ml of blood from an 11 kg dog?
    a. Femoral
    b. Cephalic
    c. Jugular
    d. Saphenous

TRUE OR FALSE

Select T (true) or F (false) for each statement below.

1. _____ The jugular vein is most commonly used for blood collection and administering IV drugs in the horse.

2. _____ When collecting blood from the neck of a pig it is important to avoid the phrenic nerve.

3. _____ Male dogs may be catheterized while fully awake, but male cats will usually require heavy sedation for this procedure.

203

4. _____ When you are performing a transtracheal wash, it is important to remove at least 90% of the fluid infused to prevent drowning of the animal?

5. _____ If you cannot administer antiseizure medication to a convulsing dog by the IV route, you can give it intrarectally or intranasally.

6. _____ The auricular vein is used for intravenous catheterization in hogs.

7. _____ Blood collection from the marginal ear vein of the cat is used to look for blood parasites.

8. _____ If an animal has pathologic changes in its lungs, then thoracocentesis is the most indicated diagnostic procedure.

9. _____ The best site for IM injections in farm animals is in the gluteal muscles.

10. _____ Stroking the perineal area of a cow will induce stimulate her to urinate.

11. _____ A Foley catheter may be used for transtracheal aspiration and for urinary catheterization.

12. _____ Coupage is a technique used to loosen mucous in the lungs.

13. _____ Anorexia describes a condition in which the animals are not eating.

14. _____ Some vaccines in cats may be administered by the intradermal route.

15. _____ Kinking a stomach tube while removing it will prevent flashback.

MATCHING KEY TERMS

1. _____ Percutaneous
2. _____ Hematoma
3. _____ Thoracentesis
4. _____ Cystocentesis
5. _____ Pneumothorax
6. _____ Pleural effusion
7. _____ Diagnostic peritoneal lavage
8. _____ Coupage
9. _____ Pancytopenia
10. _____ Phlebitis

A. Removal of fluid from the pleural cavity through a needle or catheter inserted between the ribs

B. A term referring to something passing through the skin

C. A collection of fluid between the thin layers of tissue lining the lung and the wall of the chest cavity (pleura)

D. A collection of blood outside a blood vessel caused by a leak or an injury

E. The act of striking the chest wall rhythmically with cupped hands. Cupping the hands creates an air cushion on impact so that tenacious mucous is dislodged

F. Inflammation of a vein

G. Use of a syringe and needle to obtain uncontaminated urine directly from the bladder

H. A decrease below normal in the concentration of the three major blood cell types: red cells, white cells, and platelets

I. The insertion of fluid in the peritoneal cavity. The fluid is allowed to dwell for a short period of time and then drained. Gross, microscopic, and chemical analysis is performed on the returned fluid

J. Accumulation of air between the outer lining of the lung and the chest wall, causing collapse of the lung

SHORT ANSWER FILL IN THE BLANK

1. For peripheral venipuncture, introduce the needle into the occluded vein as far _____ as possible.

2. This color tube contains EDTA anticoagulant.

   _____

3. To perform venipuncture from the right lateral saphenous vein, the animal is placed in _____ recumbency.

4. This needle size is commonly used to perform venipuncture on the medial saphenous vein.

   _____

5. This method of urine collection is needed to collect urine that is free of contamination from the distal urethra and genital tract.

_____

6. A normotensive, normovolemic animal with intact renal function should produce urine at this rate.

_____

7. Thoracocentesis is performed at this intercostal space in dogs.

_____

8. This is the route of choice for administering medications if a rapid onset of action is required.

_____

9. Intravenous and intraarterial catheters must not remain in the vessel longer than _____.

10. When giving an intramuscular injection into the semitendinosus or semimembranosus muscles, this nerve must be avoided.

_____

11. This amount of blood may be collected from the auricular vein of swine (maximum amount).

_____

12. The intercostal vessels and nerves run along this border of the ribs.

_____

PHOTO QUIZ _____

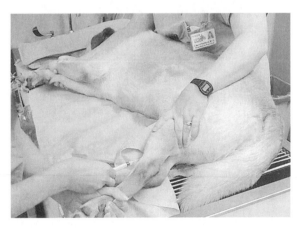

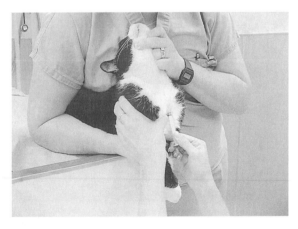

1. Name the blood vessel being used for venipuncture in this patient.

_____

2. Name the blood vessel being used for venipuncture in this patient.

_____

Chapter **20** **Diagnostic Sampling and Therapeutic Techniques**

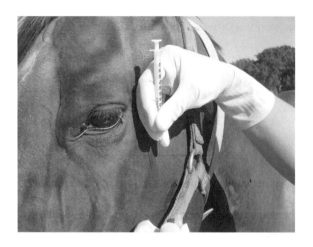

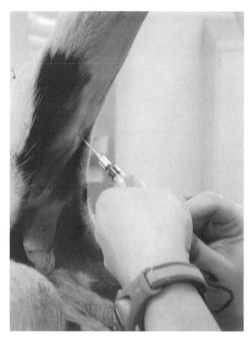

3. Name the blood vessel being used for venipuncture in this patient.

_____

4. Name the blood vessel being used for venipuncture in this patient.

_____

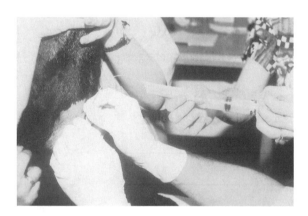

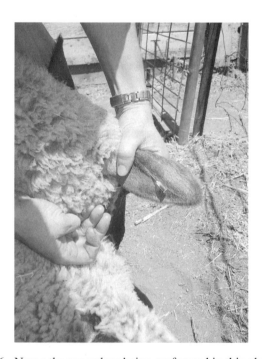

5. Name the procedure being performed in this photo.

_____

6. Name the procedure being performed in this photo.

_____

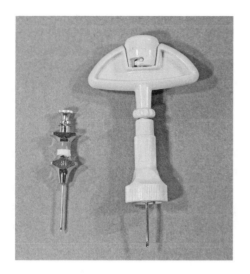

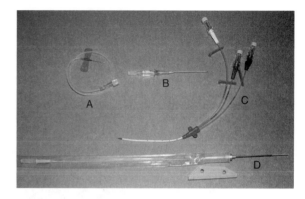

7. The bone marrow needle on the right is a

_____ style, while the one

on the left is a _____
style.

8. Identify the types of intravenous catheters.

A. _____

B. _____

C. _____

D. _____

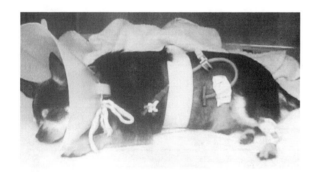

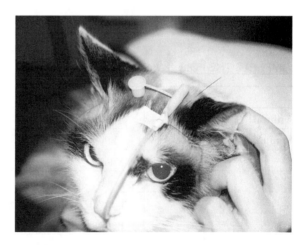

9. This patient is receiving nutritional support via a

_____ tube.

10. This patient is receiving nutritional support via a

_____ tube.

Chapter **20** **Diagnostic Sampling and Therapeutic Techniques**

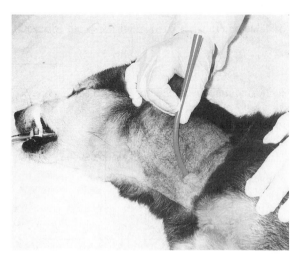

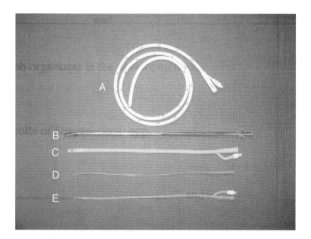

12. Identify each type of urinary catheter shown.

A. _____

B. _____

C. _____

D. _____

E. _____

11. This patient is receiving nutritional support via a

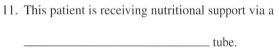 tube.

COMPLETE THE FOLLOWING CHART

General Guidelines for Selection of Urethral Catheters			
Animal	**Sex**	**Weight**	**Urethral Catheter Size**
Canine	Male	<9 kg	
	Male	9-23 kg	
	Male	>23 kg	
	Female	<9 kg	
	Female	9-23 kg	
	Female	>23 kg	
Feline	Male	All weights	3.5 Fr
	Female	All weights	3.5 Fr

WORD SEARCH

COUPAGE EFFUSION HEMATOMA
HEMOLYSIS OSMOLALITY PANCYTOPENIA
PERCUTANEOUS PHLEBITIS PNEUMOTHORAX
THORACENTESIS THROMBOSIS VASODILATION

```
I X E M L A MI T U P F E P N I Y A A M
E U U N N P U N N I O L R S B A A B B L
S D A A S E N H E T E U B E T S S T P Y
C G S E I I O O L Y U R O E I S H E N H
A S C P P N I A T F C C F S O P E E O T
S R A L C H E O A N P I E H C T MI I L
E S S S L B A P S S N R I E E A A E O A
I O U N S I E N O S M O L A L I T Y I I
S T H O R A C E N T E S I S Y L O M E H
B A MI E H E U O P Y E M S U A M R S S
T T S T O N C M S R E C N T U H A C C B
S O X A I L A O C E L O N N S F P V F L
O P H L E B I T I S N U O A T A F E A Y
C U C I S A U H U L A P T T P A H E S A
O E S D N O T O S C N A F T P A H A F O
S I S O B M O R H T R G A I N S S M E E
B E O S O P R A E L O E A F L N O O E U
Y I U A H N N X I O E M P O P P O E T O
T B C V I A F O O T A I O F X S N S A M
N Y A X G U U I E P O M H I L I L B E I
```

CROSSWORD PUZZLE

Across

1. Removal of fluid from the pleural cavity through a needle or catheter inserted between the ribs

4. A method of enteral feeding in which a tube is surgically introduced through the abdominal wall

9. Accumulation of air between the outer lining of the lung and the chest wall, causing collapse of the lung

10. Thrombocytopenia is a decrease in the number of _____ in the blood

12. Phlebitis is an inflammation of a/an _____

14. A catheter threaded through the urethra to the bladder where it is held in place with a tiny, inflated balloon

15. The act of striking the chest wall rhythmically with cupped hands. Cupping the hands creates an air cushion on impact so that tenacious mucous is dislodged

16. A decrease below normal in the concentration of red cells, white cells, and platelets

17. The formation, development, or presence of a clot

19. A response of body tissues to injury or irritation; characterized by pain, swelling, redness, and heat

20. A surgically created opening from an area inside the body to the outside

Down

2. Use of a syringe and needle to obtain uncontaminated urine directly from the bladder

3. Insertion of a needle into the abdominal cavity to remove fluids

5. Absence or loss of appetite for food

6. A term referring to something passing through the skin

7. The rupture of red blood cells resulting in the liberation of hemoglobin

8. Aspiration of fluid from a joint

11. A condition characterized by an abnormally high total number of circulating white blood cells

13. A collection of blood outside a blood vessel caused by a leak or an injury

16. A method used to make multiple copies of DNA

18. Intraosseous refers to the administration of a drug or fluids in the _____

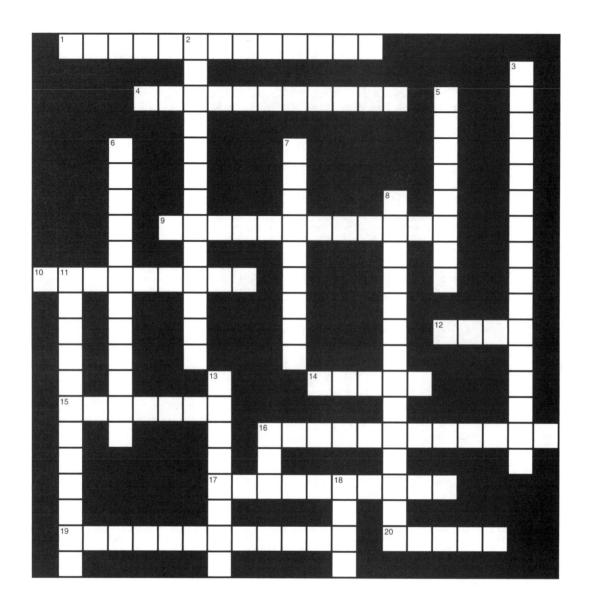

21 Small Animal Medical Nursing

LEARNING OBJECTIVES

When you have completed this chapter, you will be able to:

1. Describe general care of small animal patients, including bathing, grooming, ear cleaning, and nail trimming procedures
2. Explain the special considerations in the care of recumbent, geriatric, and pediatric patients
3. Describe the procedures for obtaining body temperature, blood pressure, pulse rate and character, and respiratory rate
4. Differentiate between sensible and insensible fluid losses and explain methods used to determine patient hydration status and calculate fluid requirements for rehydration of patients
5. List routes of administration of fluid therapy treatments and describe monitoring procedures used for fluid therapy patients
6. Describe the indications for and procedures used in blood transfusion and oxygen therapies
7. List the canine and feline blood groups and describe procedures for blood typing and cross-matching
8. List and describe the five methods of physical therapy used in small animal practice
9. Describe the indications for and procedures used in respiratory and topical therapies in small animal practice
10. List and describe common diseases of dogs and cats and provide an overview of small animal vaccines and vaccination protocols
11. Define zoonosis and identify common zoonotic conditions and methods of control of zoonotic diseases
12. List common diseases of the eyes and describe methods of diagnosis and treatment
13. List and describe common cardiac and endocrine disorders of dogs and cats and describe methods of diagnosis and treatment
14. List and describe common urogenital and gastrointestinal disorders of dogs and cats and describe methods of diagnosis and treatment
15. List and describe common orthopedic disorders encountered in small animal practice

DEFINE

1. Gastric lavage _____

_____

2. Cerumen _____

_____

3. Ceruminolytics _____

_____

4. Tympanic membrane _____

_____

5. Palpation _____

_____

6. Diastolic blood pressure _____

_____

7. Systolic blood pressure _____

_____

8. Tachypnea _____

_____

9. Hyperpnea _____

_____

10. Capillary refill time _____

_____

11. Central venous pressure _____

_____

12. Manometer _____

_____

13. Vasoconstriction _____

_____

14. Arterial blood gases _____

_____

_____

_____

15. Pulmonary thromboembolism _____

_____

16. Anticoagulants _____

_____

17. Edema _____

_____

18. Atrophy _____

_____

19. Hypoxia _____

_____

20. Arrhythmia _____

_____

21. Dyspnea _____

_____

22. Cyanosis _____

_____

23. Hemoglobin saturation _____

_____

_____

24. Fomite _____

_____

_____

25. Hypocerebellum _____

_____

26. Anaphylactic _____

_____

27. Epithelialization _____

_____

28. Disseminated intravascular coagulopathy (DIC) _____

_____

_____

_____

_____

29. Electrocardiography _____

_____

30. Echocardiography _____

_____

31. Positive inotropes _____

_____

32. Cortisol _____

_____

_____

33. Glucocorticoid _____

_____

_____

34. Mineralocorticoid _____

_____

35. Azotemic _____

_____

Chapter **21** **Small Animal Medical Nursing**

36. Ketonemia _____

_____

_____

_____

_____

37. Ketonuria _____

_____

38. Septicemia _____

_____

39. Peritonitis _____

_____

40. Cross-matching _____

_____

TRUE OR FALSE

Choose T (true) or F (false) for each statement below.

1. _____ Canine blood donors that weigh 50 lb can have 500 to 1000 ml of blood drawn every 3 weeks.
2. _____ If dextrose solution of more that 2.5% is given subcutaneously, skin may slough and abscesses may form.
3. _____ Dogs receiving dexamethasone for intervertebral disk disease may develop secondary problems, such as anorexia, abdominal pain, acute pancreatitis, and gastrointestinal hemorrhage.
4. _____ Modified-live–virus vaccines are not recommended in dogs and cats receiving immunosuppressive agents as with cancer or autoimmune disease.
5. _____ If serial readings of central venous pressure on a dog are 10 cm, 8 cm, and 9 cm, then intravenous fluid administration rate should be increased.
6. _____ Appetite stimulants may increase interest in eating but do not assure adequate intake by the patient.
7. _____ Sensible and insensible fluid loss can be calculated as approximately 60 ml/lb/day.
8. _____ All transfusion reactions occur within 1 hour of beginning the procedure.
9. _____ The pulse oximeter measures hemoglobin saturation in peripheral blood vessels.
10. _____ It is recommended that anal sacs be expressed regularly.
11. _____ Urinary acidifiers are often given to cats with FLUTD to kill microbial infections in the urine.
12. _____ Hypothermia partially contributes to a puppy's or kitten's inability to mount a good immune response during the first 2 weeks of life.
13. _____ Glaucoma results from a decreased production of aqueous fluid or excess drainage of it from the eye.
14. _____ Feline heartworm disease is more difficult to diagnose than canine heartworm disease partially because the worm burden in the cat is so much lower than in the dog.
15. _____ The deficiency of taurine commonly found in most commercial cat foods today contributes to the increased incidence of dilated cardiomyopathy in this species.
16. _____ Diabetes mellitus is diagnosed by documenting polydipsia, polyuria, and cataracts in an older animal.
17. _____ Pepto-Bismol can cause an animal's stools to be black and appear as melena.
18. _____ Urethral obstructions in cats can be fatal because severe metabolic derangements can result.

19. _____ Clinical signs of hip dysplasia almost always correlate with the severity of the disease detected radiographically.

20. _____ The overall recurrence rate for bladder stones is high in dogs, approximately 25%.

MATCHING

1. _____ Canine distemper   A. A disease of the reproductive tract
2. _____ Corneal ulcer   B. A disease of animals that is transmissible to humans
3. _____ Toxoplasma   C. Disease that causes gingivitis, conjunctivitis, rhinitis, and dermatitis
4. _____ Leptospirosis   D. Increase in intraocular pressure
5. _____ Zoonosis   E. Diagnosed by using fluorescein dye
6. _____ Uroliths   F. Excessive glucose levels
7. _____ Silver nitrate   G. A disease that can have respiratory, gastrointestinal, and neurologic signs
8. _____ Panleukopenia   H. A disease that women contemplating getting pregnant should test for
9. _____ FELV   I. A disease caused by a bacteria that may be transmitted via urine
10. _____ FIV   J. Pathologic lesion of heart muscle
11. _____ Glaucoma   K. Found in the bladder 90% of the time
12. _____ Cardiomyopathy   L. Parvovirus of cats
13. _____ Cushing   M. Used to stop bleeding
14. _____ Diabetes mellitus   N. Diseases associated with excess cortisol
15. _____ Brucellosis   O. A disorder that may cause immunosuppression and/or neoplasia

SHORT ANSWER

1. When bathing an animal, the eyes should be protected by placing _____ in

   the eyes. Likewise, the ears should be kept free from water by _____.

2. When cutting nails, the cutting surface of the nail trimmer should be held?

   _____

3. Expression of anal glands requires the following supplies:

   A. _____

   B. _____

   C. _____

4. The pulse is commonly felt in the _____.

5. Signs of volume overload include:

   A. _____

   B. _____

   C. _____

   D. _____

   E. _____

6. _____ and _____ are principle components of feline respiratory disease complex.

7. Cages that have been exposed to kennel cough should not be used for a period of _____ because of transmission of the disease to other animals.

8. Canine puppies should receive the last parvo vaccination at the age of _____.

9. _____ should be given to all puppies and kittens to help with passive transfer of antibodies.

10. Rabies vaccinations should be repeated every _____ depending on local ordinances.

11. _____ is a uterine disease of the immediate postpartum period.

12. _____ usually occurs 2 to 3 weeks postpartum and presents as weakness, trembling, and convulsions.

13. _____ is a disease of the uterus that occurs during the luteal phase (1 to 2 months after estrus).

14. _____ is usually evident in intact male dogs that present for stranguria, dysuria, hematuria, and/or difficulty in defecation.

15. The formula for subcutaneous fluids is _____ ml/kg.

16. With acute gastroenteritis, it is imperative to rest the gastrointestinal tract for _____ hours.

17. The most common viral infection of puppies is _____.

18. A diet used to treat phosphate uroliths is _____.

19. _____ is a common developmental problem of the canine coxofemoral joint.

20. Intervertebral disk disease (IVDD) is often seen in which breeds?

    A. _____

    B. _____

    C. _____

    D. _____

    E. _____

    F. _____

For the next four questions, use the information provided in the following scenario. A 2-year-old Skye terrier needs a blood transfusion immediately to save his life. The hospital where you work maintains an on-premise, canine universal blood donor. You find a previously obtained, unused bag of blood in the 5°C (41°F) refrigerator, collected using ACD anticoagulant, and dated "November 1." It is now November 10.

1. What do you do with the refrigerated blood?
   a. Discard it. It is outdated.
   b. Prepare to administer it as is.
   c. Warm it slowly to 37°C (98.6°F) in a warm-water bath.
   d. Heat it slowly to 50°C (122°F) in a hot-water bath.

2. How do you administer blood?
   a. Slowly and intravenously through a sterile blood-administration kit
   b. Rapidly and intravenously through a sterile blood-administration kit
   c. Slowly and intramuscularly through a sterile blood-administration kit
   d. Slowly and intravenously through a regular intravenous drip set

3. If you have to draw blood from the donor, from where will you draw it?
   a. Cephalic vein
   b. Femoral artery
   c. Cranial vena cava
   d. Jugular vein

4. If you used the bag of blood and had some left over, could you reuse the remaining blood on another day?
   a. Yes
   b. No

5. Possible signs of a negative blood-transfusion reaction include:
   a. Vomiting, fast heart rate, and low blood pressure
   b. Salivation, muscle tremors, and fever
   c. Dry cough and respiratory distress
   d. All of the above

6. In the case of a mild transfusion reaction, the first thing to do is slow down the administration rate.
   a. True
   b. False

7. A treatment sheet states to "hot pack" an area twice daily. What is the best way to do this?
   a. Soak a cloth in very hot water, wring lightly, apply until it cools, and repeat. Treat for up to 20 minutes.
   b. Fill an examination glove with water as hot as you can stand, apply it to the area until it cools, and repeat. Treat for up to 20 minutes.
   c. Place a 1-L bag of intravenous fluids heated to body temperature on the area until it cools.
   d. Place a heating pad set on "medium" heat on or around the affected area for 20 minutes.

8. Therapeutic exercise of a weak or nonambulatory patient can be provided by:
   a. Assisted walking using a towel or sling around the abdomen to help support the body's weight
   b. A treadmill
   c. Swimming
   d. a and c

9. Percussion (coupage) is a technique that involves striking the animal's chest to loosen bronchial secretions and thus facilitate drainage.
   a. True
   b. False

10. Whenever possible, animals with lung problems should be maintained in
    a. Sternal recumbency
    b. Right lateral recumbency
    c. Left lateral recumbency
    d. Ventral dorsal recumbency

11. How is a medicated bath performed differently from a cleansing bath?
    a. Leave the shampoo on at least 15 minutes.
    b. Cover more of the body, such as between the toes and on the face.
    c. Rinse three times for completeness.
    d. Do not dry with a towel; place the pet directly in the cage under a dryer or in an outdoor run.

12. When treating ear mites with nonivermectin, topical, otic (ear) preparations, which statement is most accurate?
    a. All animals in the house must be treated.
    b. Treatment should continue for at least 3 weeks.
    c. Gloves must be worn when instilling the medication into the ears.
    d. a and b

13. The appetite can be enhanced in patients whose eyes and nose are obstructed with discharge by:
    a. Frequent walking
    b. Clearing the accumulated discharge from the eyes and nose
    c. Placing them in an isolated ward
    d. a and c

14. As in large animals, kittens and puppies rely heavily on the ingestion of colostrum to obtain protection from infectious diseases.
    a. True
    b. False

15. Vaccines given by the _____ route can produce mild clinical disease.
    a. Subcutaneous
    b. Intramuscular
    c. Intranasal
    d. a and c

16. A vaccination may *not* protect a patient that has already been exposed to the disease.
    a. True
    b. False

17. What is the replacement volume for a 26 lb beagle that is 8% dehydrated?
    a. 940 ml
    b. 9.4 L
    c. 2080 ml
    d. 2.1 L

18. What is the maintenance fluid requirement for a 42 kg collie?
    a. 1145 ml
    b. 2500 ml
    c. 5544 ml
    d. 7500 ml

19. Calculate the drops per minute to infuse 1500 ml over 24 hours using a 15 drop/ml drip set.
    a. 2
    b. 16
    c. 24
    d. 30

CROSSWORD PUZZLE

Across

1. The tympanic membrane is also referred to as the _____ (2 words)
6. Gastric _____ involves feeding by passing a feeding tube into the stomach
9. Reduction of oxygen supply to tissue below physiologic levels despite adequate blood perfusion
10. Most commonly due to lack of insulin that is needed to shuttle glucose into most cells of the body; can be a complication of a diabetic mellitus patient
12. Positive inotropes are drugs that increase the contractility of the _____
13. Systolic blood pressure is the measurement of blood pressure when the heart is in systole or _____
16. Natural glucocorticoid produced by the adrenal cortex of the adrenal gland
18. Wasting away of a cell, tissue, organ, or part
19. The process of excessive coagulation of blood followed by lack of coagulation of blood because of clotting factors being used up
20. Inflammation of the serosa that lines the walls of the abdominal cavity and covers the abdominal organs and mesenteries
21. An object that in itself is harmless, such as clothing or instruments, but is able to harbor pathogenic or infectious agents and serve as an agent of transmission of an infection
22. The act of feeling with the fingers with light pressure to the surface of the body to determine the consistence of the parts beneath in physical diagnosis
23. Waxy secretion found in the external ear canal

Down

2. Any variation from the normal rhythm of the heart beat
3. Difficult or labored breathing
4. Instrument used to measure the pressure of liquids such as the blood
5. Fast, shallow breathing
7. The constriction of arterioles that leads to decreased blood flow to a part of the body
8. The accumulation of fluid in a space that is not normally fluid filled because of venous or lymphatic obstruction or increased vascular permeability
11. An exaggerated allergic reaction to a foreign protein or substance in the body
14. Increased blood urea nitrogen and creatinine
15. Overwhelming bacterial infection in the blood and tissues of a patient
16. A bluish discoloration of the mucous membranes or skin as a result of severe reduction of hemoglobin in the blood
17. Abnormal increase in depth and rate of the respiratory movements
24. Measurement of the electrical conductance of the heart

218

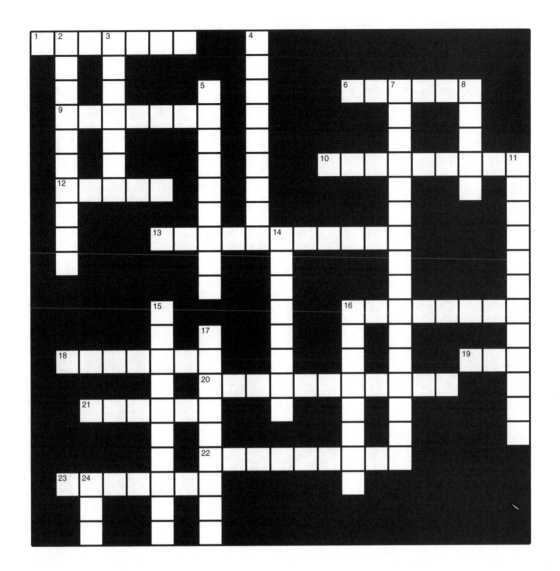

Large Animal Medical Nursing

LEARNING OBJECTIVES

When you have completed this chapter, you will be able to:
1. List the common diseases and disorders of horses and describe the causes, symptoms, treatment, and control
2. List the physiologic parameters used to monitor hospitalized equine patients
3. Describe unique requirements for care of hospitalized recumbent and infectious equine patients
4. Describe concerns related to placement and care of intravenous catheters in horses
5. List common medications used on equine patients and describe their indications
6. Describe routine laboratory studies performed on equine patients
7. List the common diseases and disorders of food animals and describe the causes, symptoms, treatment, and control
8. List the common diseases and disorders of small ruminants and describe the causes, symptoms, treatment, and control
9. List the common diseases and disorders of swine and describe the causes, symptoms, treatment, and control
10. List the common diseases and disorders of camelids and describe the causes, symptoms, treatment, and control

MATCHING 1

Match the term with the definition.

1. _____ Anestrus
2. _____ Keratoconjunctivitis
3. _____ Dystocia
4. _____ Catarrhal
5. _____ Pneumothorax
6. _____ Visceral
7. _____ Stranguria
8. _____ Proprioceptive
9. _____ Epizootic
10. _____ Septicemia

A. Difficult birth
B. Acute form of a disease such as TGE
C. An interval of sexual inactivity between two periods of estrus in female mammals that breed cyclically
D. Stimuli received within the tissues of the muscles and tendons
E. Abdominal
F. Inflammation of the cornea and conjunctiva
G. Inflammation of the mucous membranes
H. Systemic disease associated with the presence and persistence of pathogenic microorganisms or their toxins in the blood
I. The presence of air or gas in the pleural cavity
J. Straining during urination

MATCHING 2

Match the term with the definition.

1. _____ Xyphoid
2. _____ Serous
3. _____ Azotemia
4. _____ Epistaxis

A. An excess of urea and other nitrogenous wastes in the blood as a result of kidney insufficiency
B. Inflammation of the muscles
C. Watery secretion
D. A common pathologic condition in goats that may develop in does with or without exposure to a buck

5. _____ Myositis

E. Pertaining to or containing both blood and serum

6. _____ Strabismus

F. The posterior portion of the sternum

7. _____ Ketosis (acetonemia)

G. Deviation of the eye

8. _____ Pseudopregnancy

H. Presence of endotoxins in the blood, which may result in shock

9. _____ Serosanguineous

I. Nosebleed; hemorrhage from the nose

10. _____ Urolithiasis

J. Ketone bodies that accumulate in the blood

11. _____ Endotoxemia

K. Formation of urinary calculi

MATCHING 3

Match the medication(s) with the correct statement(s).

1. _____ Potent antiinflammatory properties

2. _____ Administered intramuscularly and should never be administered intravenously

3. _____ Antiinflammatory used in horses to relieve swelling and edema

4. _____ Good gram-positive and gram-negative spectrum

5. _____ Most effective NSAID for musculoskeletal pain

6. _____ Good efficacy against *Streptococcus zooepidemicus*

7. _____ Used sparingly in horses

8. _____ Effective for soft tissue and visceral pain

9. _____ Adverse effects may include immunosuppression, polyuria/polydipsia, poor hair coat, poor wound healing

10. _____ Agents that are nonsteroidal antiinflammatory drugs

11. _____ Administered orally or per rectum for anaerobic bacterial infections

12. _____ May cause hypotension and persistent paraphimosis in stallions

13. _____ May be administered IM or IV

14. _____ Good efficacy against *Streptococcus equi equi*

15. _____ Nitrile gloves should be worn during handling and administration

16. _____ Can be nephrotoxic

17. _____ Administered intravenously

18. _____ May be administered orally or by IV

19. _____ Provides up to 4 hours of sedation and analgesia

20. _____ May combat the effects of toxemia in equine patients with GI tract disease

21. _____ Approximately 20 minutes of sedation and analgesia

22. _____ Moderate gram-positive and gram-negative spectrum

23. _____ May cause fatal aplastic anemia in humans from exposure during patient administration

24. _____ No analgesic properties and only moderate tranquilization

25. _____ Efficacious against gram-negative pathogens

26. _____ Mild to moderate analgesia for musculoskeletal pain

A. Penicillin

B. Corticosteroids

C. Aminoglycoside antimicrobials

D. Detomidine

E. Metronidazole

F. Potassium penicillin

G. Phenylbutazone

H. Ketoprofen

I. Flunixin meglumine

J. Xylazine

K. Acepromazine

L. Butorphanol

M. Chloramphenicol

N. Trimethoprim-sulfa antimicrobials

O. Dimethyl sulfoxide (DMSO)

P. Procaine penicillin

Q. Ceftiofur sodium

FILL IN THE BLANK

1. _____ is a common equine respiratory disease that is very contagious and is caused by *Streptococcus equi equi*.

2. In an equine patient with strangles, if an abscess develops in an abnormal location, it is termed

   _____ strangles.

3. Difficult cases of strangles are often treated with antibiotics and *Streptococcus equi equi* is susceptible to

   _____.

4. The guttural pouches of the equine patient are located just above the _____ and

   _____.

5. When an equine patient has guttural pouch mycosis, fungal plaque forms over the _____

   carotid artery, adjacent to the nerves that control _____.

6. _____ is a highly contagious viral respiratory disease in the equine patient that is transmitted via aerosolization of the virus during coughing.

7. Incubation of equine influenza is _____ days with the patient remaining sick for 3 to 4 days.

8. The contagious virus that can produce respiratory disease, abortion, and neonatal and neurologic disease is caused

   by equine _____.

9. Brood mares should be vaccinated against equine herpes virus using an inactivated univalent vaccine during the

   _____, _____, _____, and

   _____ months of pregnancy to help avoid abortion.

10. The vaccine for equine viral arteritis is approved for use in _____ and

    _____ mares under the supervision of the USDA.

11. _____ is a persistent viral disease of horses causing anemia, fever, and weight loss.

12. Young horses are prone to _____ that can be caused by stress, a high-grain diet, musculoskeletal pain, and the administration of NSAIDs.

13. Horses should be vaccinated for rabies this often: _____.

14. _____ is a highly fatal neurologic disease in the horse, characterized by a stiff, stilted gait, hyperexcitability, seizure, and coma.

15. Equine dermatophytosis (ringworm) is most commonly caused by the fungi _____ and

    _____.

Chapter **22** **Large Animal Medical Nursing**

16. Corneal ulcerations are often the result of _____.

17. When fluorescein stain is used to detect corneal ulcerations, the defects in the surface of the cornea will turn

    _____ in color.

18. A heart rate greater than _____ beats/min indicates severe pain in the equine patient.

19. Patient monitoring forms are designed to identify _____ in the physical signs.

20. IV catheter sites in the equine patient should be monitored twice daily for _____,

    _____, and _____.

21. The resting _____ in the equine patient is highly variable and must be serially
    evaluated in the excited patient.

22. The evaluation of the total and differential WBC count is important to identify the presence of

    _____.

23. Urinalysis is essential for the evaluation of primary _____ disease.

SHORT ANSWER

1. List the symptoms you may see when an equine patient has strangles.

    A. _____

    B. _____

    C. _____

    D. _____

    E. _____

2. Name the bacterium that causes strangles in the equine patient.

    _____

3. List the lymph nodes that are typically infected and become abscessed when an equine patient has strangles.

    A. _____

    B. _____

4. List the anatomical structures that are located under the surface of the guttural pouch lining and that are vulnerable
   to damage from pathologic conditions that affect the guttural pouch.

    A. _____

    B. _____

5. What is the term for bacterial infection in the guttural pouch that is often associated with strangles?

    _____

6. What is the term for a fungal infection of the guttural pouch and what is the agent responsible for it?

A. _____

B. _____

7. What are the clinical signs of empyema that you may see in the equine patient?

A. _____

B. _____

8. What are the potential consequences to the equine patient's health when they have guttural pouch mycosis?

A. _____

B. _____

C. _____

9. List the symptoms you may see in the equine patient that has influenza.

A. _____

B. _____

C. _____

10. What are the recommended vaccination protocols for influenza in the following equine patients?

A. Horses with little exposure to other horses

_____

B. Young horses and performance horses

_____

C. Brood mares

_____

11. Equine influenza vaccine comes as an intramuscular injection or an intranasal vaccine. Explain the difference in use or response by the patient to the different vaccination routes.

_____

_____

12. What are the three ways that equine herpes virus can be transmitted?

A. _____

B. _____

C. _____

13. Vaccination against equine herpes is recommended in which categories of horses?

    A. _____

    B. _____

14. While vaccination against equine herpes virus is short-lived and inconsistent it is recommended that young horses and performance horses be vaccinated. How often should these horses be vaccinated?

    _____

15. What contagious viral disease may produce limb swelling, conjunctivitis, abortion, and respiratory disease in the horse?

    _____

16. What is the other name for the allergic airway disease known as "heaves"?

    _____

17. What are the clinical signs of heaves?

    A. _____

    B. _____

    C. _____

    D. _____

    E. _____

    F. _____

18. How is equine infectious anemia (EIA) transmitted?

    _____

19. What are the clinical signs that may be exhibited by a foal with gastric ulcerations?

    A. _____

    B. _____

    C. _____

    _____

20. List the three bacteria that may cause life-threatening diarrhea in the equine patient.

    A. _____

    B. _____

    C. _____

21. What are two possible causes of choke in the equine patient?

    A. _____

    B. _____

22. What is one significant complication that can occur in the equine patient who has choke?

_____

23. What are the four most common disorders of the brain and brainstem in the equine patient?

A. _____

B. _____

C. _____

D. _____

24. What is the most common tumor in the equine patient?

_____

25. What is the most common cause of blindness in the equine patient?

_____

26. What is the name of the disease that is an acute inflammatory disease of muscle?

_____

27. What are the clinical signs of exertional rhabdomyolysis?

A. _____

B. _____

C. _____

D. _____

E. _____

28. List the responsibilities of the veterinary technician in the equine hospital.

A. _____

B. _____

C. _____

D. _____

29. Describe the nursing care you must perform on a recumbent equine patient.

A. _____

B. _____

C. _____

D. _____

E. _____

F. _____

30. What are the two most common equine diseases that require isolation of the patient when hospitalized?

A. _____

B. _____

31. Where can IV catheters be placed in the equine patient?

A. _____

B. _____

C. _____

32. How often should a Teflon IV catheter be replaced?

_____

33. How often should an IV catheter in an equine patient be flushed with heparinized saline?

_____

34. What information is provided in a CBC?

A. _____

B. _____

C. _____

D. _____

E. _____

F. _____

35. What complications may occur after a CSF tap is performed?

A. _____

B. _____

36. Describe the possible complications of an abdominocentesis.

A. _____

B. _____

C. _____

TRUE OR FALSE

Choose T (true) or F (false) for each statement below.

1. _____ Bastard strangles are a particularly difficult disease to treat successfully.

2. _____ Horses with strangles can be reintroduced to other horses in 2 to 3 weeks after recovery from the clinical disease.

228

3. _____ The attenuated strangles vaccine will not completely prevent infection in horses, but minimizes clinical signs.

4. _____ Early stages of guttural pouch empyema can be treated with antibiotics and lavage of the guttural pouch.

5. _____ Chondroids form in the guttural pouch of a patient with guttural pouch mycosis.

6. _____ Equine patients who have recovered from a viral respiratory disease should be rested for a minimum of 3 weeks.

7. _____ The clinical signs of herpes virus are milder but hardly distinguishable from equine influenza.

8. _____ Equine herpes virus causes abortion in the mare in the third to sixth month of pregnancy.

9. _____ The most important management of heaves is to remove the offending allergens from the horse's environment.

10. _____ Horses infected with EIA can be placed in other herds without fear of disease transmission.

11. _____ Colitis in the equine patient can quickly develop into hypovolemia, shock, toxemia, electrolyte loss, and acid-base imbalance because of impaction.

12. _____ Potomac horse fever occurs predominantly in states west of the Mississippi.

13. _____ Vaccines are available for Eastern and Western equine encephalitis and for West Nile.

14. _____ Equine protozoal myelitis (EPM) causes ataxia in horses and the clinical signs are often asymmetrical.

15. _____ Equine recurrent uveitis is easily cured using long-term, antiinflammatory therapy.

16. _____ The causes of exertional rhabdomyolysis can be attributed to exertion or a change in diet.

17. _____ An increased heart rate is a sign of a healthy equine patient.

18. _____ All equine patients should be kept in an isolation facility.

19. _____ Equine patients should only be placed in slings if they are able to stand on their own.

20. _____ A blood sample for a CBC should be collected in an EDTA tube.

21. _____ A blood sample for serum chemistry should be collected in a tube without anticoagulant or in a heparinized tube.

22. _____ Horses normally have a pinkish tint to their serum.

23. _____ Normal horse urine is alkaline and contains many calcium carbonate crystals.

24. _____ CSF should be handled carefully as the fluid may have zoonotic potential.

MATCHING 4

Match the condition or organism with the correct statement.

1. _____ Responsible for diarrhea in 7- to 10-day-old piglets

2. _____ Causes neurologic signs in baby pigs, flulike signs in growing pigs, and embryonic death, abortion, or stillbirths in pregnant pigs

3. _____ Caused by coronavirus and occurs in an epizootic and enzootic form

4. _____ The most common bacterial isolate from pneumonic swine lungs

5. _____ A chronic, progressive disease of swine that results in atrophy of the nasal turbinates

6. _____ Caused by a bacterium that enters the body through the lymphatic system

7. _____ The most important primary cause of diarrhea in pigs less than 5 days old

8. _____ The most common cause of chronic pneumonia in swine

9. _____ Also known as malignant hyperthermia or pale soft exudative pork disease

10. _____ Causes enterotoxemia in 3 to 4 day old pigs

11. _____ The spirochete that causes swine dysentery

A. Transmissible gastroenteritis (TGE)

B. Atrophic rhinitis

C. Erysipelas

D. Porcine stress syndrome

E. Pseudorabies virus

F. *Mycoplasma hyopneumoniae*

G. Coccidiosis

H. *Clostridium perfringens* type C

I. Enterotoxigenic *Escherichia coli* (ETEC)

J. *Pasteurella multocida*

K. *Brachyspira hyodysenteriae*

Match the terms with the correct statement(s).

1. _____ Neonatal camelids

2. _____ Typically these camelids are used for meat, leather, fiber, and as pack animals

3. _____ Common vaccinations for camelids

4. _____ These camelids are grazers

5. _____ A parasite that migrates through the spinal cord of camelids and can cause neurologic deficits

6. _____ Orphaned camelids must receive minimum human contact and left with the herd except for feeding to avoid this problem

7. _____ These camelids are known for their superior fiber but are also a source of meat and leather

8. _____ Huacuya and suri are camelids that belong to which group?

9. _____ Estimated by adding temperature (f) and percent humidity and is important to avoiding heat stress in camelids

10. _____ These camelids prefer to browse

A. Llamas

B. Alpacas

C. Bezerk llama syndrome

D. *Clostridium perfringens* C and D and tetanus

E. Cria

F. *Parelaphostrongylus tenuis*

G. Heat index

MATCHING 6

Match the condition or organism with the correct statement(s).

1. _____ Responsible for ruminant clinical syndromes of septicemia, abortion, and neurologic disease

2. _____ Common metabolic problem of dairy cows that occurs within 48 hours of calving

3. _____ CNS disease that is a result of an underlying defect in thiamine metabolism

4. _____ Caused by *Chlamydia psittaci* in sheep and *Mycoplasma conjunctivae* in the goat

5. _____ Inflammation of the mammary gland

6. _____ Occurs in high-producing dairy cows during the first few months of lactation if they are unable to meet the high-energy demands of lactation

7. _____ Caused by the penetration of the pericardial sac by a metallic foreign body

8. _____ Treatment of choice for periparturient hypocalcemia

9. _____ Caused papilloma virus

10. _____ In goats, this condition is caused by *Clostridium perfringens*

11. _____ Metabolic disease that commonly affects pregnant ewes and does during late gestation

12. _____ Fungus responsible for ringworm in cattle

13. _____ Caused by *Dichelobacter nodosus* and *Fusobacterium necrophorum* in the sheep and goats

14. _____ Caused by *Clostridium tetani*

A. Mastitis

B. Calcium gluconate IV

C. Ketosis

D. Pericarditis

E. Warts

F. Listeria monocytogenes

G. California Mastitis Test

H. Enterotoxemia

I. Foot rot

J. Milk fever

K. Tetanus

L. Polioencephalomalacia

M. Pseudopregnancy

N. Trichophyton verrucosum

O. White muscle disease

P. *Pregnancy toxemia*

Q. *Moraxella bovis*

R. Caseous lymphadenitis

S. Infectious Keratoconjunctivitis

T. *Staphylococcus aureus*

U. Contagious ecthyma

15. _____ May occur following castration, tail docking, and dehorning in the sheep and goat

16. _____ Caused by *Corynebacterium pseudotuberculosis*

17. _____ Diagnostic tool used in mastitis testing

18. _____ Associated with the gangrenous form of mastitis in sheep and goats

19. _____ A common viral disease of small ruminants causing rusty proliferative lesions around the mouth and nose of lambs

20. _____ A common pathologic condition in goats that may develop in does with or without exposure to a buck

21. _____ Recognized worldwide as a common, frequently fatal disease of goats

22. _____ Causative agent of infectious bovine keratoconjunctivitis

23. _____ Occurs in young lambs, calves, kids, and pigs born to dames who are deficient in selenium during gestation

FILL IN THE BLANK

1. Bacterial causes of diarrhea in the calf may be caused by _____,

   _____, or _____ and _____ diseases

2. Treatment for diarrhea in the calf includes _____ and correction of

   _____ and _____ abnormalities.

3. Two common conditions that occur in the head of the bovine patient are _____ and

   _____.

4. Bloat is classified as _____, where eructation is normal but gas cannot be expelled,

   or _____, which is because of a failure of eructation.

5. Traumatic reticuloperitonitis can also be called _____ disease.

6. Common causes of acute diarrhea in the adult bovine patient include:

   A. _____

   B. _____

   C. _____

   D. _____

   E. _____

7. _____ should be suspected as a cause of diarrhea when an acute outbreak is followed by chronic diarrhea, especially if there has been new livestock introduced, or a feed or water change.

8. Interdigital necrobacillosis is also called _____.

9. Laminitis is a direct cause of _____ .

10. Two important causes of lameness and sudden death in young cattle are blackleg and malignant edema and are

    caused by _____ and _____ .

11. The most common neoplastic disease of cattle is _____ .

12. The cause of periparturient hypocalcemia is the severe decline in serum _____ levels.

13. The two major problems that may occur in the first 48 hours of a lamb's life that may cause death are

    _____ and _____ .

14. Goats should be vaccinated against enterotoxemia at a maximum interval of _____
    months.

15. Prevention of _____ and _____ in the neonatal period
    is important to successful pig rearing.

16. Camelids are _____ nasal breathers, and so _____
    mouth breathing is considered abnormal and cause for concern.

SHORT ANSWER

1. What is the most important step performed by the veterinary technician with a neonate calf?

   _____

2. Describe ways to clear the mucus from the nose, mouth, and upper airway of a neonate calf.

   A. _____

   B. _____

   C. _____

   D. _____

   E. _____

3. Diarrhea in the young calf can be caused by which viruses?

   A. _____

   B. _____

   C. _____

4. List the clinical signs of woody tongue.

   A. _____

   B. _____

   C. _____

D. _____

E. _____

5. What is the treatment for woody tongue?

   _____

6. List the clinical sign of lumpy jaw.

   _____

7. List the clinical signs of pharyngeal trauma and abscessation.

   A. _____

   B. _____

   C. _____

   D. _____

   E. _____

   F. _____

8. List two keys to prevention for pharyngeal trauma and abscessation.

   A. _____

   B. _____

9. What are the clinical signs of grain overload?

   A. _____

   B. _____

   C. _____

10. What is the best way to prevent grain overload?

    _____

11. What is the cause of primary bloat?

    _____

12. What may be the cause of secondary bloat?

    A. _____

    B. _____

    C. _____

D. _____

E. _____

13. List the clinical signs of bloat.

A. _____

B. _____

C. _____

D. _____

E. _____

F. _____

G. _____

14. What is the cause of traumatic reticuloperitonitis?

_____

15. What is the most common cause of chronic diarrhea in the bovine patient?

_____

16. What syndrome affects primarily feedlot calves and dairy calves younger than 6 months of age and is caused by a complex interaction of respiratory viruses, bacteria, and stress?

_____

17. Most lameness in cattle is caused by lesions or problems in what part of the limb?

_____

18. What is one cause of acute laminitis?

_____

_____

19. List the five point plan for mastitis control.

A. _____

_____

B. _____

_____

C. _____

_____

D. _____

_____

E. _____

_____

20. List the three main causes of dystocia.

A. _____

B. _____

C. _____

21. List the three factors that may interfere in the formation of the ewe-lamb bond.

A. _____

B. _____

C. _____

22. What vaccine should be given to small ruminants before surgery or after an injury?

_____

23. Which species is most susceptible to copper toxicity and why?

_____

_____

_____

_____

_____

24. List the pathogens that are responsible for abortion and reproductive failure in swine.

A. _____

B. _____

C. _____

D. _____

E. _____

F. _____

25. What is the most common nutritional disease of potbellied pigs?

_____

26. Most premature crias cannot nurse, so what should be done to prevent failure of passive transfer?

_____

27. Describe anatomically where it is ideal to perform venipuncture in the camelid.

A. _____

B. _____

28. Describe the five point system used to evaluate body conditioning in the camelid.

A. _____

B. _____

C. _____

D. _____

E. _____

TRUE OR FALSE

Choose T (true) or F (false) for each statement below.

1. _____ A newborn calf needs to receive colostrum within the first 12 hours after birth.
2. _____ Treatment for grain overload may include lavage of the rumen, oral antacids, and antibiotics.
3. _____ Johne disease is completely curable and has no lingering after effects.
4. _____ Diseases of the foot are not a serious condition and can be easily cured.
5. _____ Blocks can be used on the healthy claw to reduce weight bearing on a diseased claw.
6. _____ Clinical signs of lymphosarcoma due to BLV will vary greatly depending on the organs or systems involved.
7. _____ Dystocia is not common in cattle and very rarely do cattle require veterinary assistance.
8. _____ A placenta is considered retained if it has not expelled by 8 to 12 hours.
9. _____ Camelids do not regurgitate and rechew their food.
10. _____ Prematurity in the cria is life threatening and requires immediate and intensive therapy.

Match each figure with the disease shown.

A. Corneal ulceration
B. Ulcerative lesions of contagious ecthyma
C. Decubital ulcers
D. Necrobacillosis
E. Actinobacillosis (woody tongue)

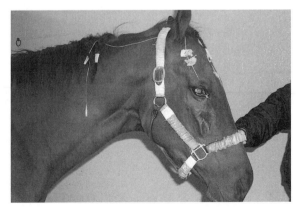

1. _____

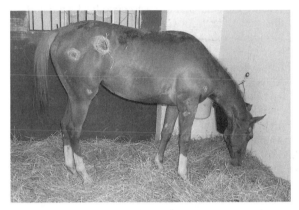

2. _____

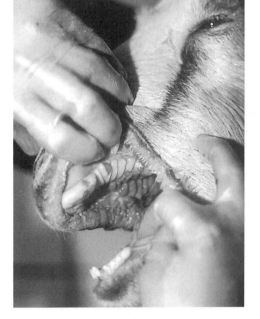

3. _____

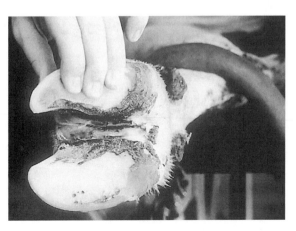

4. _____

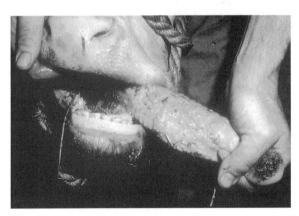

5. _____

Across

1. A drug that expels parasitic worms from the body, by either killing or stunning them
4. An outbreak of disease affecting many animals of one kind at the same time
8. To take hold of or grab as when cattle eat grass or hay
9. Along the same line as a centerline
10. The area between the anus and the dorsal part of the external genitalia, especially in the female
11. Tearing of the eyes due to excessive secretion of tears or to obstruction of the lacrimal passages
12. An act of belching
13. Originating or derived from sources within the same individual
14. Subnormal body temperature
17. Either of the angles formed by the meeting of the upper and lower eyelids
20. Occurs when one of the jaws is caudal to its normal relationship with the other jaw
21. A foot infection that gains access to the foot through the white line traveling up the sensitive lamina underneath the hoof wall forming an abscess that drains at the coronet
22. A morbid dread of water
24. A yellowish pigmentation of the skin, tissues, and certain body fluids
26. Spasmodic blinking due to involuntary contraction of the orbicularis oculi muscle
30. A bluish or purplish discoloration due to deficient oxygenation of the blood
31. Inflammation of muscle
32. To cleanse by removal (usually surgical) of lacerated, devitalized, or contaminated tissue
33. Localized or generalized itching because of irritation of sensory nerve endings
34. A small cartilaginous extension of the caudal part of the sternum
35. The period of sexual quiescence between two periods of sexual activity in cyclically breeding mammals
36. A condition marked by an abnormal increase of ketone bodies in the circulating blood

Down

1. An excess of urea and other nitrogenous wastes in the blood as a result of kidney insufficiency
2. Sensitive lamina
3. Anterior uveitis is inflammation of the _____
4. Belonging to the mucous membrane lining the uterus
5. A condition of spasm of the muscles of the back, causing the head and limbs to bend backward and the trunk to arch forward
6. Inflammation of subcutaneous, loose connective tissue
7. Dissection of a dead fetus in utero
11. A disease of the intestinal tract
15. A condition in which the penis is extended and cannot be retracted to its normal position within the preputial cavity
16. An attack of bleeding from the nose
17. Surgical puncture
18. The presence of blood or blood cells in the urine
19. The incidence of disease
23. Difficulty in swallowing
25. A distressing but ineffectual urge to evacuate the rectum or urinary bladder
27. Loss of appetite, especially when prolonged
28. Slow or difficult labor or delivery
29. The material composed of serum, fibrin, and white blood cells that escapes from blood vessels into a superficial lesion or area of inflammation

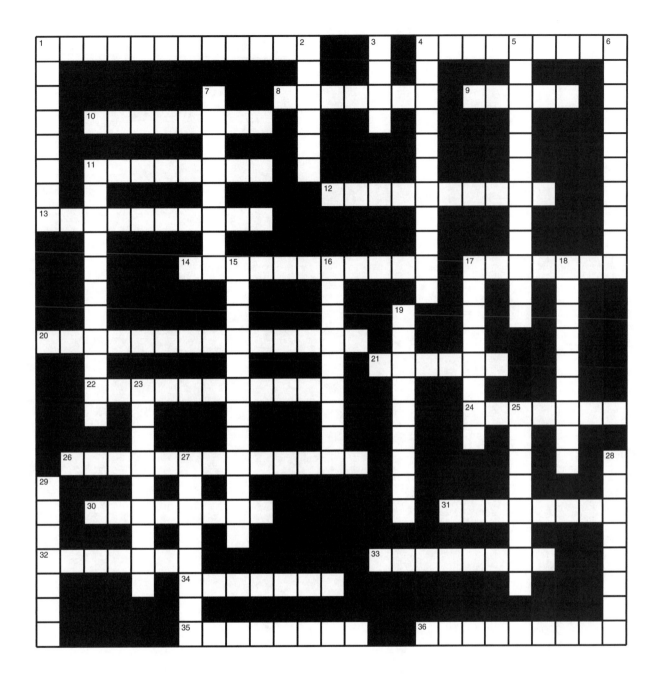

Chapter **22** **Large Animal Medical Nursing**

23 Nursing Concepts in Alternative Medicine

LEARNING OBJECTIVES

When you have completed this chapter, you will be able to:
1. Describe considerations in development of home-prepared diets for dogs and cats
2. List the commonly used nutraceuticals and describe their therapeutic uses
3. List the commonly used western herbs and describe their therapeutic uses
4. List the common ingredients found in Chinese herbal and ayurvedic herbal formulas
5. Describe the principles of aromatherapy and list common aromatherapy oils and their uses
6. Describe the basic principles of homeopathy and list forms of homeopathic preparations and considerations for their storage and administration
7. Describe the principles of flower essence therapy and list common flower essences and their uses
8. Define applied kinesiology and list the techniques used in patient assessment and treatment
9. List the theories that describe the principles of acupuncture and describe the role of the veterinary technician in acupuncture therapy
10. List and describe the physical modalities used in alternative and complementary medicine

SHORT ANSWER

1. In holistic practice, what is considered to be the foundation for achieving a state of ideal health?

   _____

2. List three ways owners may optimize nutrition for large animals.

   A. _____

   B. _____

   C. _____

3. When feeding a home-prepared diet to a carnivore, why is it recommended that vegetables be lightly steamed and chopped before feeding?

   _____

   _____

4. What must a vet tech research to determine if a commercial diet fits a client's/patient's needs?

   _____

5. Define synergy.

   _____

   _____

6. Although safer than many pharmaceuticals, herbal therapy still has risks and side effects. List two common precautions VTs need to be aware of when educating clients about herbal therapy:

A. _____

B. _____

7. Describe the difference in treatment for acute and chronic conditions if using traditional Chinese medicine (TCM).

_____

_____

8. Besides the traditional needles, how might acupuncture points be stimulated?

A. _____

B. _____

C. _____

D. _____

E. _____

9. What is the most common use for acupuncture today?

_____

10. In acupuncture, the body's energy (Qi) travels through pathways known as _____.

11. According to TCM, stagnant energy in the body manifests as _____ and deficient

energy in the body manifests as _____.

12. Briefly describe the five common theories of how acupuncture works.

A. _____

_____

_____

B. _____

_____

_____

C. _____

_____

_____

D. _____

_____

_____

E. _____

_____

_____

13. Describe moxibustion.

_____

_____

14. Compare and contrast Aqua-puncture and Electro-acupuncture.

_____

_____

_____

15. What are the main components of ayurveda?

A. _____

B. _____

C. _____

D. _____

E. _____

16. What are two common routes of administration of aromatherapy essential oils?

A. _____

B. _____

17. Explain the fundamental differences between homeopathy and allopathic medicine.

_____

_____

_____

_____

18. Define repertorizing.

_____

_____

_____

19. Name three Western herbs that are stimulating.

   A. _____

   B. _____

   C. _____

20. Name three Western herbs that are sedating.

   A. _____

   B. _____

   C. _____

21. List three types of strengthening exercises veterinary technicians can do with animals.

   A. _____

   B. _____

   C. _____

22. List three types of proprioception exercises veterinary technicians can do with animals.

   A. _____

   B. _____

   C. _____

23. List three examples of antioxidant nutraceuticals.

   A. _____

   B. _____

   C. _____

24. Define muscle paresis.

_____

25. Define deafferentation.

_____

26. How can a veterinary technician play an active role in applied kinesiology?

A. _____

B. _____

C. _____

27. Describe the use of a surrogate in applied kinesiology.

_____

_____

_____

28. Why would it be recommended to rotate a pet through 3 to 4 high quality commercial diets?

_____

_____

HERBAL THERAPY MATCHING

1. _____ Bulk herbs   A. Most common preparation for carnivores

2. _____ Capsules or tablets   B. Herbs concentrated in alcohol or glycerin

3. _____ Extracts   C. Soaked herbs held in place by gauze

4. _____ Poultice   D. Highly concentrated, use with caution

5. _____ Essential oils   E. Most common preparation for herbivores

Complete the table by listing the appropriate herbs for the following indications:

Indication	Western Herb	Traditional Chinese Medicine	Ayurvedic Herb
Liver support			
Skin issues			
GI/digestive			

Use the terms for the definitions below in the Word Search. Use common names.

```
N A T D B E W P S R N C P U L S A T I U N A N H G K
H P A T C A N I H C E E I M I I I I I I I I I I A S
I A N A I L L E W S A B S N A V E K I A E E N O M E
E L R I N I R U A T U O G N N M L R T E A L E M E U
L L B T R A R O H E R O E I A A A E S N E P E U N H
Y Y A L L I T A S L U P E H N A M T N E D R R E N G
E P H I D R A E M I M U L E E K T E M E T C E I P R
A T V E R V A I L U S C H E A U G U R I I M A M I U
C A L T R T S I H T K L I M C S A O U N U U C T I A
I U N A I R I L A V G R A N A R U P R A R A I E R V
C R A N B E R R Y S H R R R T I E A R E H V R T K I
E I E A I I A G R I M O N L N I A T E M K A A I V H
I N E D E E Y N O M I R G A E I K R E I E T N T T U
O I N N N H O A R D E H P E K N C T A K K N E N N I
M A R T A U R I N E C Y P R E S S A A D N A O N H Y
E A E M S W E Y H T M N E M R T E T E S L M N S L R
M G H A R R C E N T U A R Y E L I I E L R U O N R U
M A N I E L D N G I N K O C T A R R I E K Y H R I Y
T H U A I C E E Y H T R A U M E L T P N E Y P I A Y
Y E N E E M N G H N S N T N U N A P E I M A E R S A
G I N K G A O I I P A L O E N L O C E N E I R R R C
A E E H A E M D H I E M N O U P I K I D R N N R A N
E N U C D C E E M C A M I P Y D I M E R E U C S E R
S G E K T A N S E N E O A R A H S E A U U A R P G E
A I U N E N N A N N C W V E G E C L N G C N A E E V
U I N P K I I I V A L E R E N A M I E Y S H L P E P
O L M T R H C E T H G L I I L N A M U A E R A P Y W
R L I I E C L H C I E I V Y R N E O R U R P O E W E
S E R S U E A A I R A I N A E E N M A S A O U R A S
L W W A A L T H Y R U A T N E C U A A K M E R M S A
N S P T C E U S A N N U E H O C E H I A B A I I H A
I O A A Y R E S C U E R E M E D Y C H H I A Y N W N
A B R L N E A C E N E E T L R T Y O L A S L T A A
V N N B O S N H E V A L E R I A N N L E U A A C G M
R E L Y E G A A C A E N A H E O U E O L C A S P A T
E A E I P S A M R E H N I H E A W K U E D E V P N N
V L E T D E O O A P A N A P S S A M A E P M N A D U
S T A I E A G M N E C C D V O P I Y A T R D O T H C
T A I P R A T I B L C I I B T M H Y A T A R E N A E
C E W R E R P L E A R R H A E T H O R E E U M R E E
E T C C L C T I R P S G R V U M A I D A T K M R E U
```

1. Bach Flower Essence used for hyperactivity.

_____

2. Ayurvedic herb used to treat digestive disorders.

_____

3. Chinese herb used for pain reduction.

_____

4. Homeopathic remedy for purulent discharge.

_____

5. Bach Flower Essence used for prolonged grief.

_____

6. Chinese herb used to enhance Qi and boost the immune system.

_____

7. Aromatherapy essential oil used topically for bursitis and tendinitis.

_____

8. Western herb used to support the immune system.

_____

9. Homotoxicology product used to treat inflammation and pain. Contains arnica, aconitum, and belladonna.

_____

10. Western herb used to promote mental alertness.

_____

11. Western herb used to treat urinary tract infections.

_____

12. Bach Flower Essence used for fear of the unknown (thunderstorms).

_____

13. Ayurvedic herb used as an antiinflammatory for arthritis.

_____

14. Aromatherapy essential oil used topically to improve circulation and support nerves and intestines.

_____

15. Homeopathic remedy for bruising and/or bleeding.

_____

16. Bach Flower Essence used for submissiveness, timidness.

_____

17. Ayurvedic herb used for fatigue and skin disorders.

_____

18. Bach Flower Essence—a combination of five essences to help in times of shock, trauma, and stress.

_____

19. Nutraceutical used to support heart and eye function.

_____

Chapter **23** **Nursing Concepts in Alternative Medicine**

20. Chinese herb used to treat bronchitis and asthma.

_____

21. Bach Flower Essence used for constant barking or whining.

_____

22. Western herb used to treat anxiety and promote sleep.

_____

23. Ayurvedic herb used for wounds and rashes.

_____

24. Western herb used for detoxification and liver support.

_____

25. Aromatherapy essential oil used as a dietary supplement to support digestion and stimulate the sense of taste.

_____

CROSSWORD PUZZLE

Across

1. _____ therapy is a type of treatment performed with the hands, like massage and chiropractic
4. Flexing, extending, abduction, and adduction of the limb joints and stretching the muscles that surround the joints to increase joint nutrition, proprioception, and reducing the chance of injury
5. A form of massage that consists of a gliding stroke that follows the contour of the body
7. _____ compression is the use of manual pressure on trigger points to bring about muscle relaxation and relieve pain
9. A type of massage that consists of kneading, rhythmic lifting, squeezing, and releasing the tissue
10. A form of medicine that concentrates on the "whole" animal and animal wellness, rather than concentrating on clinical signs of disease
11. A form of massage using tapping motion of the hands or fingers
15. An abnormal relationship between two adjacent vertebrae consisting of muscles, ligaments, connective tissue, a spinal nerve, blood vessels, lymphatics, and cerebrospinal fluid
16. A type of supplement consisting of animal products to supply nutrients (steroids, enzymes, and raw materials of some organs such as the liver) to the patient to help restore health
18. A system of medicine, which is based on the principle that "like cures like"
19. A food or naturally occurring food supplement that is thought to have beneficial effects on health

Down

2. The area of medicine where diagnosis is done by palpation of the pulses in different positions
3. Applied _____ is a form of medicine that includes joint mobilizations or manipulations, myofascial therapy, cranial techniques, meridian therapy, clinical nutrition, dietary management, and reflex procedures
4. Knowing where the body is in space
6. A form of massage that manipulates the tissue to increase circulation. It is commonly used over tendons when tendonitis is present, over knots and trigger points, and over joint capsules with excessive fibrous tissue.
8. _____ therapy is a form of medicine that manually restores reduced motion in the spine and limbs
12. The type of therapy that uses essential oils to bring about a physiologic or psychological response in the body
13. A systematic and scientific manipulation of the soft tissues of the body for the purpose of obtaining or maintaining health
14. A form of medicine that combines acupuncture, herbology, and massage therapy
17. Light amplification of stimulated emissions radiation

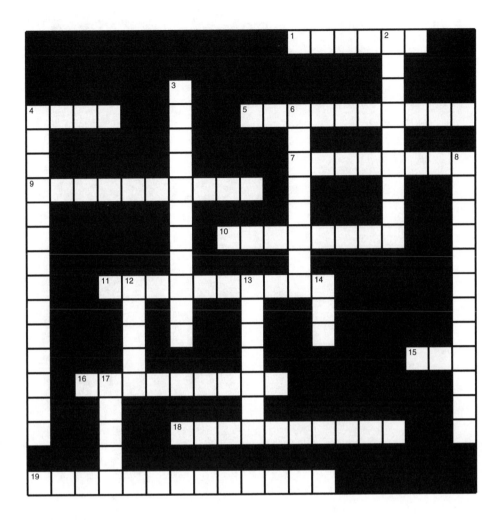

24 Physical Therapy and Rehabilitation

LEARNING OBJECTIVES

When you have completed this chapter, you will be able to:
1. Differentiate between rehabilitation and physical therapy
2. Describe the roles of the members of the animal rehabilitation team
3. Describe the goals of and indications for use of physical therapy in animals
4. List and describe the five elements of patient management in physical therapy
5. Describe legal issues related to the practice of physical therapy
6. List services commonly offered by physical therapists
7. Differentiate between passive, active, and active-assistive exercise
8. Describe the principles of hydrotherapy and explain methods to provide hydrotherapy to animal patients
9. Define proprioception and give examples of proprioceptive activities performed with animal patients
10. List supportive and assistive devices used with animal patients
11. List and describe commonly used physical therapy modalities
12. List common classifications of strokes used for myofascial manipulation
13. Describe considerations in design of training or conditioning programs for canine athletes
14. Differentiate between orthotics and prosthetics
15. Define common terms related to physical therapy and rehabilitation

MULTIPLE CHOICE

Massage Definitions
Select the definition that most nearly defines the given word.

1. Tapotement
   a. Kneading—rhythmic lifting, squeezing, and releasing of tissue
   b. Rapid shaking or slower rocking of the tissue during massage
   c. Uninterrupted flow of strokes and transition between strokes
   d. Use of tapping motion of the hands or fingers during massage

2. Pétrissage
   a. A form of tapotement used to loosen phlegm congestion in the lungs
   b. Manual technique for deactivating a trigger point
   c. The arrangement of massage strokes
   d. Kneading—rhythmic lifting, squeezing, and releasing of tissue

3. Cryotherapy
   a. Manipulation of tissue to increase circulation
   b. Cold therapy—removes heat from the body
   c. System of massage for teaching physical awareness of the body
   d. The use of stretching to prevent the loss of normal range of motion

4. Vibration
   a. Rapid shaking or slower rocking of the tissue during massage
   b. Trigger-point massage; concentrates on knots in the muscles
   c. Japanese form of massage; literally means "finger pressure"
   d. Gliding stroke that follows the contour of the body

5. Excursion
   a. The length of one massage stroke
   b. Use of tapping motion of the hands or fingers during massage
   c. Systematic and scientific manipulation of the soft tissues
   d. Abnormal relationship between two adjacent vertebrae

6. Massage
   a. Cold therapy—removes heat from the body
   b. System of massage for teaching physical awareness of the body
   c. Systematic and scientific manipulation of the soft tissues
   d. Rapid shaking or slower rocking of the tissue

251

7. Coupage
   a. A form of tapotement used to loosen phlegm congestion in the lungs
   b. Uninterrupted flow of strokes and transition between strokes
   c. Consciously sought out goal of a massage therapist
   d. The arrangement of massage strokes

8. Team
   a. Abnormal relationship between two adjacent vertebrae
   b. System of massage for teaching physical awareness of the body
   c. Systematic and scientific manipulation of the soft tissues of the body
   d. Use of tapping motion of the hands or fingers during massage

9. Shiatsu
   a. The length of one massage stroke
   b. Manipulation of tissue to increase circulation
   c. Consciously sought out goal of a massage therapist
   d. Japanese form of massage; literally means "finger pressure"

10. Subluxation
   a. Gliding stroke that follows the contour of the body
   b. Abnormal relationship between two adjacent vertebrae
   c. Trigger-point massage—concentrates on knots in the muscle
   d. A condition where the patella moves out of alignment

11. Myotherapy
   a. Manipulation of the tissue to increase circulation
   b. Cold therapy—removes heat from the body
   c. Trigger point massage—concentrates on knots in the muscles
   d. Alternating heat and cold therapy

12. Ischemic compression
   a. Manual technique for deactivating a trigger point
   b. Rapid shaking or slower rocking of the tissue
   c. Use of rapid tapping or poking motion of the fingers
   d. Where two vertebrae fuse together, cutting off blood flow

13. Continuity
   a. Scheduling multiple massage appointments at once to prevent delays
   b. Use of rapid tapping or poking motion of the fingers
   c. Manual technique for deactivating a trigger point
   d. Uninterrupted flow of strokes and transition between strokes

14. Friction
   a. The use of stretching to prevent the loss of normal range of motion
   b. The term used when an animal feels discomfort during massage
   c. Manipulation of tissue to increase circulation
   d. Systematic and scientific manipulation of the soft tissues

15. Passive range of motion
   a. The length of one massage stroke
   b. The use of stretching to prevent the loss of normal range of motion
   c. The arrangement of massage strokes
   d. Allowing the animal to move on its own, unassisted movement

16. Sequence
   a. The number of massage appointments necessary for improvement or recovery
   b. Use of tapping motion of the hands or fingers during massage
   c. The arrangement of massage strokes
   d. Alternating heat and cold therapy

SHORT ANSWER

1. Compare and contrast "rehabilitation" and "physical therapy."

_____

_____

_____

_____

2. List the seven goals of physical therapy.

   A. _____

   _____

   B. _____

   _____

   C. _____

   _____

   D. _____

   _____

   E. _____

   _____

   F. _____

   _____

   G. _____

   _____

3. What is imperative that veterinary technicians do before they practice any type of physical rehabilitation?

   _____

   _____

4. In the continuum of care of physical therapy, compare and contrast the roles of the veterinarian, the physical therapist, and the veterinary technician.

   A. Veterinarian _____

   _____

   B. Physical therapist _____

   _____

   C. Veterinary technician _____

   _____

5. How can veterinary technicians involve owners with their animal's rehabilitation?

_____

_____

_____

6. Passive exercises would be appropriate to use in situations where:

A. _____

B. _____

C. _____

7. Describe three benefits of passive exercise.

A. _____

B. _____

C. _____

8. Describe four benefits of active exercise.

A. _____

B. _____

C. _____

D. _____

9. Besides rehabilitation, how can hydrotherapy be used?

A. _____

B. _____

C. _____

D. _____

10. Describe the five inherent properties of water and how they are used in hydrotherapy.

A. _____

_____

_____

B. _____

_____

_____

C. _____

_____

_____

D. _____

_____

_____

E. _____

_____

_____

11. Compare and contrast manipulations, physiologic movement, and accessory motion.

   A. Manipulation _____

_____

_____

   B. Physiologic movement _____

_____

_____

   C. Accessory motion _____

_____

_____

12. What are supportive or assistive devices, and how can they be used in a veterinary setting?

_____

_____

_____

_____

13. Describe how ultrasound may be used in physical therapy.

_____

_____

_____

_____

14. List what must be included in the animal's medical record when documenting the use of a modality.

   A. _____

   B. _____

   C. _____

   D. _____

15. Describe how cryotherapy can be beneficial to an animal during physical therapy.

   _____

   _____

   _____

   _____

   _____

16. List contraindications and precautions when considering cryotherapy.

   A. _____

   B. _____

   C. _____

   D. _____

17. List the contraindications for Equi-Light therapy.

   A. _____

   B. _____

   C. _____

18. Explain the "SAID" principle for maximizing performance in a canine athlete.

   _____

   _____

   _____

19. What is Wolff's law?

   _____

   _____

20. Define and contrast "orthotic" and "prosthetic."

   _____

   _____

21. List the most common contributing factors for back injuries for veterinary technicians.

A. _____

B. _____

C. _____

D. _____

E. _____

F. _____

G. _____

H. _____

22. List five neurologic conditions commonly referred to physical therapists.

A. _____

B. _____

C. _____

D. _____

E. _____

Use the terms for the definitions below in the word search.

```
C P S A M N I P C R Y O T H E R A P Y G I C P I Y S
E F U S I R C T X A M P L I T U I O T T N R R P M P
E L E C T R I C A L S T I M U L A T I O N Y O Y P A
N I O T E M R G O N I O M E T L D P B I I O G N L I
P C O A E N T L T A S S T P I R A R T T A T N S E N
T M A I L S F R E Q U E N C Y T H O L O N H O H D I
O P A S S I V E B I O H O E X S O G P L O E S A X T
U I E R E S I S T A N C E T R A I N I N G R I T S R
N E T S H P I B U O Y A N C Y W R O R A S A O I Y I
S O A L I R I I H E A N N D A A O S E A B P O T S T
L N A I U R I O N N S O N O P V M I H D N Y I A P N
G Y I N A O E R I B I C N O A E Y S S Z R L O N T T
O I T G N L R E I T V S N P L F R S T P I D Y C C L
M A S S A G E T A N I D I T P O A T S B N C N O Y H
H I G T E O A U H B M C P O A R N I I E E A O H I T
V B A I N T L G Y O I I O D T M C X T A A U A E P E
S I U I H A G R N I T R I C O X E D S Y O R H S A E
A T T R V T I A L I P I E O I L N R O I T O Y I L N
N S G E S P M R D R R E C C F U U D M I S N P O P C
F B T O O A U I E I I I P G N B E T R N R O E N A O
R R T P N F G I P O M O B I L I Z A T I O N R R T A
E R R T N I R S Y N T G I O T S E N E P I A T R I Y
S C U P O O O P U S O A P R O S T H E T I C O O O B
I M S P R A T M L I G A M E N T T F Y E I H N P N I
S A S M H N N O E W A Y E F O R Y P O O W R I E I I
T S P E O O G N T T E N D O N A W X O N O N C R U N
A S I N N B T X Y H E N R T Y U N T E P I R I T T G
N A A N E P I O O U E R I N I O L E M E T E T Y E N
C G A I I D B L T F F R U T E N A T N N I P Y O T M
E T N S N M P D I H N P A I R O T O R U P L A P T H
T L A F T A I I A Z E T D P C I I E G A A O I E N I
R O S E E N L R T S A R E A Y T C U R P S I E A R O
A F E A R I E I A E A T A N R S L O R V A O D M I A
I R R M V P O E E L F M O E D T E I X S E S U E A C
N E O P E U R N A P S E C H S I O N A I O N S N I Y
I O V L N L O E H N L O R A M P N A G L D U T I D U
N U E I T A A M P L I T U D Z G S I S R T E L I V T
I E A T I T L N O R L S P R A I N O T T R E O L P O
N N E U O I D M P G N N E T S H L F I I R M T U T E
O T T D N O M O D A L I T Y S P R A I H S A N S L I
N C L E S N R L X O P R O P R I O C E P T I I L R A
D S I O P P I H Y D R O T H E R A P Y S D O I N O R
I H L P T C R N A V H I E Y T C T D O P D H E G H M
```

1. Therapeutic techniques used to decrease tissue temperature; cold therapy.

_____

2. The use of electricity to facilitate healing and reduce pain.

_____

3. A term used to describe the amount of electrical pulses per second (PPS).

_____

4. Prediction of the level of improvement and how long it will take to reach those levels.

_____

5. Exercise requiring movement from an external force, no voluntary muscle contraction from the patient.

_____

6. This type of exercise enhances muscle strength and endurance, and helps maintain flexibility.

_____

7. The use of water for therapeutic effects.

_____

8. Tool used to measure joint range of motion.

_____

9. Anatomic structure that connects bone to bone.

_____

10. The sense of touch used to assess what structures lay below the skin.

_____

11. Excessive stretch of a muscle that may cause tearing of the muscle fibers.

_____

12. Inflammation of a tendon.

_____

13. Wide group of agents that may include thermal, acoustic, or electric energy.

_____

14. Fluid-filled sacs that decrease friction between structures.

_____

15. Ability of a limb to move through a specific range of motion.

_____

16. Varying types of manual strokes applied to the body.

_____

17. Tool using sound waves to modify tissue temperature and change blood flow to surrounding tissues.

_____

18. Awareness of body position and movement in space.

_____

19. Extensive stretching of a ligament.

_____

20. Upward thrust of water created when a patient is submersed.

_____

21. Water molecules adhering to one another.

_____

22. Treatment techniques and procedures used to improve a patient's condition.

_____

23. Clinical judgments directed more towards neuromusculoskeletal deficiencies.

_____

24. Passive manipulation that produces a sustained stretch on a particular joint.

_____

25. Passive motion of any kind as a form of treatment for musculoskeletal disorders.

_____

26. Assistive device used to aid the handler in ambulation, often has long straps.

_____

27. Different current types such as AC or DC.

_____

28. Intensity of the electrical unit output.

_____

29. Rise/decay time of electrical stimulation.

_____

30. Light therapy.

_____

31. Natural vasodilator, released from hemoglobin when stimulated by a low-level laser.

_____

32. Device used to support an injured limb (e.g., sling).

_____

33. Device designed to replace a missing limb.

_____

34. Muscle tightness.

_____

35. Anatomic structures that attach muscle to bone.

_____

25 Pharmacology and Pharmacy

LEARNING OBJECTIVES

When you have completed this chapter, you will be able to:

1. Define common terms related to pharmacology and pharmacy
2. Describe the factors that affect the absorption and distribution of drugs and list mechanisms by which drugs may be biotransformed and eliminated
3. List the dosage forms of medications, the routes by which medications may be administered, and factors that affect route selection
4. Describe the classifications of drugs that affect the nervous, cardiovascular, and gastrointestinal systems and give examples of each
5. List the classifications of agents used to treat common internal parasite infections of animals and name the parasite(s) that may be treated with each
6. List the pharmacologic agents used in treatment and prevention of heartworm disease
7. List the classes of compounds used to treat common external parasite infestations of animals
8. List the classifications of antimicrobial agents used to animals and give examples of each
9. List the hormonal substances used in treatment of animals and describe indications for their use
10. Describe legal issues and requirements related to purchasing, storing, dispensing, and administering pharmacologic agents
11. Define compounding and explain legal issues related to compounding of medications
12. Explain the purpose and uses of material safety data sheets
13. Calculate quantities of medications in a variety of dosage forms for dispensing or administering to patients
14. Define inventory turnover rate and explain its importance in managing pharmacy inventory
15. Describe procedures for procuring, organizing, and pricing pharmacy inventory

MATCHING

1. _____ Dose
2. _____ Pharmacokinetics
3. _____ Distribution
4. _____ Therapeutic index
5. _____ Drug
6. _____ Elimination
7. _____ Dosage
8. _____ Excretion
9. _____ Metabolism
10. _____ Effective dose
11. _____ Pharmacology
12. _____ Parenteral
13. _____ Absorption
14. _____ Pharmacodynamics
15. _____ Half-life

A. Process of transformation that involves splitting of the molecule plus the addition of water molecules to each of the split portions

B. The ratio between the dose that is toxic and the dose that is therapeutic

C. The processes that remove a drug from the body

D. One of the processes of transformation that involves the loss of electrons

E. Is the irreversible transformation of parent compounds into daughter metabolites

F. The time required for 50% of the serum concentration to be eliminated

G. Is the dispersion of substances throughout the fluids and tissues of the body

H. The elimination of the substances from the body

I. Drug is given through the gastrointestinal tract

J. The process of a substance entering the body

K. The point of maximum therapeutic concentration of a drug

L. Local effect, substance is applied directly where its action is desired

M. A chemical that affects the living process

16. _____ Topical

17. _____ Enteral

18. _____ Peak serum level

19. _____ Oxidation

20. _____ Reduction

21. _____ Hydrolysis

22. _____ Conjugation

23. _____ Intramedullary

N. The smallest amount of a substance required to produce a measurable effect on a living organism

O. An injection into the bone marrow

P. Absorption, distribution, metabolism, and excretion of drugs

Q. Physical and chemical properties of drugs and their action of drugs in the body

R. The study of drugs

S. Substance is given by routes other than the digestive tract

T. The process of transformation that involves the gain of electrons

U. The transformation process that joins two compounds together to make another compound that is easily soluble in water

V. The total amount of toxicant received by the animal

W. The amount of toxicant per weight of an animal

TRUE OR FALSE

Choose T (true) or F (false) for each statement below.

1. _____ Free drugs must be excreted directly or metabolized to be cleared from the body.

2. _____ Pharmacokinetics is the ability of an organism to modify chemical structures to make them inactive.

3. _____ Conjugation is one of the ways to remove lipid soluble drugs.

4. _____ Biotransformation always inactivates drugs completely.

5. _____ Animals with hepatic disorders are more likely to have impaired ability to biotransform medications.

6. _____ Per Os is an example of a parenteral route of medication administration.

7. _____ An example of enteral route would be medications given as a constant rate infusion.

8. _____ If a medication is to be given QID, it is given every 6 hours.

9. _____ A constant rate infusion is when a controlled amount of medication is given during a controlled amount of time.

10. _____ Lidocaine is often administered as a topical application.

11. _____ Oxidation is one of the transformations that result in loss of electrons.

12. _____ Intraarticular injection is one that is injected into the heart.

13. _____ Inhalation is a route of absorption for medications.

14. _____ Drug excretion is primarily through the liver and the kidneys.

15. _____ Waste is removed by the kidneys and excreted through bile.

16. _____ Some drugs are eliminated through the mammary glands and into the milk.

17. _____ In production animals, drugs that appear in meat or milk are called residues.

18. _____ The blood-brain barrier helps prevent blood from entering the brain.

19. _____ Agonists are drugs causing action by attaching to specific receptors.

20. _____ Over-the-counter drugs do not require a prescription by a veterinarian.

21. _____ Sympathomimetic agents cause hypotension and bronchoconstriction.

22. _____ Epinephrine causes decreased heart rate and vasodilation of blood vessels.

23. _____ Thiopental is classified as an ultra short barbiturate.

24. _____ Ketamine is classified as a dissociative anesthetic agent.

25. _____ Opioids are derived from poppy alkaloids.

1. The following is when a medication is the most available in serum:
   a. Half-life
   b. Peak serum level
   c. Therapeutic index
   d. Pharm time

2. Neuroleptanalgesics are a combination of a tranquilizer and the following:
   a. Barbiturate
   b. Dissociative anesthetic
   c. Opioid
   d. Aspirin

3. Most euthanasia solutions contain the following:
   a. Phenobarbital
   b. Ketamine
   c. Morphine
   d. Pentobarbital

4. This type of drug is used to help suppress the coughing reflex center:
   a. Decongestants
   b. Antitussives
   c. Bronchodilators
   d. Antibiotics

5. This medication stimulates the central nervous system and is commonly used to help stimulate breathing in newborn pets post C-section:
   a. Doxapram
   b. Diazepam
   c. Xylitol
   d. Butorphanol

6. This classification of drugs is used to remove fluid by causing increased urination:
   a. NSAIDS
   b. Opioids
   c. Diuretics
   d. Antitussives

7. Vasodilators cause the following:
   a. Increased blood pressure
   b. Vasoconstriction
   c. Vasodilation
   d. Increased urination

8. Methionine causes the following:
   a. Decreased lung congestion
   b. Urinary acidification
   c. Crystalluria
   d. Increased urine pH

9. Emetics cause the following:
   a. Increased urination
   b. Laxative effects
   c. Vomiting
   d. Decreased gastric mobility

10. Gastrointestinal prokinetics do the following:
    a. Stimulate emesis by binding to the CRTZ
    b. Decrease motility of the gastrointestinal system
    c. Increase motility of the gastrointestinal system
    d. Decrease gastrointestinal transit time

11. Cholinergic agents cause the following effects:
    a. Dry mouth
    b. Constipation
    c. Tachycardia
    d. Bradycardia

12. Miotics are used to treat:
    a. Chronic heart failure
    b. Acute renal failure
    c. Glaucoma
    d. Inflammatory bowel disease

13. Keratoconjunctivitis is a condition that causes:
    a. Decreased production of tears
    b. Increased gastric motility
    c. Decreased gastric motility
    d. Increased tear production

14. Gentocin is an antibiotic that has been associated with:
    a. Hepatotoxicity
    b. Ototoxicity
    c. Blindness
    d. Osteoarthritis

15. Antiseptics are used to:
    a. Decrease growth of bacteria
    b. Increase urine production
    c. Increase gastrointestinal transit time
    d. Precipitate fats

16. The following is both an astringent and an antiseptic:
    a. Alcohol
    b. Hypochlorites
    c. Benzalkonium chloride
    d. Acetic acids

17. The following antibiotics are bacteriostatic:
    a. Penicillin
    b. Cephalosporins
    c. Amoxicillin
    d. Tetracycline

18. Side effects of tetracycline include:
    a. Staining of teeth in young animals
    b. Gingival pigment changes
    c. Alopecia
    d. Decreased sun sensitivity

19. The following classification of medication is used to treat heartworm disease:
    a. Cephalosporins
    b. Arsenicals
    c. Aminoglycosides
    d. Fluoroquinolones

20. The following are signs of overhydration:
    a. Pale mucous membranes
    b. Dry or tacky mucous membranes
    c. Crackle sounds in the lung fields
    d. Bradycardia

21. The following is an example of a colloid fluid:
    a. Lactated ringers
    b. 0.9% Saline
    c. Normosol
    d. Hetastarch

22. Sodium bicarbonate is often added to fluids to correct the following:
    a. Acute renal failure
    b. Metabolic acidosis
    c. Metabolic alkalosis
    d. Pancreatitis

23. Dextrose is added to fluids to help:
    a. Remove potassium and chloride
    b. Increase urination
    c. Correct hypoglycemia
    d. Decrease blood pH

24. Chemotherapy is used in oncology to:
    a. Decrease tumor size
    b. Prevent secondary bacterial infection
    c. Prevent secondary fungal infection
    d. Increase metastases

25. The following is used to depress the immune system:
    a. Corticosteroids
    b. Cephalosporins
    c. Antihistamines
    d. Pyrogens

CALCULATIONS

1. A dog is given diazepam for status epilepticus using constant rate IV infusion at a dose of 0.5 mg/kg diluted in D5W. If the dog weighs 15 lb, how many milligrams would be given as total dose?

2. A bird is given acyclovir for treatment of Pacheco disease at a dose of 80 mg/kg PO q8h. If the bird weighs 500 g, how many milligrams would the bird receive in a 24-hour period?

3. A cat is given aminophylline tablets at a dose of 6.6. mg/kg PO twice daily as a bronchodilator. How many milligrams would an 11 lb cat receive if this is given for 7 days?

4. A pet owner accidentally applies 2.5 ml of a dog flea product containing 45% permethrin to a 15 lb cat. What is the dosage that this cat received?

5. A dog is put on cephalosporin for pyometra at a dose of 30 mg/kg PO q8h, how many milligrams would the dog receive if he were on this for 14 days if the dog weighs 57 lb?

6. You need to create a solution of 40% ethanol and you have 1000 ml of 80% ethanol. What is the volume of the second solution?

7. You need to create a solution of 5% N-acetylcysteine and you have 50 ml of 20% N-acetylcysteine. What is the volume of the second solution?

_____

8. The dose of butorphanol in the horse is 0.1 mg/kg IV q4h. If a horse weighs 1200 lb, how many milligrams would be given to it in 48 hours?

_____

9. An anesthetized dog is to be given 0.11 mg/kg IV slowly of yohimbine to reverse the affects of xylazine. If the dog weighs 45 lb, how many milligrams of yohimbine is to be given?

_____

10. A dog with chronic hepatitis is given ursodiol at a dose of 15 mg/kg PO q12h. If the dog is on this medication for 7 days, how many milligrams would he receive if he weighed 20 lb?

_____

CROSSWORD PUZZLE

Across

3. Anthelmintics are drugs used in the treatment of
 _____
7. A drug that increases the rate of urine output
8. Nerve cells that relay information from the central nervous system to the rest of the body
9. A nutritional supplement designed for any specific clinical purpose
13. Agents used to induce vomiting
14. Agents used to increase bowel motility
15. Analgesics that remedy pain by affecting pain receptors in the brain
17. The process by which drugs are eliminated from the body
18. Any chemical agent that affects living processes
19. Drugs that alleviate pain

Down

1. To mix a dry lyophilized powder form of a drug with a diluent for administration either orally, parenterally, or topically
2. Drugs that lower body temperature from a raised state
4. Biotransformation
5. The minimum drug serum concentration during a given dose interval
6. Creatinine is a natural waste product of _____ tissue
10. The uptake of substances into or across tissue
11. Dose greater than the upper limit of the therapeutic range that causes poisonous symptoms
12. Time required for the serum concentration of a drug to decrease by 50% (two words)
16. Pharmacognosy is the aspect of pharmacology that includes the history and _____ of drugs

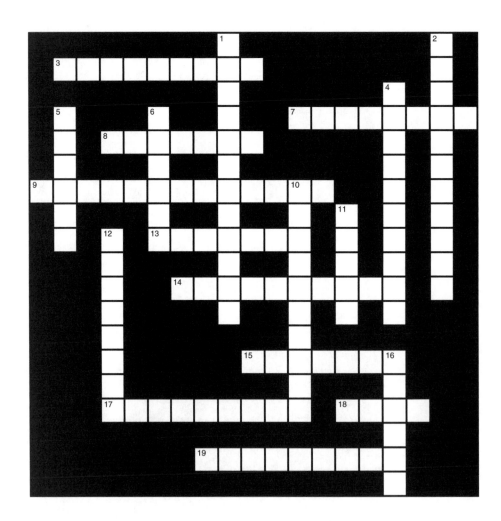

26 Pain Management

LEARNING OBJECTIVES

When you have completed this chapter, you will be able to:
1. Describe methods used to recognize pain and monitor response to analgesics in small and large animals
2. Differentiate between dysphoria and pain response and describe physiologic effects of pain on the body systems
3. Differentiate between pain and nociception and describe the phases of nociception
4. Define hyperalgesia and allodynia, and explain their role in management of chronic pain
5. Describe the concepts of preemptive analgesia and multimodal analgesia
6. List the steps in calculating constant rate infusions
7. List the classes of medications used in management of pain and give examples of each
8. List the routes of administration of local and systemic anesthetics, analgesics, and sedatives
9. List the types of adjunctive medications used in pain management
10. List and describe nonpharmacologic options of treatment of pain

MATCHING

1. _____ Are commonly used as anesthetic agents and only provide analgesia for about 30 minutes
2. _____ Transmit aching or throbbing pain
3. _____ Is when analgesics are administered into the epidural space at the lumbosacral junction
4. _____ Absence of pain achieved through u se of medication
5. _____ An unpleasant sensory experience
6. _____ Provide temporary analgesia for dental procedures
7. _____ Include morphine and fentanyl
8. _____ Analgesia is given before surgery to help reduce postoperative pain
9. _____ Help mediate inflammation and pain
10. _____ Route of anesthesia often involves the use of a patch that slowly administers medication into the skin
11. _____ Pain arises from the organ system
12. _____ Pain that arises from skin, subcutaneous tissues, muscle, bones, or joints
13. _____ Are commonly used for topical and local pain control
14. _____ Are the body's natural response to pain and help provide some analgesia

A. NSAIDs
B. Visceral
C. Endorphins
D. Analgesia
E. Preemptive
F. Somatic
G. Opioids
H. Pain
I. Dental blocks
J. Alpha-2 Adrenergic agonists
K. Transdermal
L. Epidural
M. Fibers

TRUE OR FALSE

Choose T (true) or F (false) for each statement below.

1. _____ Infusion of local analgesics is used to provide analgesia to deeper tissues.
2. _____ Examples of regional nerve blocks used in epidural, spinal, and brachial.

3. _____ Epidural analgesia provides analgesia of the head, shoulders, forelimbs, and head.

4. _____ Injecting local anesthetics directly into joint space can result in effective analgesia after orthopedic surgery.

5. _____ A tourniquet should never be left on for more than 2 hours because it can block necessary blood flow, which could result in tissue anoxia and cell death.

6. _____ COX-1 inhibition reduces inflammation, however, COX-2 inhibition can result in adverse effects, such as GI ulceration and bleeding.

7. _____ Acetaminophen can be safely used in cats.

8. _____ Gabapentin is an anticonvulsant that has been used in humans to treat chronic pain.

9. _____ Opioids are further classified as agonists that stimulate opioid receptors or antagonists that block opioid receptors.

10. _____ The most commonly used pure opioid agonists are morphine, hydromorphone, and fentanyl.

11. _____ Vocalizing and body posture are two examples of how animals show pain.

12. _____ A pet that is in pain will vocalize, withdraw, scratch, or bite when touched.

13. _____ A pet that is in pain will have a decreased heart rate and decreased blood pressure.

14. _____ Nonpharmacologic methods to control pain include the use of heating pads and comfortable bedding.

15. _____ Carprofen is a type of opioid.

16. _____ Fentanyl is classified as an NSAID.

17. _____ Animals experiencing the wind-up effect generally need more analgesia than those that do not experience this.

18. _____ Preemptive use of analgesics is when analgesics are given following a surgery.

19. _____ Opioids are metabolized in the liver and excreted in the urine.

20. _____ Fentanyl was the first opioid agent used in medicine.

21. _____ Morphine is a pure agonist with affinity for both mu and kappa opioid receptors.

22. _____ Cats may experience a paradoxical excitation reaction with opioid medications.

23. _____ Morphine is effective for visceral pain only.

24. _____ Schedule II drugs have a high abuse potential and may produce physical dependence in humans.

25. _____ Morphine is a schedule III drug.

26. _____ Naloxone is the reversal agent for opioids.

27. _____ Butorphanol has both agonist and antagonist properties.

28. _____ Opioids should never be given intraarticularly.

29. _____ Aspirin is effective for both somatic and visceral pain.

30. _____ NSAIDs require approximately 30 to 60 minutes to reach full analgesic effect.

31. _____ NSAIDs do not have antiinflammatory properties.

32. _____ NSAIDs are antipyretic.

33. _____ Acetaminophen can cause methemoglobinemia in cats.

34. _____ Buffered NSAIDs may help decrease gastric irritation.

35. _____ Local anesthetics provide long-term pain control.

36. _____ Local anesthetics have a quick onset of action.

37. _____ Lidocaine is classified as a local anesthetic.

38. _____ Lidocaine is administered topically at a 50% concentration.

39. _____ Xylaxine has long lasting analgesic properties.

40. _____ α_2-adrenergic agonists are not commonly used for their analgesic properties.

MULTIPLE CHOICE

1. Opioids are commonly used analgesics due to their:
   a. Efficacy
   b. Slow onset of action
   c. Reversibility with atropine
   d. Reversibility with yohimbine

2. Fentanyl is most commonly administered by:
   a. Transdermal patch
   b. Oral medication
   c. Intravenous route
   d. Intramuscular route

3. The following medication is an opioid antagonist:
   a. Yohimbine
   b. Atipamezole
   c. Naloxone
   d. Fentanyl

4. Amantadine is another NMDA antagonist and has been used as an adjunct to NSAIDs to treat pain due to:
   a. Acetaminophen poisoning in cats
   b. Dystocia
   c. Cancer in cats
   d. Osteoarthritis in dogs

5. An overdose of local anesthesia may result in:
   a. Diabetes insipidus
   b. Cerebral hemorrhage
   c. Liver failure
   d. Methemoglobinemia

6. This is the procedure of injecting local anesthetic in close proximity to a nerve to produce loss of sensation of pain:
   a. Nerve block
   b. Infusion
   c. Topical anesthetic application
   d. None of the above

7. This procedure involves an administration of a continuous line of local analgesic in an area proximal to the effected area:
   a. Line block
   b. Infusion
   c. Topical anesthetic application
   d. Interstate analgesia

8. The duration of lidocaine can be extended by using it in combination with a:
   a. 1:200,000 dilution of atropine
   b. 1:200,000 dilution of epinephrine
   c. 1:20 dilution of atropine
   d. 1:50 dilution of saline

9. The following is an example of an α_2-adrenergic agonist:
   a. Xylazine
   b. Naloxone
   c. Morphine
   d. Ketamine

10. The following is true about ketamine:
    a. Is an α_2-adrenergic agonist
    b. Has excellent visceral analgesic effects
    c. Is given through patch administration
    d. Has good superficial analgesic effects

11. Pain can cause the following effects in animals:
    a. Increased vocalization
    b. Decreased blood pressure
    c. Decreased heart rate
    d. Kidney failure

12. Pain is received when the following receptors are stimulated:
    a. Norepinephrine
    b. Nociceptors
    c. Muscarinic
    d. Nicotinic

13. Adverse effects of NSAIDs include:
    a. Squamous cell carcinoma
    b. Decreased size of thyroid gland
    c. Gastric ulceration
    d. Mydriasis

14. Tranquilizers are used to:
    a. Supplement the effects of opioid analgesics
    b. Antagonize the effects of opioid analgesics
    c. Block the effects of opioid analgesics
    d. Reverse the effects of opioid analgesics

15. The following is classified as a NSAID:
    a. Meloxicam
    b. Pentobarbital
    c. Codeine
    d. Lidocaine

16. The following are two types of cyclo-oxygenases:
    a. CAD and ACD
    b. COX-1 and COX-2
    c. CYC-A and CYC-2
    d. COX-alpha and COX-beta

17. The duration of analgesia of opioids may be extended if:
    a. They are given rectally
    b. With an NSAID
    c. They are given as an epidural
    d. They are given orally

18. Local anesthetics are commonly used for:
    a. Orthopedic surgeries
    b. Dental procedures
    c. GDV corrections
    d. Ovariohysterectomies

19. The following lacks analgesic qualities:
    a. Halothane
    b. Xylazine
    c. Fentanyl
    d. Morphine

20. The following is pain that is felt in another part of a body and not in the part that experienced the painful event:
    a. Acute
    b. Generalized
    c. Corsican
    d. Referred

CALCULATIONS

1. Butorphanol is to be given to an 11-lb cat at a dose of 0.4 mg/kg q.i.d. How many milligrams would be given in 24 hours?

2. A 45-lb dog recovering from surgery is to be given 0.05 mg/kg q3h. How many milligrams are given in 24 hours?

3. One half ounce of a 0.5% lidocaine solution is infiltrated into a surgical site of a 90-lb dog. How many milligrams per kilogram was administered?

4. One-quarter ounce of a topical crème containing 2.5% lidocaine and 2.5% prilocaine is rubbed on a 75-lb dog's leg. How many milligrams per kilogram was administered of each medication?

5. A 15-lb cat is to be given a dose of 0.05 mg/kg of morphine as an epidural. How many milligrams are to be given?

CROSSWORD PUZZLE

Across

4. The process of amplifying or dampening incoming pain signals after arrival in the spinal cord

8. An uneasy emotional state characterized by anxiety and abnormal behavior

9. Administering low doses of drugs in IV fluids at a fixed rate over time

12. A neurotransmitter is a chemical that is released from cells in the nervous system that "transmits" a message to another nerve cell or _____ organ

13. The sending of pain signals via nerve fibers to the spinal cord

14. The conversion of unpleasant stimuli into nerve signals at the point of injury

16. Delivered via absorption through the skin such as in a patch

17. Pain detection _____ is the point at which pain nerve fibers are stimulated enough to send pain signals to the central nervous system

18. Pain _____ is the greatest intensity of pain that can be tolerated by an individual

Down

1. Recruitment of nonpainful nerve fibers transmitting information as pain resulting in previously pleasant or neutral sensations being experienced as unpleasant

2. Term used to describe three neuralgic phases of the pain pathway

3. _____ analgesia is pain management administered before any trauma occurs to prevent expected pain

5. A drug which binds to a receptor and inhibits expression of its function

6. Medications administered intraarticular will be placed in a _____

7. Lowering of the pain threshold resulting in less stimulation being required to produce pain

10. A food or food supplement thought to have a beneficial medical effect

11. Delivered via absorption through mucous membranes such as the gums

15. The type of delirium resulting from incomplete recovery from gas anesthesia

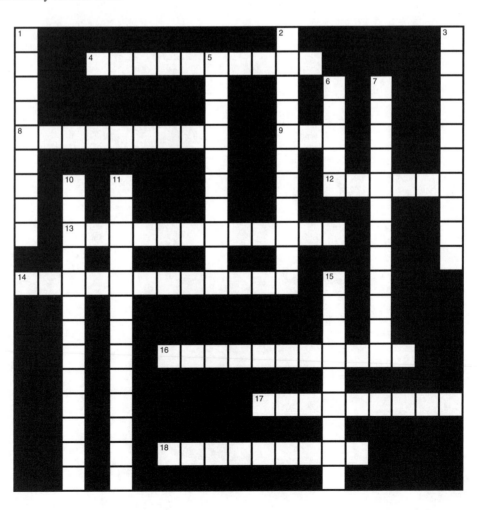

27 | Veterinary Anesthesia

LEARNING OBJECTIVES

When you have completed this chapter, you will be able to:

1. Define anesthesia and differentiate between general and local anesthesia
2. Differentiate between sedation, tranquilization, and neuroleptanalgesia
3. Explain the concept of balanced anesthesia and list the factors to consider in developing an anesthetic plan for a patient
4. List the classes of injectable medications used in anesthetic protocols and give examples of each
5. List and describe the features of the commonly used inhalant anesthetics
6. List the parts of the anesthesia machine, describe the function of each part, and list procedures used for verifying proper operation
7. Differentiate between nonrebreathing and rebreathing systems and explain the proper use, advantages, and disadvantages of each type of system
8. List the reflexes used in monitoring of anesthetic depth and describe the relationship between vital signs, patient reflexes, and anesthetic depth
9. List the stages and planes of anesthesia and describe changes in patient physiology and behavior in each stage
10. Describe the equipment needed and procedures used for placement of an endotracheal tube
11. Describe procedures used for IV, IM, mask, and chamber induction
12. Describe general consideration for patient positioning, comfort, and safety during anesthesia
13. Describe procedures used in monitoring patients during recovery from anesthesia
14. Differentiate between manual and mechanical ventilation and explain indications, procedures, and complications of ventilation
15. Describe common anesthetic problems and emergencies

MATCHING

1. _____ A compound that reversibly produces the loss of ability to perceive pain and/or other sensations

2. _____ A peculiar type of breathing pattern in which inspiration is followed by a prolonged pause and expiration is short

3. _____ The upper portion of the digestive tube, between the esophagus below and the mouth and nasal cavities

4. _____ The medical specialty concerned with the pharmacologic, physiological, and clinical basis of anesthesia and related fields

5. _____ A transient generalized muscular weakness

6. _____ Loss of sensation resulting from depression of nerve function or from neurologic dysfunction

7. _____ Irregularity of the heartbeat

8. _____ One of the two subdivisions of the trachea serving to convey air to and from the lungs

9. _____ The inability to coordinate muscle activity during voluntary movements

10. _____ Absence of gas from a part or the whole of the lungs, due to failure of expansion or resorption of gas from the alveoli

A. Alveolus
B. Analgesia
C. Analgesic
D. Anesthesia
E. Anesthetic
F. Anesthesiology
G. Apneustic respiration
H. Arrhythmia
I. Ataxia
J. Atelectasis
K. Brachycephalic
L. Bradycardia
M. Bronchiole
N. Bronchus
O. Cartilage

11. _____ Shortness of the head

12. _____ One of the finer subdivisions of the bronchi, all less than 1 mm in diameter, and having no cartilage in its wall

13. _____ Thin-walled saclike terminal dilations of the respiratory bronchioles, alveolar ducts, and alveolar sacs where gas exchange occurs

14. _____ Rhythmical or jerky oscillation of the eyeballs

15. _____ A connective tissue characterized by its nonvascularity and firm consistency; consists of chondrocytes, an interstitial matrix of fibers (collagen), and a ground substance

16. _____ Removal of waste material from the body

17. _____ Regional anesthesia produced by injection of local anesthetic solution into the peridural space

18. _____ A leaf-shaped plate of elastic cartilage, covered with mucous membrane, at the root of the tongue

19. _____ High blood pressure

20. _____ An abnormally low heart rate

21. _____ The process whereby the undigested residue of food and the waste products of metabolism are eliminated

22. _____ A loss of some types of sensation with persistence of others. A form of general anesthesia, but not necessarily complete unconsciousness

23. _____ Low blood pressure

24. _____ General anesthesia resulting from breathing of anesthetic gases or vapors

25. _____ A general term referring to topical, field block, or nerve block

26. _____ The sum of the chemical and physical changes occurring in tissue

27. _____ The part of the respiratory tract between the pharynx and the trachea; it consists of a framework of cartilages and elastic membranes housing the vocal folds

28. _____ Superficial loss of sensation in conjunctiva, mucous membranes or skin, produced by direct application of local anesthetic solutions, ointments, or gels

29. _____ A compound capable of producing analgesia without producing anesthesia or a loss of consciousness

30. _____ The air tube extending from the larynx into the thorax where it bifurcates into the right and left main bronchi

31. _____ An abnormally high heart rate

32. _____ A neurologic or pharmacologic state in which painful stimuli are no longer painful

P. Cataplexy

Q. Elimination

R. Epidural anesthesia

S. Epiglottis

T. Excretion

U. Dissociated anesthesia

V. Hypotensive

W. Hypertensive

X. Inhalation anesthesia

Y. Larynx

Z. Local anesthetic

AA. Nystagmus

BB. Metabolism

CC. Pharynx

DD. Trachea

EE. Tachycardia

FF. Topical anesthesia

TRUE OR FALSE

Choose T (true) or F (false) for each statement below.

1. _____ The respiratory system of the dog is divided into two sections: upper respiratory and the lower respiratory systems.

2. _____ The pharynx is considered part of the upper respiratory system.

3. _____ The upper respiratory tract consists of the nares, nasal cavity, sinuses, pharynx, and bronchioles.

4. _____ The veterinary technician's role in anesthesia begins with patient recovery.

5. _____ Animals under anesthesia do not require constant supervision.

6. _____ With inhalant anesthetic, the only way to adjust the level of anesthesia is through the additional drug to increase anesthetic depth or by a reversal agent to decrease anesthetic depth.

7. _____ Inhalant anesthetic machines do not produce waste gas, which may be harmful to staff members.

8. _____ With inhalant anesthetic, the O ring can be adjusted to increase or decrease anesthetic depth.

9. _____ The mechanism of action of cyclohexamine anesthetics is to sedate the chemoreceptor zone in the cerebrum and stimulate the cerebellar center.

10. _____ There is no direct reversal agent for pentobarbital.

11. _____ The direct reversal agent for medetomidine is atropine.

12. _____ Dissociative anesthetic agents are known for their inconsistencies of smooth recoveries when used alone.

13. _____ Ketamine is a barbiturate anesthetic.

14. _____ The mechanism of action of propofol is to disrupt nervous system pathways in the cerebrum and stimulate the reticular center.

15. _____ Blood (hematuria) is present in the urine in cases of urinary tract hemorrhage or urinary tract infection.

16. _____ Hemoglobin (hemoglobinuria) indicates the presence of intrinsic red blood cell damage.

17. _____ An increased number of leukocytes (leukocytosis) may indicate inflammatory processes.

18. _____ The most sensitive indicator of liver damage is creatinine and BUN levels.

19. _____ The most sensitive indicator of kidney disease is ALT and AST levels.

20. _____ The exact mechanism of action of inhalant anesthetics is not known.

21. _____ Most inhalant anesthetics have a low lipid solubility, which allows for rapid entrance into the blood stream.

22. _____ Vapor pressure is the measure of the amount of liquid anesthetic that will evaporate at $0°$ C.

23. _____ Concentration coefficient is the measure of the distribution of the inhalation agent between the blood and gas phases in the body.

24. _____ Volume factor is the measure of the distribution of the inhalation agent between the blood and gas phases in the body.

25. _____ Minimum alveolar concentration is the highest concentration that produces no response to 100% of the patients exposed to a painful stimulus.

26. _____ Ketamine is used to reverse the effects associated with opiates.

27. _____ The effects of a_2-agonists, such as medetomidine and xylazine, may be antagonized with a_2-antagonists, atipamezole, or yohimbine (respectively).

28. _____ The pop-off valve should be open at all times.

29. _____ The chemical reaction between carbon dioxide and the granules in the carbon dioxide absorber granules causes the granules to change color.

30. _____ An otoscope has a smooth blade and a light source and can be used to visualize the oropharyngeal structures.

31. _____ Sizes of endotracheal tubes most commonly used in cats range from 13 to 25 mm and 15 to 28 mm for dogs.

32. _____ When inserting small tubes, a stylet may be used to prevent the tube from bending.

33. _____ Caution should be used when using local anesthetics during intubation because their overuse has been associated with methemoglobinemia in cats.

34. _____ To determine the proper length of tube needed, the distance from the incisors to the xyphoid cartilage should be measured.

1. Which one of the following is part of the veterinary technician's role during anesthesia?
   a. Surgery
   b. Patient monitoring
   c. Planning anesthetic use
   d. Diagnosing anatomic disorders

2. Which of the following parameters are commonly monitored on a patient under anesthesia?
   a. Estrus phase
   b. Heart rate
   c. Ocular temperature
   d. Glucose level

3. When preparing to intubate an animal, the following structure should be visualized:
   a. Esophagus
   b. Pharyngeal cavity
   c. Trachea
   d. Alveoli

4. Which of the following would be normal for a dog's temperature?
   a. 96.8
   b. 98.6
   c. 105
   d. 102

5. The normal heart rate for a cat is _____ beats per minute:
   a. 300
   b. 80
   c. 180
   d. 60

6. Which of the following statements is true?
   a. The exact mechanism of action of barbiturates is direct suppression of the cerebral center zone.
   b. Barbiturates have been shown to inhibit the release of acetylcholine, norepinephrine, and glutamate.
   c. Barbiturates provide analgesia.
   d. Barbiturates can be reversed with ketamine.

7. Which of the following drugs are α_2-adrenergic agonists?
   a. Pentobarbital
   b. Propofol
   c. Xylazine
   d. Ketamine

8. Anticholinergics are used to control:
   a. Dry mouth and eyes
   b. Bradycardia
   c. Sedation level
   d. Tachycardia

9. Preanesthetics are used to:
   a. calm an excited animal
   b. increase side effects of anesthetic drugs
   c. increase the amount of anesthesia required
   d. increase discomfort that would be expected postoperatively

10. Atropine is derived from:
    a. Deadly nightshade
    b. Biturate salt
    c. Para-aminobenzoic acid
    d. Salicylic acid

11. Which of the statements is true about atropine?
    a. Is an anticholinergic agent
    b. Is a cholinergic agent
    c. Effects the neurotransmitter at the chemoreceptor
    d. Effects the nicotinic receptors.

12. Which of the following is an α_2-adrenergic antagonist:
    a. Pentobarbital
    b. Atipamazole
    c. Xylazine
    d. Ketamine

13. Tiletamine is commercially available only in combination with:
    a. Pentobarbital
    b. Detomidine
    c. Zolazepam
    d. Atropine

14. Barbiturates are contraindicated in:
    a. Greyhounds
    b. Golden retrievers
    c. Obese animals
    d. Cats

15. Greyhounds
    a. Have a normally bradycardic heart rate
    b. Are classified as sight hounds
    c. Have been shown to be sensitive to atropine
    d. Can be treated with barbiturates without worry

16. The MAC of isoflurane is:
    a. 1.5 in dogs and 1.2 in cats
    b. 3.5 in dogs and 6 in cats
    c. 0.5 in dogs and 0.5 in cats
    d. 1 in dogs and 2 in cats

17. The MAC of sevoflurane is:
    a. 1.5 in dogs and 1.2 in cats
    b. 2.09 to 2.4 in dogs and 2.58 in cats
    c. 5 in dogs and 8 in cats
    d. 6 in dogs and 2 in cats

18. Halothane is contraindicated in patients with a pre-dilection towards:
    a. Diabetes insipidus
    b. Insulin responsive metabolic disorder
    c. Obesity
    d. Malignant hyperthermia

19. The general recommendation is that oxygen tanks should be changed when the tank gauge reads a pressure below:
    a. 300 psi
    b. 500 psi
    c. 100 to 200 psi
    d. 1000 psi

20. Overfilled reservoir bags may also increase the risk of:
    a. Atelectasis
    b. Sedation
    c. Alveoli rupture
    d. Aspiration pneumonia

21. Nitrous oxide is sometimes used in combination with oxygen because:
    a. The amount of anesthetic needed is reduced
    b. Sedation level is greater
    c. Analgesia level is greater
    d. The amount of anesthetic needed is increased

22. These granules are used in the carbon dioxide absorber canister:
    a. Carbon monoxide
    b. Silica gel desiccant
    c. Soda lime
    d. Sodium chloride

23. Additional anesthetic liquid should be added when the level:
    a. Is less than one-half full
    b. Completely empty
    c. Is one-quarter full
    d. Three-fourths of the way full

24. The pressure manometer should not exceed:
    a. 15 to 20 cm of water
    b. 100 cm of water
    c. 150 to 200 cm of water
    d. 110 mm Hg

25. Granules in the carbon dioxide absorber canister should be removed when they:
    a. Completely dissolve
    b. Swell up like popcorn
    c. Produce steam
    d. Change color

26. The reservoir bag:
    a. Should have a minimum volume of 600 ml/kg body weight of a patient
    b. Allows the patient's respiration to be monitored
    c. Can be used to deliver nitrous oxide only to the patient or to critical care patients
    d. Should never be squeezed

27. This endotracheal tube contains an eye that prevents complete blockage from mucous:
    a. Magill
    b. Magic
    c. Murphy
    d. Maui

28. The following is often used to pass a tube:
    a. Tongue depressor
    b. Otoscope
    c. Laryngoscope
    d. Stylus

29. Endotracheal tubes that are too long:
    a. May lead to anesthesia of only one lung lobe
    b. Are never a problem
    c. Are preferred
    d. May go into the animal's stomach

30. Endotracheal tubes:
    a. Protect the patient's airway
    b. Increase the amount of waste gas production
    c. Prevent inhalation of anesthesia
    d. Make anesthetic gas delivery less efficient

31. Overinflation of the endotracheal tube cuff could result in:
    a. Damage to the trachea from pressure
    b. No problems
    c. Increase anesthetic qualities
    d. Damage to the esophagus

32. The following is a stress triad:
    a. Neutrophils (increase), lymphocytes (decrease), and eosinophils (decrease).
    b. Neutrophils (increase), lymphocytes (increase), and eosinophils (increase)
    c. Neutrophils (decrease), lymphocytes (decrease), and eosinophils (decrease)
    d. Neutrophils (decrease), lymphocytes (increase), and eosinophils (increase)

33. Which of the following statement is correct:
    a. A red top tube contains anticoagulants
    b. A lavender top tube is used to check for zinc
    c. A red top tube is used to prepare serum samples
    d. A red tube has EDTA in it

34. A low PCV (packed cell volume) indicates:
    a. Anemia
    b. Dehydration
    c. Increased red blood cell production
    d. Polycythemia

35. The following statement(s) are true concerning platelets:
    a. Platelets are produced by the liver
    b. Low numbers of platelets may indicate liver dysfunction
    c. Initiate the coagulation process
    d. Platelets aggregate to form the initial hemostatic plug

PHOTO QUIZ

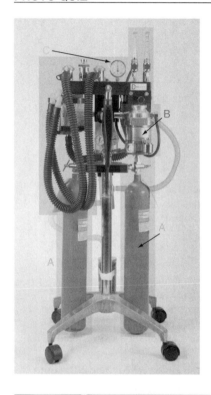

1. Identify the parts of the anesthesia machine.

   A. _____

   B. _____

   C. _____

2. Identify the parts of the anesthesia machine.

   A. _____

   B. _____

   C. _____

   D. _____

   E. _____

   F. _____

   G. _____

   H. _____

CROSSWORD PUZZLE

Across

1. Atelectasis is the collapse of a portion or all of one or both _____
4. A brand name of a self-inflating reservoir bag used to provide manual ventilation (two words)
6. Lacking strength; weak
9. A nonrebreathing circuit with a reservoir bag and corrugated tubing in which the fresh gas inlet is located near the patient and the pressure relief valve is located away from the patient; Mapleson D circuit
11. Inability to coordinate movement
12. A temporary absence of spontaneous breathing
15. Neuromuscular _____ are drugs that relax and paralyze muscles, and which cause cessation of breathing due to paralysis of the muscles of respiration
17. Pertaining to old age
18. The amount of air that moves in and out of the lungs in a minute; the tidal volume multiplied by the respiratory rate
21. Pneumomediastinum means the presence of air in the space between the lungs which contains the _____ and great vessels
22. Involuntary muscle twitching
23. Blue discoloration of the mucous membranes
25. High body temperature
29. Low tissue oxygen levels
30. Flow of stomach contents into the esophagus and mouth unaccompanied by retching
31. Swallowing an excessive volume of air
34. A state of unconsciousness from which the patient cannot be aroused
36. Severe abdominal pain of sudden onset caused by a variety of conditions, including obstruction, twisting, and spasm
38. A positive _____ is a drug that increases the force of contraction of the heart muscle
40. Hematuria means blood in the _____
41. Status epilepticus is continuous _____ activity
42. Slow heart rate

Down

2. A rhythmic, involuntary oscillation of both eyes
3. The patient species, breed, age, sex, and reproductive status
5. Eructate
7. A drug that liquefies respiratory secretions promoting elimination
8. A nonrebreathing circuit with a reservoir bag and corrugated tubing in which the fresh gas inlet is located near the bag and the pressure relief valve is located near the patient; Mapleson A circuit
10. Pertaining to the time immediately following birth
12. To listen to sounds made by internal organs, especially the heart and lungs
13. Absence of pain
14. Lacking any muscle tone
16. Another word for asphyxiation
19. An antiemetic is a drug used to treat or prevent _____
20. Rapid respiratory rate
21. Elevated carbon dioxide levels in the blood
24. Decreased responsiveness to stimulation
26. Low blood pressure
27. Constriction of the pupil of the eye
28. A drug that induces sleep
32. Any abnormality in the electrical activity of the heart
33. Yellow discoloration of the skin and mucous membranes
34. Weight loss, loss of muscle mass, and general debilitation that may accompany chronic diseases
35. Near death
37. Thick and sticky
38. Also referred to as gastrointestinal stasis
39. Adrenocortical pertains to the cortex or _____ layer of the adrenal gland

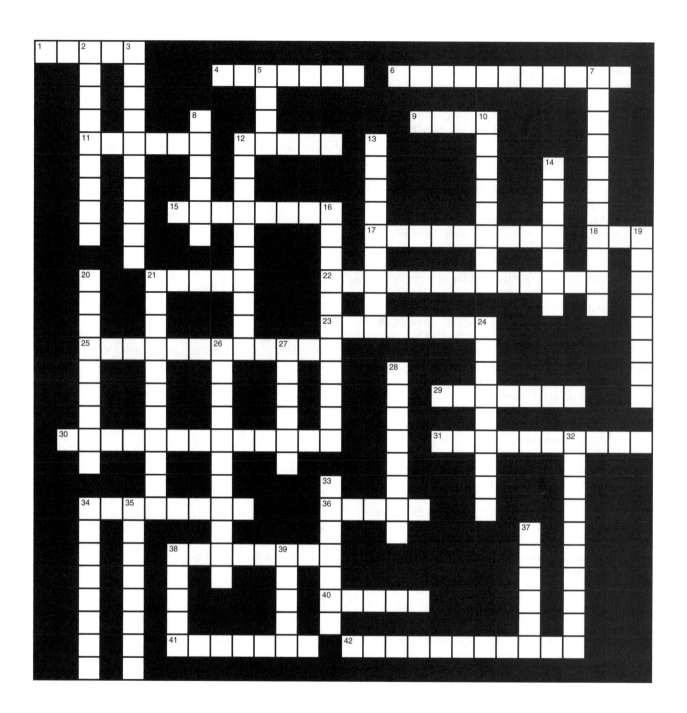

28 Surgical Instruments and Aseptic Technique

LEARNING OBJECTIVES

When you have completed this chapter, you will be able to:

1. Name and describe the commonly used surgical instruments
2. State advantages of surgical stapling and list common surgical stapling devices
3. List commonly used instruments and equipment for ophthalmic, orthopedic, and arthroscopic procedures
4. List surgical instruments and supplies routinely included in general and emergency surgical packs for small and large animals
5. Describe procedures for cleaning, packing, and sterilizing instruments
6. Describe procedures for folding and packing cloth surgical drapes and gowns
7. Differentiate between sterilization and disinfection
8. List and describe physical and chemical methods of sterilization and methods of quality control of sterilization methods
9. State safe storage times for sterile packs
10. List and describe common antiseptic and disinfectant agents
11. Describe requirements for preparation of the operating room and maintenance of operating room sterility
12. Describe preparation requirements for patients, including skin preparation, patient positioning, and draping
13. Describe preparation requirements for the surgical team and explain the procedures that may be used for hand scrubbing before surgery
14. Describe the procedure for donning surgical attire
15. Describe procedures for opening sterile items

DEFINE

1. Antisepsis _____

_____

2. Asepsis _____

_____

3. Sterilization _____

_____

4. Flash sterilization _____

_____

_____

5. Hemostatic forceps _____

_____

6. Ingress port _____

_____

7. Needle holders _____

_____

8. Orthopedic surgery _____

_____

9. Osteochondral chip fragments _____

_____

10. Prosthesis _____

_____

11. Residual activity _____

_____

12. Rongeurs _____

_____

13. Sterile field _____

_____

_____

_____

14. Strike through _____

_____

15. Thumb forceps _____

_____

16. Towel clamps _____

_____

PHOTO MATCHING

Match the following to the instruments shown.

1. _____ Brown-Adson thumb forceps
2. _____ No. 3 scalpel handle
3. _____ Bandage scissors
4. _____ Backhaus towel clamps
5. _____ Snook ovariohysterectomy hook
6. _____ Ophthalmic instrument pack
7. _____ No. 4 scalpel handle

8. _____ Rat-tooth thumb forceps
9. _____ Metzenbaum dissecting scissors
10. _____ Olsen-Hegar needle holders
11. _____ Mosquito hemostats
12. _____ Balfour retractors
13. _____ Periosteal elevators
14. _____ Suture removal scissors

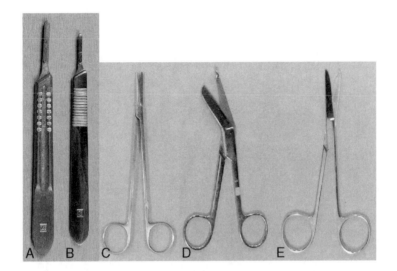

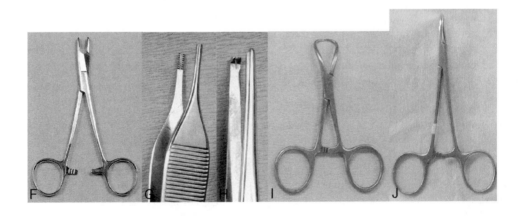

283

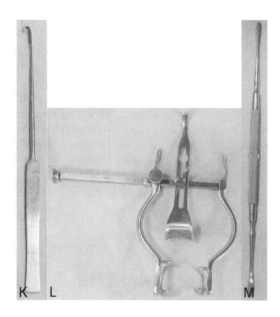

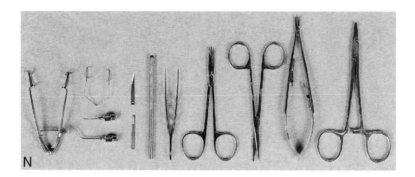

MULTIPLE CHOICE

1. Which of the following does not contribute to contamination progressing to infection when you are referring to the surgical site?
   a. Degree of tissue damage in the wound
   b. Number of infectious agents
   c. Gender of the patient
   d. General health of the patient

2. Which type of thumb forceps is used primarily on skin and/or fascia?
   a. Brown-Adson
   b. Dressing
   c. Adson
   d. Balfour

3. Stapling equipment is named by abbreviation of:
   a. Their designed function
   b. The brand of staples
   c. How they are sterilized
   d. The manufacturer

4. Retractors used most commonly in orthopedic surgery include:
   a. Balfour and Gelpi
   b. Gelpi and Weitlaner
   c. Weitlaner and Balfour
   d. Adson and Gelpi

5. Ophthalmic packs contain which of the following specialized instruments?
   a. Staples
   b. Rongeurs
   c. Gigli wire
   d. Needle holders

6. Arthroscopes are primarily used to:
   a. View the chest cavity in dogs and horses
   b. Remove osteochondral chip fragments in dogs and horses
   c. Remove osteochondrotic lesions in cats and cattle
   d. They are not used in animals

7. Fluid delivery systems are any of the following *except:*
   a. Pressurized bag design
   b. Automated pump system
   c. Hydroflex
   d. Trickle bag design

8. Which of the following is not used in cleaning/caring for instruments?
   a. Ultrasonic cleaner
   b. Povidone-iodine solution
   c. Neutral pH detergent
   d. Instrument milk

9. Which of the following is not an exogenous source of contamination?
   a. Bacteria
   b. Surgical instruments
   c. Patient's skin
   d. Surgical team
   e. The surrounding air

10. An emergency sterilization technique is:
    a. Hydrogen peroxide gas plasma
    b. Ethylene oxide
    c. Flash sterilization
    d. Cold sterilization

11. The three types of methods used for sterilization include:
    a. Filtration, antibacterial soap, radiation
    b. Filtration, radiation, povidone-iodine
    c. Filtration, povidone-iodine, heat
    d. Filtration, heat, radiation

12. Autoclaves:
    a. Always sterilize the materials placed in them
    b. Do not have special instructions on how to pack them
    c. Introduce the steam into the middle of the chamber and force it around the materials using fans
    d. Do not sterilize the load unless the steam has penetrated the packs completely

13. The following are all used as sterilization indicators in autoclaves *except:*
    a. Chemical sterilization indicators
    b. Culture tests
    c. Masking tape
    d. Fusible melting pellet

14. Antiseptic and disinfectant compounds include:
    a. Chlorhexidine, bleach, formaldehyde, iodine
    b. Chlorhexidine, ethylene oxide, bleach, iodine
    c. Chlorhexidine, bleach, ethylene oxide, formaldehyde
    d. Chlorhexidine, ethylene oxide, formaldehyde, iodine

15. Which of the following is not true when prepping a patient for surgery?
    a. The area is clipped at least 2 to 4 cm in every direction from the proposed incision.
    b. Sterile, water-soluble lubricant may be placed in wounds before clipping around them.
    c. Long hair growing near the periphery of the clipped area does not need to be cut short.
    d. Areas that appear infected should be clipped last so as not to spread infection.

16. Traumatized skin during prep is caused by:
    a. The vacuum sucking up the skin
    b. The sterile, water soluble lubricant
    c. Rough clipping
    d. Clipping the hair in the direction of its growth

17. One-step preps:
    a. Are packaged in two parts that easily assemble
    b. Contain sponges used to spread the solution starting from the outside edge and working into the proposed incision site
    c. Require a 30-second application and dry within 1 minute
    d. Contain isopropyl alcohol, which will be flammable until it dries

18. When a patient is placed into a position for surgery, which term is not used to describe the position?
    a. Lateral recumbency
    b. Rostral recumbency
    c. Dorsal recumbency
    d. Sternal recumbency

19. Which of the following is not acceptable surgical attire?
    a. Shoe covers
    b. Surgical caps
    c. Surgical gown
    d. Street clothes

20. Surgical caps and masks are worn by:
    a. All hospital staff
    b. Only the surgeon in the surgical suite
    c. All hospital staff in the surgical suite
    d. Only the surgeon and assistant needed during the surgery

21. Equine surgery usually does not require:
    a. An overhead hoist system
    b. Leg bands
    c. A padded induction room
    d. A V-folding surgical table

22. In handing supplies to the surgeon, a nonsterile assistant must:
    a. Open all sterile items for the surgeon
    b. Make sure to reach over the sterile field
    c. Move the hand or arm over the top of the pack while opening it
    d. Open all the folded edges of the pack at the same time

23. The sterile area on a person is considered to be:
    a. Any part of the gown including the sleeves
    b. The front of the gown, from below the shoulders to the waist
    c. The front and back of the gown, from below the shoulders to the waist
    d. The sleeves and the whole front of the gown

24. Sterile drapes are used for keeping the:
    a. Surgery site free of blood
    b. Animal warm
    c. Animal in place
    d. Surgery field sterile

FILL IN THE BLANK

Strike-through	Aqueous solutions	Stirrups
Mayo instrument stand	Cold sterilized	Disinfection
Arthroscope	Surgical lasers	Electroscalpels
General surgical pack	Cold tray	Gigli wire
Instrument milk	Steinmann pins	K-wire
Accordion fashion	Glutaraldehyde	Scrub-in

1. _____ is used to cut bone during orthopedic surgeries.

2. When fluid penetrates a surgical drape or gown creating a pathway for organisms to invade the sterile surface, it is called _____.

3. Some types of wounds are closed without using complete sterile technique. Such types of wounds include abscesses and the surgical instruments are _____ rather than sterilized via steam or gas.

4. _____ is the destruction of vegetative forms of bacteria but not the spores.

5. Cold sterilized instruments are usually located in a _____ and are used for dirty or nonsterile surgeries.

6. Most surgeries require some of the same instruments. Therefore a _____ is usually used that contains these instruments. Specialized instruments are then wrapped separately and opened only if needed.

7. _____ is one of the solutions that instruments are soaked in when they are in cold sterilization.

8. When an assistant is asked to help during a sterile procedure, they will need to _____ to keep the field sterile.

9. Instruments need to be cleaned and then soaked in _____ to help keep them well lubricated and working properly.

10. The surgical pack and other instruments used in surgery are placed on a _____ for use during surgery, which is then placed close to the surgical patient and within easy reach of the surgeon.

11. _____ can be used to cut or coagulate tissue and help to minimize bleeding.

12. During orthopedic surgery, the affected leg is hung up using strips of tape called _____.

13. _____ may be used to cut or destroy tissue. One of the most common types used in veterinary medicine are carbon dioxide.

14. Gowns and drapes need to be sterilized for surgery. In order for them to fit into an autoclave and then be sterilely used, they are wrapped in _____.

15. _____ cannot be used in living tissue unless greatly diluted due to the higher levels of iodine than iodophors.

16. The _____ can be used as both a diagnostic and surgical tool in veterinary surgery. It is used mostly to examine joints.

17. Intermedullary pins are also called _____ and are placed in the medullary cavity of long bones for fracture fixation.

18. _____ is used to pin small bone fragments due to their smaller size.

TRUE OR FALSE

Choose T (true) or F (false) for each statement below. If false, please state why.

1. _____ Only sterile assistants may open sterile items for the surgeon.

   _____

2. _____ When a nonsterile assistant hands the surgeon or assistant sterile items, he or she can reach over the sterile field.

   _____

3. _____ To open a plastic/paper pouch, scalpel blade, or suture pack, the edges of the wrapper should be peeled back slowly and symmetrically, keeping the package opening directly away from the body.

   _____

4. _____ If a sterile item slips below the tabletop during surgery, it is contaminated and should no longer be used.

   _____

5. _____ Sterile surgical drapes are used to maintain a sterile field around the surgical site and can be placed by any personnel that has scrubbed-in.

   _____

6. _____ The sterile area on a person is considered to be the front of the gown, from just below the shoulders to the waist or the level of the table. This includes the armpits and neckline.

   _____

7. _____ When scrubbing the hands in preparation for surgery, the scrub should contact all the surfaces of the fingers, hand, and forearms and the soap should be in contact with the skin for 5 minutes.

   _____

Chapter **28** **Surgical Instruments and Aseptic Technique**

8. _____ Strict hand scrubbing is not as important if you are going to be putting on sterile gloves.

_____

9. _____ During surgery the surgeon and any sterile assistant are the only ones required to wear surgical caps and masks.

_____

10. _____ The skin of the surgery patient is prepped in the following order: clipping of the hair as close to the skin as possible, initial skin preparation using chlorhexidine or povidone-iodine scrub, and rinse with alcohol. Sterile gloves are then worn and sterile gauze is used to do the final sterile skin preparation.

_____

11. _____ One-step preps are easy to apply, much faster than traditional scrubbing techniques and have a rapid onset.

_____

12. _____ Right lateral recumbency means the animal is lying on its right side, dorsal recumbency means the animal is on its stomach, and ventral recumbency means the animal is on its back.

_____

13. _____ Most operating rooms are designed to make cleaning them easy; therefore the operating room should be simple and uncluttered.

_____

14. _____ Since sterility is so important, all operating rooms should be cleaned daily, with more intense cleanings scheduled weekly to keep dust and bacteria from building up.

_____

15. _____ Arthroscopic equipment can be sterilized with gas, ethylene oxide, or cold sterilization. For multiple uses in 1 day, the equipment is gas sterilized in between each surgery.

_____

16. _____ Cold trays are used to hold instruments that are being cold sterilized. These instruments should only be used for minor procedures such as abscesses and superficial lacerations.

_____

17. _____ Aldehydes, chlorides, phenols, alcohols, chlorhexidine, and iodophors are considered either antiseptics, disinfectants, or both.

_____

18. _____ External tape is used to indicate exposure to gas sterilization on both the outside and inside of the pack.

_____

19. _____ Autoclaves are used routinely for sterilization of packs and singly wrapped instruments. It is important that items be packed loosely to allow steam penetration to all the items and their contents.

_____

20. _____ Autoclaving a pack will make sure it's contents are both clean and sterile.

_____

21. _____ Filtration is used to sterilize gloves and some suture materials while radiation is used to sterilize pharmaceuticals.

_____

22. _____ Aseptic technique is important during surgery to help prevent or control the number of infectious agents introduced into the wound/surgery site.

_____

23. _____ During every surgery some bacterial contamination will occur at the surgical site no matter how good the sterile technique is.

_____

24. _____ Microorganisms can be introduced into the surgical site via endogenous or exogenous routes. The exogenous route cannot be controlled because it comes from within the patient.

_____

25. _____ Instruments with hinges or locking mechanisms should be treated with instrument milk after each cleaning to help lubricate them and keep them working properly.

_____

MATCHING 1

Match the instrument with the type of small animal pack it should go into (there can be more than one answer for each instrument).

1. _____ No. 3 scalpel handle
2. _____ Mayo scissors
3. _____ Periosteal elevator
4. _____ Towel clamps
5. _____ Bone curette
6. _____ Ronguers
7. _____ Stainless steel bowl
8. _____ Sterilization indicator
9. _____ Metal ruler
10. _____ Sponges
11. _____ Lap sponge
12. _____ Adson thumb forceps
13. _____ Crile forceps
14. _____ Needle holder
15. _____ Army-Navy retractor
16. _____ Senn retractor
17. _____ Allis forceps
18. _____ Wire-suture scissors
19. _____ Snook hook
20. _____ Steinmann pins
21. _____ Towels
22. _____ Michel clips and applicator

A. General surgical pack
B. Emergency pack
C. Orthopedic pack

MATCHING 2

Match the safe storage time with the appropriate wrapper (there may be more than one correct answer).

1. _____ Single-wrapped muslin
2. _____ Double-wrapped muslin
3. _____ Single-wrapped crepe paper
4. _____ Single-wrapped muslin sealed in 3-ml polyethylene
5. _____ Heat-sealed paper and transparent plastic pouches

A. 3 weeks in open cabinet
B. 1 week in closed cabinet
C. At least 9 months in open cabinet
D. At least 8 weeks in closed cabinet
E. At least 1 year in open cabinet

MATCHING 3

Match the stapling equipment with its common usage.

1. _____ TA
2. _____ GIA
3. _____ EEA
4. _____ LDS
5. _____ Skin stapler

A. Gastrointestinal resection
B. Skin or fascia closures
C. Lung resection
D. Blood vessel ligation
E. Gastrointestinal anastomosis

PUT IN CORRECT ORDER

Number the following procedures in the order in which they should be performed when setting up for and assisting in surgery.

A. _____ Sterile prep of the surgery site
B. _____ Clipping the hair of the patient
C. _____ Cap and mask placement
D. _____ Donning of sterile gloves via open gloving
E. _____ Opening a sterile pack by a nonsterile assistant
F. _____ Attaching the animal to the surgery table
G. _____ Initial prep of the surgery site
H. _____ Gowning up
I. _____ Start of surgery
J. _____ Scrubbing of the arms and hands

SHORT ANSWER

Describe the following techniques:

1. Gowning

_____

_____

_____

_____

2. Closed gloving

_____

_____

3. Open gloving

_____

4. Assisted gloving

_____

5. Removing gloves aseptically

_____

6. Opening a sterile pack

_____

_____

_____

_____

_____

FILL IN THE BLANK

Fill in the blanks to solve the super clue in the center (hyphens have been given a space).

1. These tissue forceps are considered to be traumatic and should only be used on tissue to be removed.

2. This method of gloving decreases the chance of contamination.

3. Before the large surgical drape is placed over the patient, these are placed around the area to be incised.

4. These thumb forceps have a broad curved surface that is good for needle handling but traumatic for tissues.

5. These are often placed in the intramedullary canal of long bones to repair fractures.

6. Instruments "sterilized" with this method should only be used in minor procedures, and they must be cleaned for at least 3 hours.

7. The contact time for this surgical scrub solution is not as critical as with povidone-iodine.

8. This method of sterilization has replaced ethylene oxide sterilization because it is safer for the environment and personnel.

9. If this happens to a gown or drape, it is no longer sterile.

10. If left on the arthroscope, residues of this chemical sterilization agent can cause chemical synovitis.

11. Repeated contact with this surgical scrub may rarely lead to the development of thyroid dysfunction.

12. These instruments achieve sterilization by producing steam under pressure.

Super Clue: This chemical disinfectant is commonly used to preserve tissues for histopathological assessment.

_____

1. _ _ _ _ _   _ _ _ _ _ _   □_ _ _ _ _ _ _

2. _ _ _ _ _ _   _ _□_ _ _ _ _

3. _ _ _ _ _ _ _   _□_ _ _ _

4. _ _ _ _ _ _ _   _ _ _□_   _ _ _ _ _ _

5. _ _ _ _ _ _□_ _   _ _ _ _

6. _ _ _ _   _ _ _ _ _☐_ _ _ _ _ _ _

7. _ _ _ _ _ _ _ _ _☐_ _ _

8. _ _ _ _ _ _ _   _☐_ _ _ _ _   _ _ _   _ _ _ _ _ _

9. _ _ _ _ _ _ _ _ _ _ _ _☐

10. _ _ _ _ _ _ _ _ _☐_ _

11. _ _ _ _ _ _ _ _ _☐_ _ _

12. _ _ _ _ _ _ _☐

SHORT ANSWER

1. You are asked to order four pairs of new towel clamps and have a choice between two types. Name the type you choose and give one reason for your choice.

   _____

   _____

2. What is the difference between sterilization and disinfection?

   _____

   _____

3. List four types of sterilization indicators used in autoclaves.

   A. _____

   B. _____

   C. _____

   D. _____

4. Name the two methods of gloving for surgery.

   A. _____

   B. _____

5. Why are masks worn during surgery? Be specific.

   _____

CROSSWORD PUZZLE

Across

2. _____ activity is the continued bactericidal activity that persists after an antiseptic or disinfectant has been applied
5. Synthetic material used to replace some tissue or part of the body
9. The stylus or removable plug used during the insertion of a tubular instrument
10. _____ sterilization is an emergency sterilization in which the instrument is placed unwrapped in an autoclave and taken directly to surgery following sterilization
12. A machine that uses pressurized steam to sterilize objects
14. The destruction of all disease-producing organisms and spores on an object
17. Lying down
18. Free from any living microorganisms
19. The destruction of the vegetative forms of bacteria but not the spores

Down

1. Hinged part of a needle holders, tissue forceps or hemostatic forceps (2 words)
3. A substance that destroys or inhibits microorganisms; typically used on inanimate objects
4. A condition of sterility, where no living organisms are present
6. Part of an instrument, usually located near the rings or handles, which allows the instrument to be maintained in one position after it has grasped or retracted the tissue
7. Refers to disinfecting the hands of the personnel who will be involved in a sterile procedure
8. Arising from within the body
11. A substance that prevents infection by inhibiting the growth of infectious agents
13. Arising from outside the body
15. A _____ port on a tubular instrument is used to infuse a solution into a cavity, such as a joint
16. The area covered by sterile drapes and the sterile region of properly attired personnel is the sterile _____

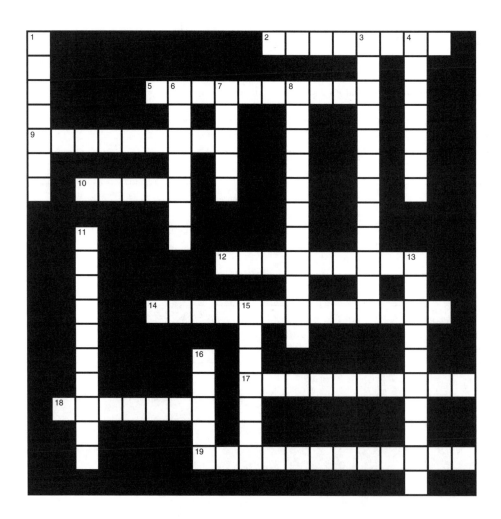

29 Surgical Assistance and Suture Material

LEARNING OBJECTIVES

When you have completed this chapter, you will be able to:
1. Describe the role of the veterinary technician in surgical assistance for large and small animal patients
2. Describe the method of placing and securing surgical drapes on the patient and special requirements for surgical draping for orthopedic or neurologic surgeries
3. Discuss considerations for placement of instruments on the instrument table and considerations for maintaining sterility of the gloved and gowned surgical team
4. Describe proper handling of skin, hollow organs, muscle, and bone tissue during surgery
5. Describe procedures and special considerations for retracting tissues during surgical procedures
6. Describe indications for and complications of sponge hemostasis
7. Differentiate between monopolar and bipolar electrosurgery modes and describe care, use, and safety issues related to electrosurgical units
8. Describe commonly used hemostatic and cauterizing agents
9. List the principles and procedures related to incision irrigation and lavage and surgical drains
10. List and describe commonly used suture material and needles and methods for their preparation

FILL IN THE BLANK

1. The function of draping is to _____.

2. Once a surgical drape has been placed on the patient it can only be adjusted _____ from the sterile surgical site.

3. The preparation of the patient's skin for surgery results in _____ but not

   _____.

4. Instruments used for manipulation of contaminated tissue should be placed _____ other instruments on the stand.

5. Surgical procedures involving the intestines require complete _____ of the

   luminal contents to prevent _____.

6. One must avoid prolonged use of self-retracting instruments to prevent _____ tissue trauma.

7. Hemostatic forceps should be clamped _____ to the bleeding vessel.

8. Electrocoagulation should only be used on vessels smaller than _____ mm.

9. Absorbable suture loses tensile strength within _____ days.

10. Synthetic absorbable suture is broken down by _____.

11. Chromic gut is broken down by _____ reaction and _____.

12. The diameter (size) of suture is classified by this agency: _____.

13. Oversized suture do not strengthen a wound and may lead to _____ and

    _____ of tissue.

14. To better visualize the liver and diaphragm, gently lift the _____.

15. Move the _____ to better visualize the deep structures of the right
    abdominal cavity.

16. Move the adjacent duodenum to better visualize the _____ and the

    _____.

DEFINE

1. Fenestration: _____

   _____

2. Iatrogenic: _____

   _____

3. Aseptic: _____

   _____

4. Sterile: _____

   _____

5. Disinfect: _____

   _____

6. Traumatic: _____

   _____

7. Atraumatic: _____

   _____

8. Hemostasis: _____

   _____

9. Lavage: _____

   _____

10. Dehiscence: _____

    _____

11. Wicking: _____

    _____

1. List five methods to position and secure a patient to the surgical table.

   A. _____

   B. _____

   C. _____

   D. _____

   E. _____

2. What common complications can occur if the patient is inappropriately secured to the surgical table?

   A. _____

   B. _____

3. Why might the surgeon request to have the warm-air circulation turned on only *after* the patient is draped?

   _____

4. Which nerves are of the most concern during fracture repair surgery?

   A. _____ located in the front limb

   B. _____ located in the hind limb

5. What are the advantages to using a scalpel blade to make the surgical incision?

   A. _____

   B. _____

   C. _____

6. Place the following surgeries in the order they should be performed: _____

   A. Pyometra removal

   B. Cruciate repair

   C. Routine spay

7. Intrasurgical assistance includes the following:

   A. _____

   B. _____

   C. _____

8. List two reasons that surgical instruments should be "snapped" into the open palm of the surgeon when they are passed.

A. _____

B. _____

9. List reasons *not* to use scissors when performing the skin incision.

A. _____

B. _____

C. _____

10. List several ways to cover exposed skin in the fenestrated area for orthopedic or neurologic procedures.

A. _____

B. _____

C. _____

D. _____

11. List several safety concerns/precautions when using electrosurgical devices.

A. _____

B. _____

C. _____

D. _____

12. What are the four main purposes served by surgical lavage?

A. _____

B. _____

C. _____

D. _____

13. In what instances might a veterinarian elect to place a surgical drain?

A. _____

B. _____

14. List the three different methods of attaching suture to the needle.

A. _____

B. _____

C. _____

15. Suture needles vary in shape and:

    A. _____

    B. _____

    C. _____

16. Which type of suture needle should be avoided when suturing hollow organs?

    _____

17. Suture material can be sterilized by:

    A. _____

    B. _____

    C. _____

18. List the qualities of an ideal suture.

    A. _____

    B. _____

    C. _____

    D. _____

    E. _____

    F. _____

    G. _____

    H. _____

19. Suture may be classified by four characteristics.

    A. _____

    B. _____

    C. _____

    D. _____

20. List the attributes of monofilament suture.

    A. _____

    B. _____

C. _____

D. _____

E. _____

21. List the attributes of multifilament suture.

A. _____

B. _____

C. _____

D. _____

22. Tissue reaction caused by suture material is undesirable because:

A. _____

B. _____

23. Arrange the following suture in order from least to most tissue reactive:

_____

A. Natural multifilament

B. Gut

C. Synthetic multifilament

D. Metallic

E. Synthetic monofilament

24. Arrange the following suture in size from largest to smallest: _____

A. 0

B. 7-0

C. 2-0

D. 5-0

E. 2

F. 000

25. Which nonabsorbable suture completely loses tensile strength within 6 months due to the inflammatory response it

evokes? _____

26. Why is hemostasis during surgery important?

A. _____

B. _____

C. _____

27. List three techniques that can be employed to augment hemostasis.

A. _____

B. _____

C. _____

PHOTO QUIZ

1. Label the suture diagrams below according to their characteristics: monofilament or multifilament.

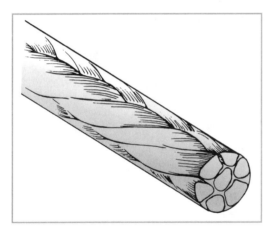

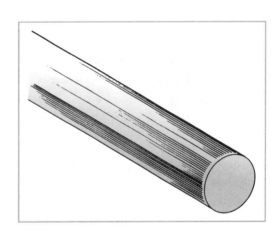

A. _____   B. _____

MATCHING

Match the procedure in column A with the wave type in column B.

Column A

1. _____ Primarily cutting

2. _____ Primarily coagulation

3. _____ Simultaneously cutting and coagulation

Column B

A. Interrupted damped sine

B. Continuous undamped sine

C. Modulated pulsed sine

Match the type of electrosurgical device with its characteristics.

4. _____ Requires a ground plate

5. _____ All blood and fluid must be blotted away before using

6. _____ Coagulating current does not run through the body

7. _____ Useful in microvascular surgery

8. _____ Used only for coagulation

9. _____ Can be used for cutting and coagulation

10. _____ Can be used in a wet surgical field

M. Monopolar

B. Bipolar

Match the hemostatic agent with its mechanism of action.

11. _____ Soak up blood and provide a lattice for forming a clot

12. _____ Only activates clotting of whole blood

13. _____ Triggers clot formation via platelet aggregation and release of coagulation factors

14. _____ Nonabsorbable; forms a mechanical plug

A. Bovine dermal collagen

B. Bone wax

C. Gelatin sponges

D. Cellulose gauze

Match the procedure with the type of lavage tip that should be used.

15. _____ Orthopedic surgery

16. _____ Thoracic surgery

17. _____ Abdominal surgery

18. _____ Removal of small quantities of liquid

19. _____ Reduce incidence of plugging with soft tissue

A. Single tip

B. Multiple-fenestrated tip

Match the drain with its characteristics.

20. _____ Penrose drain

21. _____ Suction must be applied

22. _____ Holes in the tissue around the drain must be kept open and clean

23. _____ Drain can act as an avenue for infection

24. _____ Multiple openings are present in the tube walls

P. Passive drain

A. Active drain

Match the suture type with its quality.

25. _____ Stainless steel

26. _____ Biosyn

27. _____ Dexon

28. _____ PDS

29. _____ Silk

30. _____ Vicryl

31. _____ Prolene

32. _____ Cotton

33. _____ Polyester

N. Nonabsorbable

A. Absorbable

SHORT ANSWER

1. Why is it necessary to leave sutures in 2 to 3 days longer when the incision was made using a laser as opposed to a scalpel?

_____

_____

2. Why is it important to preserve soft tissue attachment when manipulating fractures?

_____

_____

3. Why do most instruments used to hold or manipulate skin have teeth or hooks?

_____

4. Severe complications can occur if gauze sponges are left in the body. Describe several precautions that can prevent this from happening.

   A. _____

   B. _____

   C. _____

   D. _____

5. Describe how chemical cauterizing agents work.

_____

_____

6. Antibiotics are not routinely added to lavage fluids. Why?

_____

_____

7. Why should all lavage fluid be removed from the body?

_____

_____

8. Describe the ideal draping process for an equine surgery.

_____

_____

_____

_____

_____

_____

_____

30 Small Animal Surgical Nursing

LEARNING OBJECTIVES

When you have completed this chapter, you will be able to:

1. Describe the preoperative, intraoperative, and postoperative responsibilities of the veterinary technician in surgical assistance
2. Describe indications and use of prophylactic antibiotics for surgical patients
3. Describe signs of blood loss in the postoperative patient
4. Discuss concerns related to hypothermia in anesthetized patients and describe methods for increasing patient body temperature intraoperatively and postoperatively
5. Describe postoperative abnormalities that can occur in surgical incisions
6. Describe the procedure for removal of skin sutures
7. Discuss general considerations for care of bandages and drains
8. List and describe indications, preoperative, intraoperative, and postoperative considerations for common elective procedures in dogs and cats
9. List and describe indications, preoperative, intraoperative, and postoperative considerations for common nonelective procedures in dogs and cats
10. List considerations related to client education for discharged surgical patients

FILL IN THE BLANK

1. Surgically fusing a joint is called _____.

2. _____ is the time required for blanched mucous membranes to return to normal color.

3. Entrapment of tissues such that the blood supply to the tissue is occluded and the tissue becomes ischemic is referred to as _____.

4. _____ is an accumulation of purulent material within the lumen of the uterus.

5. The breakdown of a surgical incision such that the tissue layers separate from each other is called

   _____.

6. _____ is the involution of one intestinal segment into another.

7. _____ is commonly referred to as false pregnancy.

8. A temporary or permanent loss of intestinal motility due to a functional cause is called

   _____.

9. _____ is an area of thickened cartilage due to an abnormality in cartilage maturation.

10. _____ is the term used to describe a declaw procedure.

11. _____ is caused by the inflammation of the subcutaneous tissue as a result of infection or immune cause.

12. Removal of the uterus and ovaries is called _____.

13. _____ or incision into the stomach.

14. Extrusion of the viscera from the abdominal cavity is called _____.

15. _____ is a permanent opening made in the urethra to allow urine passage.

16. The veterinary technician's role in surgical assistance is an important part of _____ and

    _____ management.

17. Food is withheld before surgery to prevent vomiting and _____.

18. Inadequate animal _____ or inappropriate _____ can hinder surgical technique.

19. Prophylactic _____ are sometimes used to decrease the risk of infection in surgeries.

20. Surgical restraint involves _____ and/or general _____.

21. During a laparotomy, the line of incision is from the _____ to the

    _____.

22. Incision monitoring should be done for _____ after surgery or until the sutures are removed.

23. PCV and TP values can drop up to _____% because of anesthetic and surgery, even if no blood loss occurs.

24. The treatment selected for treating hemorrhage depends on the animal's _____ and

    ability to maintain a _____.

25. The more surface area exposed during surgery, the _____ and

    _____ the body temperature is expected to drop.

26. Soft tissue pain typically lasts _____ to _____ days after surgery.

27. Pain medications should be given according to _____, not on an as needed basis.

28. Sutures are typically removed _____ to _____ days postoperatively.

29. If a bandage is placed too tightly, it can result in _____ compromise and skin

    _____.

30. The _____ sets forth the breed standard for tail docking and dewclaw removal.

31. Tail docking and dewclaw removal in the puppy should occur between days _____

    and _____.

32. Tail docking is performed for _____ reasons.

33. When performing an onychectomy, the tourniquet is placed _____ to the elbow to

    prevent _____ damage.

34. The bandages from an onychectomy should be removed within _____ postoperatively.

35. Early complications of an onychectomy include _____ and postoperative

    _____.

36. Warm _____ is used to flush the abdomen during a celiotomy.

37. If intestinal leakage occurs after a celiotomy, _____ can occur.

38. The digestive tract requires food for cellular _____ and proper

    _____.

39. Gastric dilation volvulus is dilation of the stomach with ingesta and gas with _____
    of the stomach.

40. Gastropexy is performed on the _____ ventrolateral aspect of the body wall near

    the _____.

41. Gastropexy prevents further _____ but does not prevent

    _____.

42. Renal dysfunction after an ovariohysterectomy is usually caused by accidental _____.

DEFINE

1. Ablation: _____

2. Anemia: _____

3. Abdominocentesis: _____

   _____

4. Anastomosis: _____

5. Bacterial translocation: _____

   _____

6. Celiotomy: _____

7. Cushing disease: _____

_____

8. Decubital ulcers: _____

_____

9. Friable: _____

10. Hematoma: _____

11. Hernia: _____

_____

12. Hydrometra: _____

13. Necrosis: _____

14. Nymphomania: _____

_____

15. Ostectomy: _____

16. Pneumothorax: _____

17. Seroma: _____

18. Thoracocentesis: _____

19. Trocarization: _____

MATCHING

Match the procedure in column A with its description in column B.

Column A	Column B
1. _____ Celiotomy	A. A devitalized section of intestine is removed
2. _____ Onychectomy	B. Tack the stomach to the wall of the abdominal cavity
3. _____ Splenectomy	C. Incision into the intestines
4. _____ Urethrostomy	D. Removal of a mass or lump
5. _____ Gastropexy	E. Claw removal
6. _____ Enterotomy	F. Incision into the abdominal cavity
7. _____ Lumpectomy	G. Incision into the stomach
8. _____ Gastrotomy	H. Creating a new opening in the urethra
9. _____ Anastomosis	I. Removal of the spleen
10. _____ Orchidectomy	J. Removal of ovaries and uterus
11. _____ Ovariohysterectomy	K. Castration

1. Preoperative assessment for a surgical candidate includes:

   A. _____

   B. _____

   C. _____

   D. _____

2. Proficiency in surgical assistance will:

   A. _____

   B. _____

   C. _____

3. List the indications for prophylactic antibiotics.

   A. _____

   B. _____

   C. _____

   D. _____

   E. _____

   F. _____

   G. _____

4. General surgery can result in several physiologic problems including:

   A. _____

   B. _____

   C. _____

   D. _____

   E. _____

5. List two elements that will cause abdominal structures to dry out during surgery.

   A. _____

   B. _____

6. Name the three layers of closure for an abdominal surgery.

   A. _____

   B. _____

   C. _____

7. During the first 24 hours after surgery the skin incision should be examined for:

   A. _____

   B. _____

   C. _____

   D. _____

   E. _____

8. Manipulation of the intestines and pancreas can lead to:

   A. _____

   B. _____

   C. _____

9. Animals with substantial blood loss may experience:

   A. _____

   B. _____

   C. _____

   D. _____

10. If intraabdominal hemorrhage occurs, you would expect to see:

    A. _____

    B. _____

    C. _____

11. If hemorrhage is suspected, treatment strategies include:

    A. _____

    B. _____

    C. _____

    D. _____

E. _____

F. _____

12. List several ways to maintain an animal's body temperature during surgery.

   A. _____

   B. _____

   C. _____

   D. _____

   E. _____

13. Why are heat lamps and electric heating pads contraindicated during or after surgery?

   _____

14. At what point can heating sources be discontinued in the recovering patient?

   _____

15. What are the intraoperative signs of pain?

   A. _____

   B. _____

   C. _____

   D. _____

16. List the postoperative signs of pain.

   A. _____

   B. _____

   C. _____

   D. _____

   E. _____

   F. _____

   G. _____

   H. _____

   I. _____

   J. _____

17. Painful surgical procedures include:

A. _____

B. _____

C. _____

D. _____

E. _____

18. The characteristics of intestinal devitalization include:

A. _____

B. _____

C. _____

D. _____

E. _____

19. Ointments and creams should not be put directly on incisions because:

A. _____

B. _____

20. List eight contributing factors to incision irritation.

A. _____

B. _____

C. _____

D. _____

E. _____

F. _____

G. _____

H. _____

21. Seroma formation can occur under the following conditions:

A. _____

B. _____

C. _____

22. Wound dehiscence can be caused by:

A. _____

B. _____

C. _____

D. _____

E. _____

F. _____

G. _____

23. A bandage must be changed if it:

A. _____

B. _____

C. _____

D. _____

24. Noxious tasting agents used to prevent licking should not be placed directly on the incision because they can:

A. _____

B. _____

C. _____

25. Why are dewclaws removed from some breeds of dogs?

A. _____

B. _____

26. What are some indications for tail removal in adult dogs?

A. _____

B. _____

C. _____

D. _____

27. List three common techniques used to perform an onychectomy.

A. _____

B. _____

C. _____

Chapter **30** **Small Animal Surgical Nursing**

28. What are the classic signs of GDV?

A. _____

B. _____

C. _____

29. What are the major indications for a feline castration?

A. _____

B. _____

C. _____

D. _____

30. In addition to preventing unwanted breeding, a canine orchidectomy can be indicated for the following medical disorders:

A. _____

B. _____

C. _____

D. _____

E. _____

CRITICAL THINKING

1. Antibiotics should be used judiciously for animals undergoing surgery. Discuss why.

_____

_____

_____

2. Why is it important to track trends in physiologic parameters preoperatively, intraoperatively, and postoperatively?

_____

_____

_____

3. Why does an animal's temperature drop once it has been anesthetized?

_____

_____

_____

4. Describe the differences between elective and nonelective surgery.

_____

_____

_____

_____

5. Why is it so important to treat pain before it occurs?

_____

_____

_____

6. Why are catheters placed in the front legs or jugular vein of animals suffering from GDV?

_____

_____

_____

CROSSWORD PUZZLE

Across

1. Any large internal organ in any of the body cavities
5. A blood clot
8. Accumulation of purulent material within the lumen of the uterus
10. Dystocia refers to difficulty giving _____
11. Bacterial _____ is movement of bacteria from a normal location to an undesirable location
14. Onychectomy refers to removal of a _____
16. Abnormal protrusion of an organ or other body structure through a defect or natural opening in a covering, muscle, or bone
20. Orchidectomy refers to removal of the _____
22. _____ ulcers are pressure sores that result from an animal lying on a bone prominence for too long
24. Lacking sensation
25. The breakdown of a surgical incision such that the tissue layers separate from each other
26. Incision into a small intestinal lumen
27. Suturing two tubular organs together (i.e., intestinal loops) so that substances inside the lumen of the sutured organs can freely move from one to the other
28. Too much growth

Down

2. A temporary or permanent loss of intestinal motility due to a functional cause
3. Incision into the urinary bladder
4. The common term for an ovariohysterectomy
6. Low red blood cell count
7. _____ disease is also known as hyperadrenocorticism
9. Celiotomy is an incision into the _____ cavity
12. A measure of cell counts in the blood
13. Crystals in a urine sample
15. Surgically fusing a joint
17. Tissue death
18. False pregnancy
19. Incision into the stomach
21. Ostectomy refers to the removal of a portion of _____
23. A product of protein metabolism that is normally filtered by the kidneys for excretion

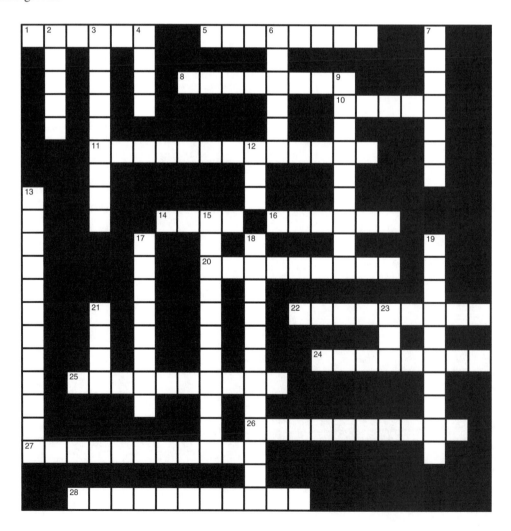

Chapter **30** **Small Animal Surgical Nursing**

Copyright © 2010 by Saunders, an imprint of Elsevier Inc.

31 Large Animal Surgical Nursing

When you have completed this chapter, you will be able to:

1. Describe the preoperative procedures needed for equine patients
2. Discuss the responsibilities of the veterinary technician during equine surgery
3. Describe postoperative monitoring, medication administration, bandage care, and grooming for equine patients
4. List commonly performed surgical procedures in equine patients
5. Describe indications, preoperative, intraoperative, and postoperative considerations for common surgical procedures in equine patients
6. List and describe common emergency situations and procedures in equine patients
7. List commonly performed surgical procedures in bovine patients
8. Describe indications, preoperative, intraoperative, and postoperative considerations for common surgical procedures in bovine patients
9. List commonly performed surgical procedures in small ruminants
10. Describe indications, preoperative, intraoperative, and postoperative considerations for common surgical procedures in small ruminants

MATCHING 1

Match the term with the correct definition.

1. _____ Fixation of the pylorus
2. _____ Muscle damage
3. _____ Removal of a retained testicle
4. _____ Fixation of the abomasum
5. _____ Fixation of the omentum
6. _____ Permanent rumen fistula
7. _____ Incision into the rumen
8. _____ Surgical incision into the abdomen
9. _____ Incision in the vaginal wall

A. Rumenotomy
B. Pyloropexy
C. Laparotomy
D. Rhabdomyolysis
E. Colpotomy
F. Abomasopexy
G. Rumenotomy
H. Omentopexy
I. Cryptorchidectomy

MATCHING 2

Match the terms with the correct statement(s).

1. _____ Newborn foals commonly affected
2. _____ Commonly occurs after breeding
3. _____ Congenital hernia
4. _____ Occurs subsequent to trauma
5. _____ Relatively common in foals
6. _____ Stallions commonly affected
7. _____ Occurs postsurgically
8. _____ May spontaneously close

A. Inguinal hernia
B. Umbilical hernia
C. Acquired body wall hernia

MATCHING 3

Match the condition with the correct statement.

1. _____ A result of overflexion of certain joints
2. _____ Inflammation of the laminas
3. _____ Nondescent of a testicle
4. _____ Bacterial infection of the guttural pouch
5. _____ A horse with a testicle outside the abdominal cavity but not in the scrotum
6. _____ Fungal plaque in the guttural pouch
7. _____ Paralysis of the left arytenoid cartilage, which prevents abduction during inspiration
8. _____ Develop in the appendicular skeleton in a medial to lateral direction
9. _____ Accumulation of air in the guttural pouches
10. _____ Urine drips from the umbilicus
11. _____ Hardware disease
12. _____ Thickening of the interdigital skin

A. Patent urachus
B. High flanker
C. Interdigital hyperplasia
D. Cryptorchidism
E. Flexural limb deformities
F. Angular limb deformities
G. Guttural pouch tympany
H. Traumatic reticuloperitonitis
I. Left laryngeal hemiplegia
J. Laminitis
K. Guttural pouch empyema
L. Guttural pouch mycosis

FILL IN THE BLANK

1. The most common approach to the abdominal cavity in the equine patient is through a

   _____ incision.

2. Abdominal wall hernias can be labeled as _____, _____,

   or _____.

3. Urinary calculi may develop in the _____ or the _____.

4. The most commonly used agents for epidural anesthesia in the horse are _____,

   _____, or _____.

5. Following the placement of a cast on an equine patient, the cast should be monitored for

   _____, _____, and _____.

6. Activated dialdehyde solution is used to disinfect _____ instruments and cameras for a

   minimum of _____ minutes.

7. The mean arterial blood pressure of the anesthetized horse should be above _____

   mm Hg to prevent _____ and _____.

8. The majority of abdominal procedures in the food animal patient are performed via a

   _____ laparotomy.

9. The toxic dose of lidocaine is _____.

10. A rumenotomy is performed via a _____ flank incision.

11. Abomasal displacement is a common problem in high-producing dairy cows fed _____,

    _____ diets.

12. An LDA, RDA, or AV can be easily diagnosed by the auscultation of distinct "ping" in the paralumbar fossa area

    since there is _____ trapped in the organ.

13. Cattle bear most of their weight on the front _____ and hind

    _____ claws.

14. The _____ feet are more commonly affected with interdigital hyperplasia.

15. After claw amputation, the bandages should be changed every _____ days and the

    entire healing process takes about _____ weeks.

16. The two blocks that can be used for ocular surgery are _____ and

    _____.

17. Male small ruminants are at risk to develop obstructive _____ because of the feeding
    of excessive grain in the diet.

18. Optimal time for disbudding/dehorning kids is _____ days in buck kids and

    _____ days in doe kids.

SHORT ANSWER

1. What is the main purpose of grooming an equine patient before surgery?

    _____

    _____

2. Describe the area to be clipped on the equine patient who will have colic surgery under general anesthesia.

    _____

    _____

3. What is the most commonly performed perineal surgery?

    _____

4. List the clinical signs of urinary calculi.

    A. _____

    B. _____

    C. _____

5. In an equine patient with a half-limb cast, where are the most common locations for sores to develop?

   A. _____

   B. _____

   C. _____

6. List the three joints that are affected in flexural limb deformities.

   A. _____

   B. _____

   C. _____

7. When a horse develops severe lameness in one foot only, what is the possible cause of the lameness?

   _____

8. What are the two most commonly used antibiotics in the food animal patient?

   A. _____

   B. _____

9. Describe patient positioning for the large animal patient that will be placed in lateral recumbency.

   A. _____

   B. _____

   C. _____

10. What are the clinical signs of a mandibular fracture in the food animal patient?

   A. _____

   B. _____

   C. _____

   D. _____

11. Describe the technique to perform a line block for flank anesthesia in the food animal patient.

   _____

   _____

12. Describe the landmarks used in the bovine patient when performing an inverted L block.

   A. _____

   B. _____

13. What are the two techniques used to perform paravertebral analgesia?

    A. _____

    B. _____

14. What nerves are blocked when performing paravertebral anesthesia?

    A. _____

    B. _____

    C. _____

15. What transverse processes are used as landmarks when performing distal paravertebral anesthesia?

    A. _____

    B. _____

    C. _____

16. What transverse processes are used as landmarks when performing proximal paravertebral anesthesia?

    A. _____

    B. _____

    C. _____

17. What observable signs confirm for the veterinary technician that the paravertebral anesthesia is effective?

    A. _____

    B. _____

    C. _____

18. Describe the process when performing regional analgesia of the foot/distal limb for the bovine.

    _____

    _____

    _____

19. When placing a tourniquet for regional analgesia of the foot/distal limb for the bovine patient, what is the maximum time the tourniquet be left on?

    _____

20. During dystocia or forced fetal extraction, what nerves can be damaged resulting in calving paralysis?

    A. _____

    B. _____

21. A caudal epidural provides a loss of sensation to what areas?

_____

22. Describe how to locate the sacrococcygeal space.

_____

_____

23. What is the most common approach to perform a cesarean section in the standing bovine patient?

_____

24. Describe the placement of obstetrical chains in the limbs of the calf.

_____

25. What three cattle breeds seem most prone to the occurrence of prolapsed vaginas?

A. _____

B. _____

C. _____

26. What agent is administered that stimulates uterine involution?

_____

27. What cattle breed seems to be predisposed to ocular squamous cell carcinoma?

_____

28. What block is performed in adult cattle before dehorning?

_____

TRUE OR FALSE

Choose T (true) or F (false) for each statement below.

1. _____ Adult horses are held off feed for approximately 24 hours before surgery.
2. _____ Adult cattle should be held off feed for 36 to 48 hours and water should be removed 12 hours before surgery where the patient will be placed in lateral or dorsal recumbency.
3. _____ Padding is not important for the large animal patient undergoing general anesthesia since most of them take less than 1 hour.
4. _____ Abomasal displacements are most likely to occur in the 8 weeks after calving.
5. _____ RDA is an emergency in the bovine patient because it often includes abomasal volvulus.
6. _____ Radial nerve paralysis is most commonly seen following a period of dorsal recumbency.
7. _____ Vaginal prolapse occurs in the last 2 months of gestation in cows with multiple fetuses.
8. _____ Congenital entropion is considered to be inherited and therefore the affected animals should not be bred.

Across

4. An incision through the abdominal wall
6. A lateral deviation of the spinal column
7. Surgical fixation of the abomasum to the body wall
9. Osteochondrosis is a disease of joints, which results in unhealthy or incomplete maturation of _____ resulting in joint effusion and sometimes lameness
10. A permanent rumen fistula
11. Rhabdomyolysis results in the breakdown of striated muscle, which leads to excretion of _____ in the urine

Down

1. Colpotomy: An incision through the wall of the _____
2. Surgical fixation of the pylorus to the body wall
3. A nervous or musculoskeletal problem that prevents any movement of the affected body part
5. The inhibition of bacterial multiplication
8. Incomplete paralysis (i.e., some function is still possible).

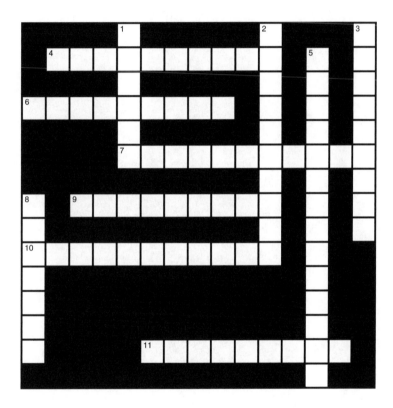

32 Dentistry and Oral Surgery

LEARNING OBJECTIVES

When you have completed this chapter, you will be able to:

1. Describe legal issues related to performance of dental services by veterinary technicians and list professional organizations related to veterinary dentistry
2. Identify terminology used in veterinary dentistry to designate location and direction and describe the modified triadan system for numbering of teeth
3. Describe normal occlusion in dogs and cats and common malocclusions and treatment methods used in orthodontics in small animals
4. Discuss aspects of the complete medical history as they relate to veterinary dentistry
5. List and describe procedures used in extraoral and intraoral examinations in small and large animals
6. Describe equipment and supplies used for dental radiography
7. Differentiate between paralleling, bisecting angle, and occlusal techniques in dental radiography
8. Differentiate between stomatitis, gingivitis, and periodontitis and explain grading of periodontal disease
9. Describe equipment and procedures for periodontal débridement using power and hand scalers
10. Explain methods for sharpening of dental instruments
11. Discuss the rationale and procedures used in polishing teeth
12. Discuss topics and methods for client education related to veterinary dentistry
13. Discuss indications for restorative dentistry and endodontics and describe common procedures performed on small animals
14. Discuss indications, procedures, and potential complications of exodontics
15. List and describe common equine dental problems and treatments

FILL IN THE BLANK

1. All teeth of humans, carnivores, and pigs are _____ teeth that have a relatively small, distinct crown compared to the size of their well-developed roots. The apices (singular: apex) of the roots are open for only a limited time during eruption and development of the teeth, and therefore the teeth do not continually grow or erupt.

2. _____ (Brachyodont or Hypsodont) teeth can erupt continually throughout the life of horses and lagomorphs.

3. Name the two types of hypsodont teeth. _____ and _____

4. _____ (Rostral or Distal) is a term that, when referring to cranial anatomy, refers to a structure that is closer to the front of the head in comparison to another structure.

5. _____ (Caudal or Cranial) is a term used to describe a structure that is toward the back of the head when compared to another structure.

6. _____ (Vestibular or Facial) is a term that describes the tooth surface facing the lips or vestibule (acceptable alternatives are buccal and labial).

7. _____ (Vestibular or Facial) is a term that describes the vestibular surface of teeth visible from the front (incisors).

8. _____ (Lingual or Palatal) refers to the surface of the mandibular teeth adjacent to the tongue.

9. _____ (Lingual or Palatal) refers to the surface of maxillary teeth adjacent to the palate.

10. _____ (Mesial or Distal) refers to the portion of the tooth in line with the dental arcade, which is closest to the most rostral portion of the midline of the dental arch.

11. _____ (Mesial or Distal) refers to the portion of the tooth that is closest to the most caudal portion of the midline of the dental arch.

12. _____ (Occlusion or Diastema) refers to the spatial relationship of teeth within the mouth.

13. Nine percent of dogs have another lymph node that is palpable in the subcutaneous tissue dorsal to the

    maxillary third premolar tooth. This node is referred to as the facial or _____ (buccal, distal, lingual, rostral, palatal) lymph node, and is often bilateral when present.

14. _____ (Buccal or Distal) mucosa refers to the mucosa that begins at the mucocutane-

    ous junction and lines the cheeks and lips. _____ (Cementum or Alveolar) mucosa refers to the mucosa that lies against the bone of the upper or lower jaw, which meets with the gingiva at the mucogingival junction.

15. The _____ (periodontium or mucosa) describes the attachment structures of the teeth and includes gingival connective tissue alveolar bone, periodontal ligament, and cementum.

16. The most common lubricant for a root canal treatment is _____ (saline or sodium hypochlorite).

17. The two types of bone loss are _____ and _____ (alveolar, palatal, buccal, horizontal, vertical).

18. A _____ (rostral or distal) crossbite (referred to as anterior crossbite in humans) occurs when closed-mouth examination reveals one or more maxillary incisors are positioned lingual to the mandibular incisors.

19. A _____ (cranial or caudal), (called posterior crossbite in humans) crossbite occurs when one or more maxillary premolar or molar teeth are positioned lingual to the opposing mandibular premolar or molar.

20. The most common oral tumor in cats is _____ (osteosarcoma or squamous cell carcinoma).

21. Maxillary canine teeth erupt _____ (mesial or buccal) to the persistent deciduous teeth.

22. _____ (Stone or Alginate) is the material used for full mouth impressions.

23. Diffuse inflammation of the entire oral cavity is seen commonly in cats and occasionally in dogs. When inflammation

    is confined to the gingiva, it is referred to as _____ (gingivitis or stomatitis). When the

    inflammation extends beyond the mucogingival junction, it is called _____ (gingivitis or stomatitis).

24. Horses have _____ (24 or 28) deciduous teeth and 36 to 44 permanent teeth, depending on the presence or absence of canine and first premolar teeth.

25. The upper jaw in a horse is wider than the lower jaw, a term referred to as _____ (anisognathism or prognathism).

26. Infundibular decay in horses is most likely to affect the _____ (maxillary or mandibular) first molar tooth.

27. _____ (Primary or Tertiary) dentin may be seen on the occlusal surface of worn teeth as a brown dot.

28. When implementing the modified triadan system to number each tooth; label each tooth listed below.

    A. Upper left second incisor _____

    B. Lower right third premolar _____

    C. Upper left second molar _____

    D. Upper right canine _____

    E. Lower right third molar _____

    F. Lower left first premolar _____

    G. Upper right fourth premolar _____

    H. Lower left first molar _____

    I. Upper left first molar _____

    J. Lower right second premolar _____

29. _____ scalers are the instruments used to scale the crowns of the teeth. The flat face may be either straight or curved lengthwise; the straight lateral surfaces are flat and converge to form a pointed back and tip. When envisioning the cross section of a _____, the instrument is characteristically triangular in shape with _____ internal angles between the face and lateral surfaces.

30. _____ should make up the bulk of the filling agent. It is a _____ rubberlike material that can be vertically and laterally condensed to adapt to the shape of the root canal.

31. The opposite of parrot mouth is referred to as _____, which occurs when the maxilla is relatively shorter than the mandible (as a result of maxillary brachygnathism or mandibular prognathism).

TRUE OR FALSE

Choose T (true) or F (false) for each statement below.

1. _____ Most mammals are diphyodont, meaning that they have one set of teeth.

2. _____ An underjet bite can be a normal occlusion in some dog breeds.

3. _____ Every dental procedure should begin with a comprehensive oral examination to evaluate extraoral structures of the face, head and neck, and intraoral structures, including the soft tissues of the oral cavity, the teeth, and their supporting structures.

Chapter **32** **Dentistry and Oral Surgery**

4. _____ The mandibular gland is easily distinguished from the mandibular lymph nodes because it is softer, larger than, and caudomedial to the mandibular lymph nodes.

5. _____ Two prominent bony structures, which are the hamular processes of the bilateral pterygoid bones, can be palpated just lateral to the midline of the soft palate. If one or both hamular processes are difficult to palpate, this may be due to the presence of a nasopharyngeal mass.

6. _____ The normal sulcus depth is 0 to 3 mm in dogs and 0 to 1 mm in cats. Probing depths greater than normal are documented on the chart as periodontal pockets.

7. _____ Recession is measured in millimeters from the CEJ to the level of the gingival margin.

8. _____ Although we often refer to the mandibular lymph "node," in reality, the area contains anywhere from 1 to 50 nodes. Other nodes that drain the head (retropharyngeal, parotid) are not normally palpable.

9. _____ The major salivary glands of the dog and cat are the paired mandibular, sublingual, zygomatic, and parotid glands.

10. _____ Gingival hyperplasia occurs when the free gingival margin migrates coronally, toward the crown of the tooth. Hyperplasia is measured in millimeters from the bottom of the sulcus to the gingival margin, which is covering a portion of the tooth crown.

11. _____ A bifurcation is the furcation between two-rooted teeth and should be assessed from the buccal and lingual/palatal surfaces.

12. _____ Dental caries (commonly referred to by the lay term of "cavities") result from demineralization of the enamel and dentin because of acids produced by certain oral bacteria. These lesions occur most commonly on occlusal (flat) surfaces of the molar teeth.

13. _____ The radiodensity of the components of the teeth and supporting structures varies widely; therefore, the terms radiopaque and radiolucent are used to describe the relative radiographic appearance of oral/dental structures.

14. _____ The periodontium is composed of four supporting structures of the tooth: (1) periodontal ligament; (2) gingival connective tissue; (3) alveolar bone forming the tooth socket; and (4) cementum covering the surface of the root.

15. _____ Plaque is composed of food particles, glycoprotein, bacteria, and saliva.

16. _____ Endotoxins are believed to be attached to the tooth surface, loosely embedded in cementum, and unattached in the sulcular space. The goal of periodontal débridement is to prevent or arrest the infection and restore the oral soft tissues to health.

17. _____ One difference between ultrasonic and sonic scalars is the frequency at which they are run.

18. _____ The transducer in a magnetostrictive ultrasonic scaler is either a metal stack or a ferrite rod. The transducer in a piezoelectric ultrasonic scaler is a quartz crystal or ceramic disk.

19. _____ The difference between the Gracey curette and the Universal is the angle of the cutting edge surfaces.

20. _____ When using an area-specific curette, the proper cutting edge is the lower edge, as determined by holding the terminal shank perpendicular to the floor. The terminal shank of an area specific curette is kept parallel to the long axis of the tooth during a vertical scaling stroke. The handle of the universal scaler is kept parallel to the long axis of the tooth during a vertical scaling stroke.

21. _____ Sharpening stones typically used for dental instruments include Arkansas, India, ceramic, and a synthetic composition, each differing in coarseness.

22. _____ To minimize risks of thermal damage, use adequate paste, refilling the cup for each tooth, especially when polishing large dog teeth. To further minimize adverse effects, use the handpiece on a low rpm (revolutions per minute) level, just enough to maintain torque and steady rotation.

23. _____ Grade I periodontal disease refers to inflammatory changes confined to the gingiva (gingivitis), which is an easily reversible sign suggesting the need for a routine dental cleaning. Grade II periodontal disease is an early form of periodontitis where evidence of attachment loss is present, and root débridement or subgingival curettage may be required. Grade III periodontal disease is considered moderate periodontitis where 25% to 50% of the attachment structures of the tooth have been lost; root débridement, gingival curettage, and periodontal surgery are often required. Grade III teeth have a fair to guarded prognosis. Grade IV periodontal disease is considered severe periodontitis. With attachment loss of 50% or greater, these teeth often require extraction.

24. _____ Metal crowns are more commonly placed than tooth-colored crowns because of their greater strength and requirements for less tooth removal than crowns with a porcelain exterior fused to metal.

25. _____ The tooth pulp consists of nerves, blood vessels, lymphatics, and connective tissue.

26. _____ H-files are used in a push-pull motion and are more susceptible to file breakage than K-files. K-files are inserted to the apical extent of the canal, turned one-quarter turn, and removed, allowing for shaping of the apical portion of the canal.

27. _____ Obturation refers to filling the canal.

28. _____ Composite fillings cannot be placed next to eugenol because eugenol interferes with the hardening of the composite. Glass ionomers are a commonly used intermediate filling material. A light-cured composite filling material is often used as the final restorative at the surface of the access site and fracture site.

29. _____ The local anesthetic of choice in oral surgery is 0.5% bupivacaine because of its ability to provide not only intraoperative but also postoperative pain relief of 1 to 3 hours duration.

30. _____ A simple extraction is defined as when a tooth falls out on its own and a surgical extraction entails using an elevator to break down the periodontal ligament.

31. _____ A flap with no releasing incisions is called an envelope flap. A flap with one releasing incision is a triangle flap, and a flap with two releasing incisions is called a pedicle flap.

32. _____ The AVDC condones veterinary technicians and noncertified personnel performing simple extractions.

33. _____ The etiology of feline tooth resorption is still unknown, but recent research suggests that vitamin D levels in commercial cat food may play a role.

34. _____ A Class I malocclusion occurs when one side of the jaw is longer then the other.

35. _____ In a class II malocclusion, the mandible is relatively shorter than the maxilla, which can be a result of an abnormally long maxilla (maxillary prognathism) or an abnormally short mandible (mandibular brachygnathism).

36. _____ Interceptive orthodontics involves the extraction of persistent deciduous or adult teeth that are causing or will cause problems associated with malocclusion. The most important factor determining success with this treatment is early detection of the problem.

37. _____ All teeth with exposed pulp tissue should be treated either by endodontic treatment (conventional root canal, vital pulp therapy) or by extraction.

38. _____ Ninety-two percent of discolored teeth show evidence of partial or complete pulp necrosis on exploratory pulpotomy.

39. _____ The most common malignant tumors in dogs are malignant melanoma, squamous cell carcinoma, fibrosarcoma, and osteosarcoma.

40. _____ Masticatory muscle myositis is an immune-mediated disease where the immune system forms antibodies toward a specific component of myosin found only in muscles of mastication.

41. _____ The tape muzzle is created using one piece of tape (adhesive side outward) around the muzzle itself, which is attached to a second piece that wraps around the head below the ears. The muzzle should be tight enough to minimize motion, but loose enough to prevent irritation of the soft tissue and to allow the tongue to move between the incisor teeth to allow for drinking and eating food of a slurry consistency.

42. _____ At eruption, the occlusal surface of equine teeth are not fully covered by cementum, compared with dogs and cats which have cementum covering only the root.

43. _____ The terms brachygnathic and prognathic should always be used with a preceding descriptive adjective to identify the upper or lower jaw.

44. _____ In horses the left and right mandibles are separated by a symphysis as in dogs and cats.

45. _____ Common presenting problems of horses with severe dental disease include weight loss, dropping of food (quidding), head shaking, and tilting of the head during mastication.

46. _____ Maxillary brachygnathism (or mandibular prognathism) is a developmental disorder where the lower jaw is relatively shorter than the upper jaw.

47. _____ Digital technology reduces radiation exposure by 50% to 90% when compared with the use of D- and E-speed film.

DENTAL INSTRUMENTS

1. You are setting up for a root canal for the next patient. Please place an X by the instrument or materials needed for this procedure.

Barbed broaches _____	H-files _____
Root tip picks _____	Elevators _____
K-files _____	Root canal cement _____
Burrs _____	Consil _____
Gutta percha _____	Glass ionomer _____
Doxirobe _____	Paper points _____
Sodium hypochlorite _____	Composite _____
Alginate _____	Orthodontic wire _____
Needle holders _____	Scissors _____
Light curing gun _____	.05% bupivacaine _____
Periosteal elevator _____	Rongeurs _____
Addison-Brown forceps _____	Suture _____
Plugger and spreader _____	Extraction forceps _____
Pathfinder files _____	Gates Glidden rotary files _____
Alveolar bone curette _____	Lateral condenser files _____
Bead sterilizer _____	Dental x-ray unit _____
Scalpel blade _____	Dental luxator _____
Gauze sponges _____	Endodontic irrigation needles _____

2. You are setting up for a surgical extraction for the next patient. Please place an X by the instrument or materials needed for this procedure.

Barbed broaches _____	H-files _____
Root tip picks _____	Elevators _____
K-files _____	Root canal cement _____
Burrs _____	Consil _____
Gutta percha _____	Glass ionomer _____
Doxirobe _____	Paper points _____
Sodium hypochlorite _____	Composite _____
Alginate _____	Orthodontic wire _____
Needle holders _____	Scissors _____
Light curing gun _____	.05% bupivacaine _____
Periosteal elevator _____	Rongeurs _____
Addison-Brown forceps _____	Suture _____
Plugger and spreader _____	Extraction forceps _____
Pathfinder files _____	Gates Glidden rotary files _____
Alveolar bone curette _____	Lateral condenser files _____
Bead sterilizer _____	Dental x-ray unit _____
Scalpel blade _____	Dental luxator _____
Gauze sponges _____	Endodontic irrigation needles _____

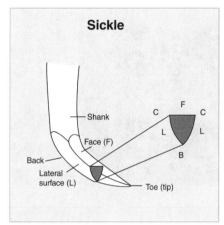

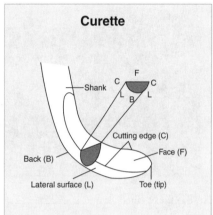

1. Describe where you would normally use each instrument.

   A. Sickle scaler _____

   B. Curette _____

   Where should you not use each instrument to prevent damage to the patient or instrument?

   C. Sickle scaler _____

   D. Curette _____

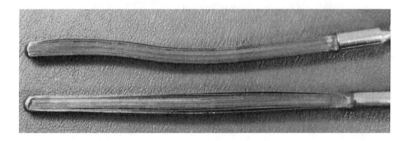

2. A. Identify these instruments. _____

   _____

   B. What do you note about the condition of these instruments?

   _____

   _____

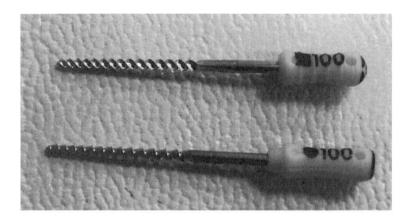

3. A. Describe these files. _____

   B. What procedure would they be used in? _____

   _____

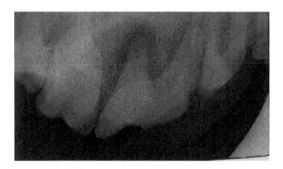

4. A. Describe this lesion. _____

   _____

   _____

   B. Using the modified triadan system, what tooth number is being described?

   _____

   C. What procedures might be recommended for this patient?

   _____

   _____

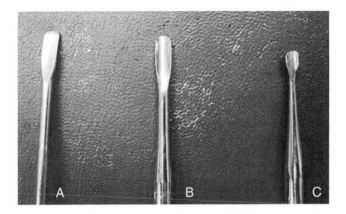

5. Identify these instruments.

A. _____

B. _____

C. _____

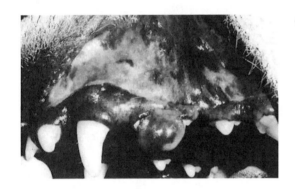

6. A. Describe this lesion. _____

B. What might be the recommendations for this patient?

_____

_____

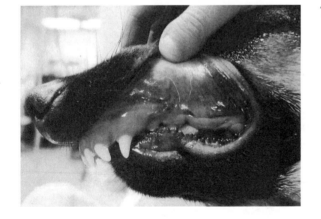

7. A. Describe this bite. _____

B. How would you classify this malocclusion?

_____

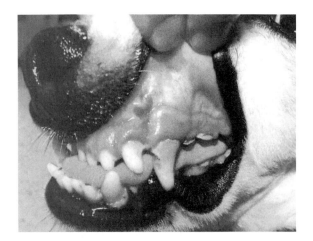

8. A. Describe this bite. _____

   B. How would you classify this malocclusion?

   _____

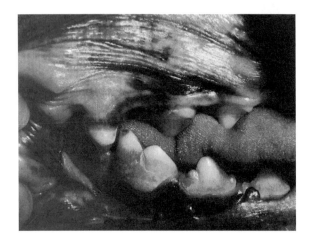

9. A. The lower right first molar or 409 is located anatomically incorrect. How would you describe this abnormality?

   _____

   B. In what breed(s) is this commonly seen?

   _____

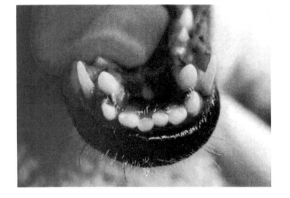

10. A. Describe the oral abnormality.

   _____

   B. What problems might occur if the abnormality is not resolved quickly?

   _____

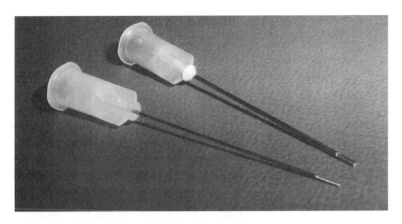

11. A. Name this instrument?

_____

B. In what procedure(s) is it used?

_____

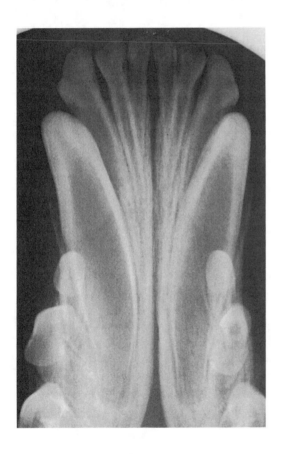

12. A. Is this a dog under 1 year of age or more than 5 years?

_____

B. How can you tell?

_____

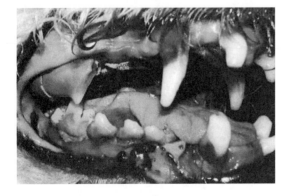

13. What stage of oral disease (1-4) is likely occurring in this dog?

_____

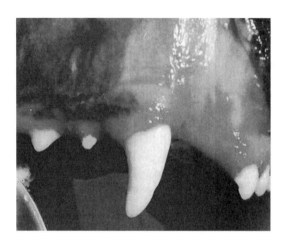

14. A. How would you describe the inflammation along the gum line?

_____

B. What stage of oral disease is likely occurring?

_____

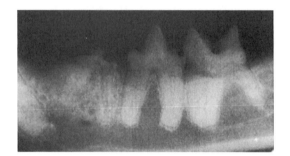

15. A. How would you describe this lesion?

_____

B. Is this a dog or cat?

_____

16. How would you describe this lesion or abnormality?

_____

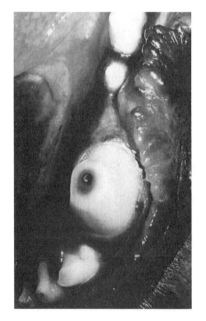

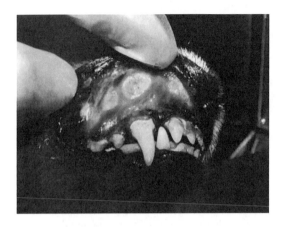

17. Identify this lesion.

_____

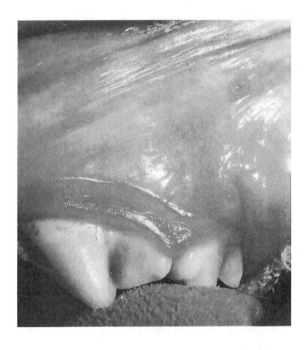

18. Identify this line or junction.

_____

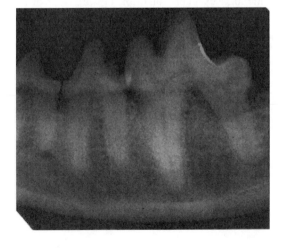

19. Identify this longitudinal space or canal on this radiograph of the mandible.

_____

CROSSWORD PUZZLE

Across

1. Pemphigus _____ is a vesicular autoimmune disease of the skin and oral mucosa, which also causes pyrexia, depression, and anorexia
3. Extraction of teeth, either via closed or surgical techniques
7. A pathologic condition where the normal sulcus depth increases because of a loss of attachment of junctional epithelium and periodontal ligament
8. A positional term in dentistry referring to the surface of mandibular teeth adjacent to the tongue
12. Hard tissue that covers the root of brachyodont teeth
13. Tooth type with a long reserve crown and roots that allow for continued growth and/or continued eruption
16. Tooth decay due to bacterial acid production and demineralization of tooth substance
17. Prognathism is a condition where the jaw is _____ than normal
18. A positional term in dentistry that describes the surface of maxillary teeth adjacent to the palate
19. Hard tissue of high mineral content that covers the crown of a tooth
22. A term referring to the primary or baby teeth
23. An accumulation of food particles, saliva, minerals, and bacteria, which appears as a white/tan, easily removable film on the teeth
25. A place where bacteria or other organisms can lodge and replicate
27. The flat surface of a hand scaler that lies between both cutting edges
30. A positional term referring to below the gum line (i.e., toward the root)
32. Tooth wear associated with tooth-to-tooth contact
33. A term used to describe a mass that is movable and compressible, such as an abscess
36. The area where the upper and lower lips meet
37. Plaque which has become calcified and is firmly adhered to the teeth
38. Root _____ is a technique of hand scaling to remove superficial layers of cementum for root débridement

Down

2. Periapical _____ is a term in dental radiography referring to decreased radiodensity at the tip of a tooth root, which is suggestive of tooth root pathology
4. A positional term referring to the part of a tooth that meets with, or occludes with, the teeth of the opposite dental arcade
5. Malocclusion where no jaw length discrepancy exists but one or more teeth are in an abnormal position
6. The nasolacrimal duct travels from the medial _____ of the eye to the rostral nasal passage; responsible for drainage of tears
9. Hard tissue that makes up the bulk of a mature tooth
10. The large bilateral muscle of mastication on the top of the head that functions to close the mouth
11. The lamina _____ is the cortical plate of alveolar bone surrounding the tooth
14. The distance the tip of a power scaler is moving back and forth in one cycle as adjusted by the power knob
15. The portion of the tooth above the gingival margin
18. The soft tissue within the center of a tooth, consisting of cells, vessels, and nerves
20. The incorrect alignment of jaws or specific teeth within the jaws
21. The term used to describe chewing and breakdown of food material by the teeth
22. Paste, liquid, or powder used to help maintain good oral hygiene
24. The large bilateral muscle of mastication positioned ventral to the zygomatic arch, which functions to close the mouth
26. The gap between teeth, as seen between incisors and cheek teeth of a rabbit
28. A hand instrument designed with a rounded toe for subgingival scaling
29. A _____ fistula is an abnormal communication between the mouth and nasal passage, usually caused by severe periodontal disease or palatal trauma
31. The smooth convex bulge on the palatal side of the incisor teeth
34. The tip of the root of a tooth
35. A pathologic exaggeration of the upward slope of the distal mandibular cheek teeth of the horse

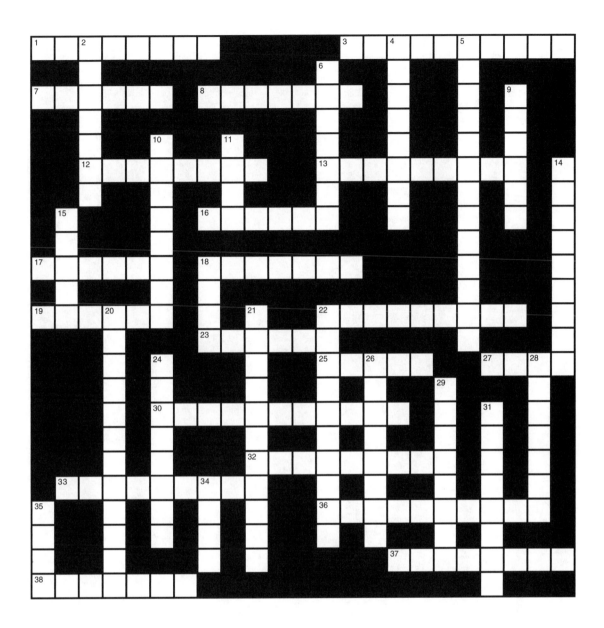

33 Emergency Nursing

LEARNING OBJECTIVES

When you have completed this chapter, you will be able to:

1. Discuss the role of the veterinary technician in equine emergency medicine
2. List equipment, supplies, and medications that may be needed to respond to equine emergencies
3. Discussion considerations for transport of horses to emergency facilities
4. List minimum data collected during assessment of equine emergency patients
5. Describe initial management of equine emergencies
6. Describe initial assessment, diagnostic, and treatment procedures for common equine gastrointestinal, orthopedic, and respiratory emergencies
7. Describe procedures for assessing dehydration in equine patients
8. Describe procedures for placement and maintenance of intravenous catheters in equine patients
9. Discuss considerations in development and implementation of an equine fluid therapy plan in emergency situations
10. Describe indications for use of blood and blood products and procedures for their use

MULTIPLE CHOICE

1. The clinical signs of pneumothorax typically include:
   a. Brick red mucous membranes
   b. Rapid, shallow breathing
   c. Hypersalivation
   d. Poor mentation

2. Which of the following is indicated in the treatment of ventricular fibrillation?
   a. Sodium bicarbonate
   b. Epinephrine
   c. Electrical defibrillation
   d. Atropine

3. Bone marrow catheters can be used in lieu of intravenous catheters in which type of patient?
   a. Obese cats
   b. Exotic pets
   c. Geriatric pets
   d. Fractious animals

4. Clinical signs to avoid after placement of an abdominal pressure wrap are:
   a. Increased respiratory effort
   b. Increased urine production
   c. Increased rectal temperature
   d. Decreased bleeding

5. Abdominal pain is sometimes associated with which of the following observations in the dog?
   a. Lateral recumbency
   b. Miotic pupils
   c. "Praying" body position
   d. Decreased urine production

6. Nonsteroidal antiinflammatory drugs (NSAIDs) may have negative side effects on which major system?
   a. Cardiopulmonary
   b. Respiratory
   c. Gastrointestinal
   d. Neurologic

7. A common RBC morphology abnormality associated with DIC:
   a. Echinocytes
   b. Schistocytes
   c. Anisocytosis
   d. Acanthocytes

8. The most consistent laboratory finding in DIC is:
   a. Neutropenia
   b. Anemia
   c. Thrombocytopenia
   d. Hypoproteinemia

9. Serial neurologic assessments should be done hourly on the postarrest patient. This can be achieved by:
   a. Monitoring for CP deficits
   b. Pupillary light response testing
   c. Changes in pulse quality
   d. Monitoring body temperature

10. Which of the following is an effective treatment for a traumatic hemoabdomen?
    a. Abdominal centesis
    b. Abdominal pressure wrap
    c. Blood transfusion
    d. Aggressive fluid therapy

11. Shock can be defined as:
    a. Increased metabolic rate
    b. Impaired oxygen delivery to the tissues
    c. Vasoconstriction and decreased heart rate
    d. Vasodilation and hypothermia

12. Which drug may be beneficial in restoring blood pressure when appropriate fluid therapy fails?
    a. Dopamine or dobutamine
    b. Furosemide
    c. Mannitol
    d. Dexamethasone sodium phosphate

13. Following resuscitation from shock, reperfusion may initiate:
    a. Bone marrow suppression
    b. Hypertension
    c. Hypotension
    d. Production of oxygen free radicals

14. A vagus-mediated arrest can occur in patients experiencing:
    a. Internal bleeding
    b. Rib fractures
    c. Severe vomiting
    d. High fever

15. Endotracheal intubation and ventilation with an Ambu bag with room air provides:
    a. 100% oxygen
    b. 43% oxygen
    c. 21% oxygen
    d. No oxygen at all

16. Acute renal failure is a common secondary complication in the postarrest patient. What is the *best* way to monitor renal function?
    a. Serial body weighing
    b. Placement of a urinary catheter for quantifying urine output
    c. Electrolyte analysis
    d. Monitor central venous pressure

17. DIC often results in multiple organ failure due to:
    a. Vasodilation
    b. Peripheral edema
    c. Capillary microthrombi formation
    d. Hypertension

18. Physiologic consequences of septic shock include:
    a. Vasodilation and increased vascular permeability
    b. Increased cardiac output
    c. Severe vasoconstriction and bradycardia
    d. Cerebral hypoxia

19. During triage of a hit-by-car, internal hemorrhage can be confirmed by:
    a. Poor pulse quality
    b. Serial PCV/TS analysis
    c. Abnormal respiratory patterns
    d. Increased capillary refill time

20. Hypercoagulation may lead to:
    a. Fever
    b. Hypertension
    c. Thrombosis
    d. Pupillary dilation

21. Peripheral pulses are not palpable when the mean arterial pressure is less than:
    a. 100 mm Hg
    b. 85 mm Hg
    c. 60 mm Hg
    d. 50 mm Hg

22. A potent diuretic commonly used in the treatment of pulmonary edema:
    a. Dobutamine
    b. Furosemide
    c. Dexamethasone sodium phosphate
    d. Nitroglycerin

23. How can a cardiac arrest be confirmed?
    a. Palpation of a pulse
    b. Cardiac auscultation
    c. Checking PLR
    d. No voluntary respirations

24. Abnormal ECG findings associated with urinary obstructions are typically:
    a. Spiked T waves
    b. Absence of p waves
    c. Shortened QRS complexes
    d. Both a and b

25. Effectiveness of chest compressions during CPCR can be assessed by:
    a. Simultaneous monitoring blood pressure
    b. Ultrasound
    c. Capnography
    d. Simultaneous monitoring for presence of pulses

26. The presence of ECG complexes with no cardiac contractions to generate a pulse is termed:
    a. Sinus bradycardia
    b. Electrical mechanical association (EMD)
    c. Ventricular fibrillation
    d. Asystole

27. The recommended dose/setting for electrical defibrillation is:
    a. 2 to 4 joules/kg
    b. 10 to 20 joules/kg
    c. 40+ joules/kg
    d. <15 joules/kg for most companion animals

28. The average adult horse has a fluid requirement of:
    a. 50 to 60 ml/kg/24-hour period
    b. 20 to 30 ml/kg/24-hour period
    c. 10 to 20 ml/kg/24-hour period
    d. 60 to 90 ml/kg/24-hour period

29. Foals have a higher total body water percentage and therefore a higher maintenance requirement of approximately:
    a. 50 to 60 ml/kg/24-hour period
    b. 100 ml/kg/24-hour period
    c. 60 to 75 ml/kg/24-hour period
    d. 200 to 400 ml/kg/24-hour period

30. Which of the following infectious diseases should be isolated from the main hospital treatment area?
    a. Leptospirosis
    b. Heartworm disease
    c. Canine parvovirus
    d. Feline leukemia

31. Which hemodynamic test can be a useful tool in assessing a patient's response to fluids?
    a. ECG
    b. Intraocular pressure
    c. Body temperature
    d. Central venous pressure

32. A fractious cat presents in severe respiratory distress. What is the best way to *immediately* provide oxygen?
    a. Nasal cannula
    b. Flow-by oxygen
    c. Oxygen mask
    d. Small oxygen chamber or tank

33. Despite three separate thoracocentesis procedures, a hit-by-car canine patient remains tachypneic. This patient may have:
    a. Hemothorax
    b. Diaphragmatic hernia
    c. Pneumothorax
    d. Collapsed lungs

34. Laryngospasms immediately following anesthetic recovery of a horse can be a potentially life-threatening complication attributed to:
    a. Extreme extension of the head and neck during surgery
    b. Hypoxia
    c. Premedications
    d. Anesthesia overdose

35. A free radical scavenger, which can be beneficial in the treatment of a reperfusion injury:
    a. Mannitol
    b. Furosemide
    c. Dopamine
    d. Dobutamine

36. The standard dose of plasma for the dog and cat is typically:
    a. 15 to 20 ml/kg
    b. 5 to 10 ml/kg
    c. 1 to 2 ml/kg
    d. 20 to 40 ml/kg

37. A closed urinary catheter is placed to monitor renal function. What is the approximate minimal acceptable urine production per hour for the dog and cat?
    a. 2 ml/kg/hr
    b. 0.5 to 1.0 ml/kg/hr
    c. 5 ml/kg/hr
    d. 7 to 10 ml/kg/hr

38. What is typically found on a urine sediment within a few hours of ethylene glycol ingestion?
    a. White blood cells
    b. Bacteria
    c. Calcium oxalate crystals
    d. Nothing—sediment is typically normal for the first 24 hours of ingestion

39. What is typically the most life-threatening abnormal electrolyte abnormality associated with urinary obstructions?
    a. Hypernatremia
    b. Hypokalemia
    c. Hyperkalemia
    d. Hyponatremia

40. How long after a transfusion should a patient's hematocrit be reassessed?
    a. 4 hours
    b. 12 hours
    c. 30 minutes
    d. 24 hours

41. Capnography uses infrared technology to estimate the carbon dioxide concentration of expired air. How is this beneficial to an animal scheduled for general anesthesia?
    a. It can confirm endotracheal intubation
    b. It can monitor the efficacy of oxygenation
    c. For the detection of airway occlusion
    d. Both a and c

42. Which of the following will impede the pulse oximeter's ability to obtain an accurate reading?
   a. Hyperthermia
   b. Hypothermia
   c. Excessive anesthetic depth
   d. Pleural effusion

43. Clinical signs of ethylene glycol toxicity include:
   a. Hyperactivity
   b. Ataxia, vomiting, seizures
   c. Fever, anorexia
   d. Acute blindness

44. Common laboratory findings in the patient suspected of ethylene glycol toxicity include:
   a. Neutropenia
   b. Neutrophilia
   c. Elevated creatinine
   d. Low albumin

TRUE OR FALSE

Choose T (true) or F (false) for each statement below.

1. _____ Urinary obstruction is less common in female dogs as compared to male dogs.

2. _____ Endotracheal tubes should be sterilized before placement in a crash cart.

3. _____ An emergency thoracocentesis can be performed without analgesia.

4. _____ A horse with a history of abdominal pain may present with abrasions along the head and face suggesting severe pain.

5. _____ Multiple "mini" crash carts or kits should be accessible in all operating rooms, dental suites, and examination rooms.

6. _____ Fluid administration rates are roughly equivalent for both shock and dehydration.

7. _____ All blood products, including frozen plasma, require a blood filter to prevent the administration of clots.

8. _____ Horses can be mildly sedated and nonsteroidal antiinflammatory drugs (NSAIDs) administered to relieve pain for easier transport to a veterinary facility.

9. _____ Transfusion reactions can occur even if a compatible blood type is administered.

10. _____ Only 25% of crystalloid fluids will remain in the intravascular space after 1 hour.

11. _____ Direct pressure is the immediate action to the presence of arterial bleeding.

12. _____ Maintenance fluids are calculated based on a patient's body condition score.

13. _____ The A-a gradient calculation can quantitate a patient's oxygen exchange. This calculation is generally used if the patient is not receiving oxygen.

14. _____ Removing an abdominal pressure bandage placed for internal bleeding should be removed slowly over a course of several hours.

15. _____ Apomorphine is contraindicated in cats.

16. _____ Rectal palpation is a diagnostic procedure performed in equine patients suffering from severe, recurrent, or persistent abdominal pain.

17. _____ The ideal total administration time for a blood transfusion is within 12 hours to prevent contamination.

18. _____ Restriction of intravenous fluids in the head trauma victim in shock is recommended to prevent an increase in cerebral edema.

19. _____ Foals should be hauled separately from the dam and with an assistant.

20. _____ Pain left untreated can have harmful physiologic consequences.

21. _____ Mannitol is contraindicated if an active intracranial bleed is suspected.

22. _____ A splint placed on a canine bone fracture should incorporate the joints above and below the fracture site for adequate stabilization.

23. _____ Spinal cord swelling can interfere with an accurate neurologic examination for up to 7 days after the initial injury or insult.

24. _____ Regardless of active bleeding, closure of all open wounds is a priority in emergency patients to minimize infection.

25. _____ Opioids can potentiate cardiac and respiratory suppression.

26. _____ DIC is always secondary to trauma or a disease process.

27. _____ Colic horses should have a nasogastric tube passed and gastric reflux removed immediately before loaded into a trailer for transport.

28. _____ Dobutamine is contraindicated for use in the postarrest patient because it may decrease cardiac contractility and cardiac output.

29. _____ Horses with hind limb fractures should be transported facing the back of the trailer to facilitate balance and to help alleviate pain.

30. _____ Treatment of shock focuses primarily on improving perfusion to the tissues.

31. _____ Septic shock is the most common form of shock in small animals.

32. _____ Treatment of DIC involves primarily support care and resolution of its primary cause.

33. _____ Normal equine stomach content is usually light green and is often foamy and typically less than 2 liters is obtained during gastric lavage.

SHORT ANSWER

1. Name a syndrome that can often parallel septic shock.

   _____

2. Name two devices useful in the detection of arrhythmias.

   A. _____

   B. _____

3. Snake evenomation can be diagnosed by the presence of _____ on a blood smear.

4. Female urinary catheterization in the dog can be accomplished by digital palpation of anatomic landmarks or by direct visualization of the urethral orifice called the _____.

5. List reasons for suction equipment to be easily accessible in the triage area for respiratory emergencies.

   A. _____

   _____

   B. _____

   _____

   C. _____

   _____

6. List two indications for administration of epinephrine.

   A. _____

   B. _____

7. Name four alternative drug administration routes if intravenous access is not accessible.

   A. _____

   B. _____

C. _____

D. _____

8. What is a flail chest?

_____

What are the potential complications?

A. _____

B. _____

C. _____

9. What are the common clinical signs of increased intracranial pressure?

A. _____

B. _____

C. _____

D. _____

10. Name the three clotting tests that in-house coagulation time machines can analyze.

A. _____

B. _____

C. _____

11. Name two drugs commonly used to reduce cerebral edema.

A. _____

B. _____

12. Rodenticide toxicity interferes with the clotting synthesis and can cause active bleeding within how many hours

after ingestion? _____

What is the treatment for most rodenticide toxicity patients? _____

13. List six common clinical signs that may suggest a patient is having a transfusion reaction.

A. _____

B. _____

C. _____

D. _____

E. _____

F. _____

What are the treatments used for transfusion reactions?

G. _____

H. _____

I. _____

Delayed hemolytic reactions to blood transfusions can occur days or weeks later. What are three signs of hemolysis?

J. _____

K. _____

L. _____

14. Horses have seven different blood types represented by which capital letters?

_____

15. Name the by-products of clot lysis often quantified to help diagnose DIC.

A. _____

B. _____

C. _____

16. List some common therapies for horses that strain during rectal examination.

A. _____

B. _____

C. _____

17. Name two devices commonly used to provide continuous monitoring of the cardiovascular system in the postarrest patient.

A. _____

B. _____

18. There are many clinical signs associated with DIC. Name two common abnormal findings associated with the integumentary system.

A. _____

B. _____

Where are these typically found?

C. _____

D. _____

E. _____

F. _____

19. What are the shock crystalloid fluid rates for the dog? Cat?

A. Dog _____

B. Cat _____

20. Platelet function can be assessed by which in-house tests? _____

21. Recumbent horses should be heavily sedated or anesthetized before loading. Once sedated:
A. How can the horse be protected during the ride?

_____

_____

B. Recumbent horses are best hauled in

_____

_____.

22. During triage, which monitoring parameters are necessary to evaluate in order to assess a patient's response to intravenous fluids?

A. _____

B. _____

C. _____

D. _____

E. _____

23. List the four general categories of shock.

A. _____

B. _____

C. _____

D. _____

24. Following fluid resuscitation for shock, production of oxygen free radicals can cause inflammation and vessel injury. What is this syndrome called?

_____

25. Potassium penicillin should not be administered to the presurgical horse within 15 minutes of induction because of

_____

_____.

26. What is the definition of cardiopulmonary arrest?

_____

27. New acronym CPCR, in place of old acronym CPR, places emphasis on which system during resuscitation efforts?

_____

28. What are some useful tools to help identify a patient's volume status?

A. _____

B. _____

C. _____

D. _____

29. What does the pulse oximeter measure? _____

What does it *not* measure? _____

30. Assisted ventilation should not exceed _____ cm H_2O during CPCR, unless directed otherwise by a veterinarian.

31. Administration of how many milliliters per pound of whole blood does it typically take to raise the patient's

hematocrit by 1 percent? _____

32. Horses that have abdominal pain should be assessed for signs of colic. List five common clinical signs of mild abdominal pain.

A. _____

B. _____

C. _____

D. _____

E. _____

List five clinical signs common with moderate to severe abdominal pain.

F. _____

G. _____

H. _____

I. _____

J. _____

K. True or False: Gastrointestinal motility can be significantly decreased by the administration of sedation; therefore, auscultation of the abdomen should be performed prior.

_____

33. Which CPCR drugs can be administered by the intratracheal route?

A. _____

B. _____

C. _____

D. _____

34. Chest compressions during closed-chest CPCR promotes blood flow by what two methods?

A. _____

B. _____

35. Why is it necessary to blood type all cats before a blood transfusion (time permitting)?

_____

_____

36. List common "QATS" or useful quick assessment tests for incoming emergency patients.

A. _____

B. _____

C. _____

D. _____

E. _____

List the significance of each.

F. _____

G. _____

H. _____

I. _____

J. _____

37. Name three common sampling sites for obtaining an arterial blood gas.

    A. _____

    B. _____

    C. _____

38. What is normal buccal bleeding time?

    A. 90 seconds
    B. Less than 60 seconds
    C. Greater than 5 minutes
    D. Less than 4 minutes

39. A blood smear should be analyzed as part of an emergency patient's initial profile. Explain.

    _____

    _____

    _____

    _____

40. Normal end-tidal CO_2 levels range from 30 to 40 mm Hg. If a patient was hypoventilated during anesthesia, would

    you expect to see values less than or greater than 30 to 45 mm Hg? _____

    If the patient was being hyperventilated, would you expect to see values greater than or less than 30 to 45 mm Hg?

    _____

41. A hit-by-car presents in cardiopulmonary arrest and intravenous access cannot be established. Name four routes for rapid administration of epinephrine, lidocaine, and atropine for CPCR.

    A. _____

    B. _____

    C. _____

    D. _____

    How are the drugs dosed for each different route?

    E. _____

    F. _____

    G. _____

    H. _____

42. What is the Fio_2? _____

43. The Pao_2 is typically _____ times the Fio_2.

44. How can pulse deficits be detected on a physical examination?

_____

45. By definition, hypertension is a systolic pressure greater than _____ mm Hg.

46. Pulses should be palpable if the MAP is greater than _____ mm Hg.

47. Clinical signs of increased intracranial pressure are listed below. Please separate signs into the two categories, early clinical signs or later clinical signs.

   Bradycardia _____

   Dilated pupils _____

   Coma _____

   Change in mentation _____

   Miosis _____

   Tachycardia _____

   Change in respiratory patterns _____

   Seizures _____

48. What is a DPL? _____

   When is this necessary?

_____

_____

49. Thoracocentesis is typically performed with the patient in sternal recumbency with the entry point into the chest at which anatomic landmarks?

_____

50. Resistance to urethral catheterization may be encountered in anatomical areas where the urethra narrows. List the three areas in the dog.

   A. _____

   B. _____

   C. _____

51. When is emesis contraindicated in the toxicity patient? _____

52. Name two household remedies for the induction of vomiting.

   A. _____

   B. _____

53. Adsorbents bind toxins to prevent absorption. Name a commonly used veterinary adsorbent.

_____

MATCHING

Match the correct answer from Column B to the questions in Column A.

Column A

1. _____ Portable ventilation device
2. _____ Gas movement in the GI tract that produces noise
3. _____ Malperfusion of blood flow
4. _____ Temporary suspension of respiration and circulation
5. _____ Severe abdominal pain
6. _____ Microscopic clumping of red blood cells
7. _____ An instrument used to visual the airway
8. _____ Widespread pathogenic bacterial infection
9. _____ An instrument that reads the percent of oxygen saturation
10. _____ A secondary, often fatal disease process

Column B

A. Agglutination
B. Laryngoscope
C. AMBU bag
D. Shock
E. DIC
F. Syncope
G. Colic
H. Pulse oximeter
I. Sepsis
J. Borborygmi

FILL IN THE BLANK

Please choose the appropriate fluid type for each question listed below.

Choose (A) for crystalloid fluid.

Choose (B) for colloid fluid.

Choose (C) for both crystalloid and colloid fluid.

1. _____ Used aggressively for the treatment of acute renal failure

2. _____ Fluid of choice for the patient with severe vomiting and diarrhea

3. _____ Treatment for head trauma

4. _____ Treatment for shock

5. _____ Treatment for hypoproteinemia

6. _____ Used primarily to increase urine output

7. _____ Correction of electrolyte disturbances

8. _____ Rapid expansion of vascular volume with small amounts of fluid

9. _____ To correct dehydration

10. _____ Safe for rapid administration in shock

FILL IN THE BLANK

Use the list provided below.

Serum	White blood cells
Platelets	Hemoglobin
Plasma	Oxygen

1. RBCs contain _____ , which has the primary function of carrying

   _____ .

2. Immune system cells responsible for mediating inflammation and fighting infection are called

   _____ .

3. Small cellular components active during clotting are called _____ .

4. What is the fluid compartment containing albumin and globulin called? _____

5. The fluid component of blood after clotting has occurred is referred to as _____ .

CASE DISCUSSION 1

A 10 kg, 12-week-old male Schnauzer puppy named Manny comes to the hospital with acute vomiting and diarrhea. He is estimated to be about 7% dehydrated.

1. What laboratory tests can be analyzed to assess the severity of his dehydration?

   A. _____

   B. _____

   C. _____

2. The patient's hematocrit is elevated and the total protein low. Explain.

   _____

   _____

3. Calculate the amount of fluids in milliliters needed to correct for dehydration. Show the formula.

   _____

   _____

4. The owner reports that Manny is vomiting and having diarrhea several times an hour. You estimate that he is losing 50 ml every 2 hours. Calculate the drip rate in milliliters per hour that the IV pump should be set at over the next 4-hour period in which he will need to receive the 700 ml needed to correct for dehydration, maintenance, and compensation for fluid losses over 4 hours.

   _____

   _____

   _____

5. After the 4-hour period, Manny appears much more alert and rehydrated, although he continues to have vomiting and diarrhea. What should his fluid rate be turned down to?

_____

_____

6. What is the most appropriate fluid of choice during the first 4 hours?

_____

7. Why should the total solids be rechecked after the 4-hour rehydration period?

_____

_____

8. Manny's total protein is 4.0 mg/dl. Should IV fluids be discontinued? What are his fluid therapy options?

_____

_____

_____

_____

CASE DISCUSSION 2

A 3-year-old male, castrated domestic short-haired cat presents for stranguria and anorexia of 48 hours duration. The owners report that today the cat went to the litter box 10 to 12 times without producing urine and that he walks stiff and is not interested in eating food. On presentation, physical examination reveals dry, gray mucous membranes, a rectal temperature of 97.9° F, weak femoral pulses, and a heart rate of 100 beats/min. No murmur was ausculted. The urinary bladder is palpated to be about the size of a fist with intense vocalization by the pet upon touching the abdomen.

1. What is the most likely diagnosis?

_____

2. This patient is in pain and vocal. Why is the heart rate low?

_____

3. What is the best plan for emergency stabilization? List in the order of importance.

A. _____

B. _____

C. _____

D. _____

E. _____

F. _____

G. _____

H. _____

4. What are the treatment options for hyperkalemia?

    A. _____

    B. _____

5. If urethral catheterization is unsuccessful, how can the bladder be temporarily evacuated?

    A. _____

    B. _____

6. Relief of the urinary obstruction can cause the kidneys to temporarily increase urine production. What is this

    phenomenon called? _____

    How does this need to be treated?

    A. _____

    B. _____

    C. _____

CIRCLE ALL THAT APPLY

1. Clinical signs associated with overhydration:

    Tachypnea

    Decreased body weight

    Pulmonary edema

    Poor pulse quality

    Polyuria

    Chemosis

    Slow capillary refill time

    Nasal discharge

    Cough

2. Clinical signs associated with poor perfusion:

    Hyperemic mucous membranes

    Increased capillary refill time

    Poor pulse quality

Hyperthermia

Dull mentation

Bounding pulses

Tachycardia

Cyanotic mucous membranes

Hypothermia

3. Common clinical signs of a horse in respiratory distress:

Flaring nostrils

Hyperactive or hypersensitive

Exaggerated abdominal or thoracic excursions

Inspiratory stridor

Expiratory stridor

Nasal discharge

Cyanosis

Abduction of the elbows and extension of the head and neck

4. Abdominocentesis is commonly performed to diagnose:

Hemorrhage

Pancreatitis

Uroabdomen

Liver disease

GDV

Renal disease

Peritonitis

Ascites

Neoplastic effusions

5. Urinary obstructions occur secondary to which of the following? Circle all that apply.

Stones

Bacterial infection

Pyometra

Inflammation

Trauma

Neoplasia

Infectious diseases

6. First aid and stabilization of the fractured or injured equine limb is crucial before transport to the hospital. External fixation of an unstable limb should occur before movement or transport. What are the recommended stabilization techniques for the injuries indicated below?

A. Ground to distal metacarpal injuries:

Hyperextension of the fetlock

Application of a distal limb cast

Removal of shoe

Application of a manufactured splint called the Kimzey Leg

B. Distal metacarpus to distal radial injuries:

Application of a Robert-Jones bandage with two splints at 90-degree angles

Application of a Robert-Jones bandage with one splint only at a 45-degree angle

C. Distal radius to elbow injuries:

Application of a Robert-Jones bandage

Application of a Robert-Jones bandage and a lateral splint fixed to the scapula to prevent abduction

D. Olecranon fractures:

Application of a stacked bandage extending the entire length of the limb

Application of a stacked bandage extending the entire length of the limb in addition to a dorsally applied splint extending at least the length of the carpus

INCREASE OR DECREASE

Choose either: (I) Increase, or (D) Decrease, for the following questions:

1. What is the expected result from excessive fluid administration on the following?

A. Central venous pressure _____

B. Body weight _____

C. Urine specific gravity _____

358

D. Packed cell volume _____

E. Total protein _____

F. Heart rate _____

2. Laboratory findings in the DIC patient:

   A. Antithrombin III levels _____

   B. Platelet count _____

   C. FDP values _____

   D. D-Dimer values _____

MATCHING

Match the drug in Column A with its appropriate indication for use in Column B.

Column A

1. _____ Atropine
2. _____ Lidocaine
3. _____ Naloxone
4. _____ Furosemide
5. _____ DMSO
6. _____ Diazepam
7. _____ Dexamethasone sodium phosphate
8. _____ Flunixin meglumine
9. _____ Sodium bicarbonate
10. _____ Pentobarbital

Column B

A. Equine cardiac arrest
B. Ventricular tachycardia
C. Euthanasia
D. Cerebral edema
E. Anaphylaxis or shock
F. Bradycardia
G. Electrical mechanical dissociation
H. Seizures
I. Endotoxemia
J. Diuresis

CASE DISCUSSION 3

The receptionist informs you that a 4-month-old kitten is en route to the hospital after apparently being attacked by the neighborhood dog. The owner reported the pet was in respiratory distress.

1. To prepare for the emergency, select from items listed below and categorize them according to the emergency ABCs (mark A, B, or C). Note: not all items listed will be used.

   _____ Jugular catheter

   _____ Laryngoscope with small blade

   _____ Thoracocentesis material

   _____ Lactated Ringers solution

   _____ Oxygen chamber

   _____ Clippers

   _____ Several small sized endotracheal tubes

   _____ Surgical scrub

   _____ Heating pad

   _____ Suction

   _____ 22- to 20-gauge IV catheter

   _____ Bandage material

   _____ AMBU bag

   _____ Gauze ties

_____ Lidocaine   _____ Sponge forceps and gauze squares

_____ Nasal oxygen catheter   _____ Small syringe

_____ Tape   _____ Spinal needle

_____ Saline flush

MATCHING

Match the correct blood component (Column A) to the proper clinical indication listed in Column B.

Column A

1. _____ Fresh whole blood
2. _____ Packed RBCs
3. _____ Cryoprecipitate
4. _____ Fresh frozen plasma
5. _____ Stored whole blood
6. _____ Frozen plasma

Column B

A. Severe bleeding, suspected coagulopathy such as DIC or von Willebrand's factor deficiency, severe anemia and hypoproteinemia

B. Anemia and hypoproteinemia

C. Severe coagulopathy, hypoproteinemia, DIC, factor deficiency, or hemophilia

D. Coagulopathy, hypoproteinemia, acute volume expansion needed

E. Hypoproteinemia

F. Anemia with normal plasma volume

FILL IN THE BLANK

Central venous pressure refers to blood pressure in central veins, and is a useful tool in assessing the efficacy of fluid therapy. If normal ranges are typically 0 to 5 cm H_2O, answer the following questions with either (A) less than normal, (B) normal, or (C) greater than normal range.

A. _____ CVP values on a patient with a pneumothorax

B. _____ CVP values on a dehydrated patient

C. _____ CVP values on a patient with pleural effusion

D. _____ CVP values on a patient showing signs of overhydration

E. _____ CVP values on a patient with congestive heart failure

F. _____ CVP values on a patient in hypovolemic shock

SHORT ANSWER

1. The zero mark of the CVP manometer is approximately at what anatomical landmark?

2. Measuring the CVP would be most beneficial to which of the following patients?

   A. Renal failure patients requiring aggressive fluid therapy

   B. Pediatric patients

   C. Hypertensive patients

CROSSWORD PUZZLE

Across

1. Accumulation in the blood of nitrogenous waste products (urea) that are usually excreted in the urine
5. Rumbling noise caused by propulsion of gas and ingesta through the intestines
8. A harsh, high-pitched respiratory sound
11. A _____ shadow is an ultrasound beam interaction with a highly reflective surface, such as bone, foreign material, or gas causing a high degree of attenuation of the beam and blocking of the pathway of the beam to deeper tissue
13. A detailed description of the distinguishing features of the patient
14. The determination of priorities for action in an emergency

Down

2. A clot consisting of fibrin, platelets, red blood cells, and white blood cells that forms in a blood vessel or in a chamber of the heart and can obstruct blood flow
3. The _____ flow is the nonturbulent flow of a viscous fluid in layers near a boundary
4. A bluish discoloration of the skin and mucous membranes resulting from inadequate oxygenation of the blood
6. A sequestrum is a piece of dead _____ that has become separated during the process of necrosis from the surrounding bone
7. Deficient in the amount of oxygen reaching body tissues
9. A deficiency of blood to a body part or organ due to function constriction or actual obstruction of a blood vessel
10. A backward or return flow such as from the small intestine into the stomach
12. Acute abdominal pain

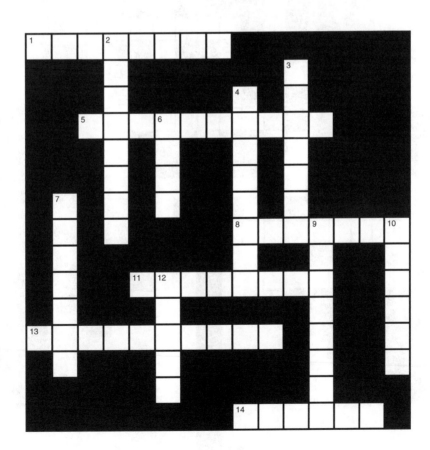

CROSSWORD PUZZLE

Across

2. The determination of priorities for action in an emergency
5. A bluish discoloration of the skin and mucous membranes resulting from inadequate oxygenation of the blood
6. A backward or return flow such as from the small intestine into the stomach
7. Deficiency of blood to a body part or organ due to function constriction or actual obstruction of a blood vessel
9. Shadow—Ultrasound beam interaction with a highly reflective surface such as bone, foreign material, or gas causing a high degree of attenuation of the beam and blocking of the pathway of the beam to deeper tissue
11. Rumbling noise caused by propulsion of gas and ingesta through the intestines
12. The _____ flow is the nonturbulent flow of a viscous fluid in layers near a boundary

Down

1. A harsh, high-pitched respiratory sound
3. Accumulation in the blood of nitrogenous waste products (urea) that are usually excreted in the urine
4. A sequestrum is a piece of dead _____ that has become separated during the process of necrosis from the surrounding bone
5. Acute abdominal pain
8. Deficient in the amount of oxygen reaching body tissues
10. A clot consisting of fibrin, platelets, red blood cells, and white blood cells that forms in a blood vessel or in a chamber of the heart and can obstruct blood flow

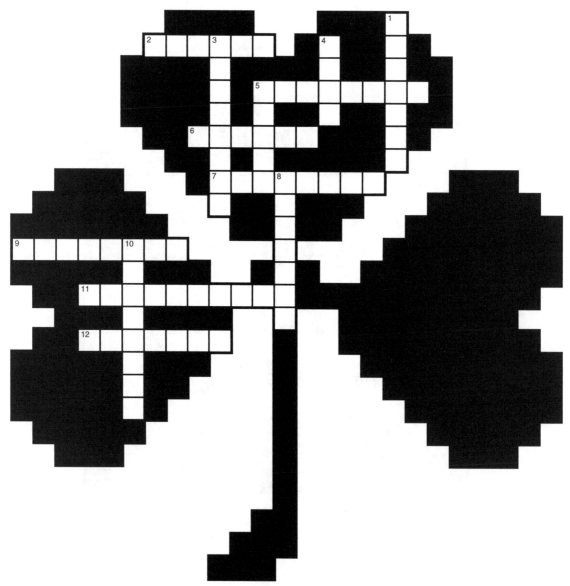

Chapter **33** **Emergency Nursing**

LEARNING OBJECTIVES

When you have completed this chapter, you will be able to:
1. Describe the process of wound healing
2. List and describe the factors that affect wound healing
3. Discuss initial management of wounds in small and large animals
4. Describe procedures for lavage and débridement of wounds in small and large animals
5. Differentiate between first intention, second intention, and third intention healing
6. Discuss indications for bandaging of wounds and describe the general structure of bandages
7. Describe common types of bandages, slings, splints, and casts used for small and large animals and provide indications for their use
8. Describe procedures for monitoring of animals with casts, bandages, splints, or slings
9. Discuss considerations for bandaging of abrasions, lacerations, puncture wounds, and degloving injuries
10. Describe classification of burns and discuss management of burn patients

DEFINITIONS

Define the following:

1. Abrasion _____

_____

2. Claw Block _____

_____

3. Contamination _____

_____

4. Débridement _____

_____

5. Epithelialization _____

_____

6. Eschar _____

_____

7. Exudate _____

_____

8. Hydrocolloid _____

_____

363

9. Hydrophillic _____

_____

10. Hypertonic _____

_____

11. Lag Phase _____

_____

12. Myofibroblast _____

_____

13. Thrush _____

_____

14. Vasoconstriction _____

_____

FILL IN THE BLANK

Carpal flexion sling   Ehmer sling   External coaptation
Nonadherent dressing   Occlusive dressing   Robert Jones bandage
Semi permeable dressing   Velpeau sling   Mineral oil

1. _____ configures to hold the carpus in flexion, thus reducing tension on the flexor surface.

2. An animal needs to keep weight off the coxofemoral joint; therefore a _____ is placed.

3. A _____ is placed to hold the forelimb against the chest and prevent weight bearing on the limb.

4. When used on a wound, a _____ allows for air transfer but not fluid.

5. After orthopedic surgery on a rear limb, a _____ is placed to help protect the limb initially.

6. A granulating wound needs a _____ placed to keep it from sticking to the wound.

7. _____ requires less changing and accelerates epithelialization compared with an exposed wound.

8. _____ is used on the outside of a limb to join or maintain two ends together, such as a broken bone or cut tendon.

9. Hair dipped in _____ can be removed from the edges of a wound with scissors. This helps keep the hair from getting into the wound.

Choose the one most correct answer for each question.

1. The process of wound healing:
   a. Is a simple biologic event that is well understood
   b. Is regulated at the molecular level and is well understood
   c. Is described in three phases: inflammatory, repair, and maturation
   d. Is a dynamic process and more than one phase is occurring at a time

2. The initiation of wound healing is started by:
   a. Platelets
   b. Macrophages
   c. Endothelial cells
   d. Fibroblasts

3. Vasoconstriction is a part of the inflammatory healing process but only lasts:
   a. A few seconds
   b. 1 to 5 minutes
   c. 5 to 10 minutes
   d. 10 to 15 minutes

4. The lag phase is:
   a. When wound strength is maximal
   b. Found during the first 10 days of healing
   c. Found during the first 24 hours of healing
   d. When wound strength is minimal

5. The repair phase:
   a. Begins as soon as a blood clot forms on the wound
   b. Is active by 5 to 10 days after injury
   c. Has very reduced wound strength
   d. Is also known as the lag phase

6. Epithelialization is found during which wound healing phase?
   a. Inflammatory
   b. Repair
   c. Débridement
   d. Maturation

7. Visible wound contraction occurs within:
   a. 24 to 48 hours
   b. 3 to 5 days
   c. 4 to 5 days
   d. 5 to 9 days

8. Which of the following is not true?
   a. Old animals heal slowly.
   b. Malnourished animals heal slowly.
   c. Sharp surgical incision causes slower healing.
   d. Corticosteroids cause slower healing.

9. Which of the following about wound lavage is not true?
   a. It is necessary to remove debris and loose particles
   b. It reduces the number of bacteria in the wound
   c. It can be done before any sampling of the wound for culture
   d. It should be performed with a warm, sterile, balanced solution

10. Lavage is accomplished mostly by mechanical action using:
    a. A 35 ml syringe and high pressure
    b. A 35 ml syringe and moderate pressure
    c. A 60 ml syringe and high pressure
    d. A 60 ml syringe and moderate pressure

11. The four methods of wound closure are:
    a. Primary wound closure, first-intention healing, appositional healing, delayed primary closure
    b. First-intention healing, appositional healing, delayed primary closure, second-intention healing
    c. Primary wound healing, delayed primary closure, second-intention healing, third-intention healing
    d. First-intention healing, delayed primary closure, second-intention healing, third-intention healing

12. A cat sustains a wound created by road rash 10 hours ago. There is a large amount of asphalt material and other debris in the wound. Which would be the best option for wound closure?
    a. First-intention healing
    b. Second-intention healing
    c. Third-intention healing
    d. Appositional healing

13. A horse that was spooked in the pasture runs into the barbed wire and sustains a superficial injury to the right forelimb. What is of concern with this injury?
    a. Broken bones
    b. Proud flesh formation
    c. Tetanus exposure
    d. Nothing—treat the wound exactly the same as with small animals

14. An abscess is considered what type of wound?
    a. Clean, sharply incised
    b. Mildly contaminated
    c. Significantly contaminated
    d. Granulation tissue

15. Bandages are considered helpful in all the following *except*:
    a. As a type of primary wound healing
    b. Protecting the wound from additional trauma/contamination
    c. Preventing hematoma formation
    d. As a form of débriding a wound

16. Why are the middle two toes left exposed in most limb bandages?
    a. Assessment of toenail growth
    b. Assessment of color, warmth, and swelling
    c. Make it easier for the animal to walk
    d. They are not generally left exposed

17. Which of the following usually requires anesthesia when placing on a horse?
    a. Lower limb wound bandage
    b. Lower limb support bandage
    c. Splint application
    d. Cast application

18. In which species is a claw block placed?
    a. Horse
    b. Cat
    c. Cow
    d. Dog

19. In which species is a modified Thomas splint still commonly used?
    a. Horse
    b. Cat
    c. Cow
    d. Dog

20. Which of the following is the most correct statement?
    a. Sores are generally not an issue for cattle having a cast placed on the limb.
    b. Horses and cattle require very different ways of placing casts and bandages.
    c. Orthopedic felt is used in cattle between the hooves.
    d. Cattle are often not as cooperative as horses and more restraint is required.

SHORT ANSWER

1. How does a wound get created?

_____

_____

2. Describe the wound healing phases.

    A. _____

    _____

    _____

    _____

    B. _____

    _____

    _____

    _____

    C. _____

    _____

    _____

    _____

D. _____

_____

3. List the seven things considered when choosing a type of wound closure.

    A. _____

    B. _____

    C. _____

    D. _____

    E. _____

    F. _____

    G. _____

4. Daisy, a Labrador mix, becomes scared by fireworks; jumps through a glass window; and sustains multiple, mostly clean, sharply incised cuts from the broken glass. The owners are able to get her into their veterinarian within 1 hour of the incident. What steps would you take in the normal course of care for addressing these wounds?

    A. _____

_____

    B. _____

_____

    C. _____

_____

    D. _____

    E. _____

_____

_____

5. Looking at Daisy again, if she then ran around the neighborhood for a few hours and got fairly dirty before making it into the veterinary clinic, how would you need to change the treatment of the wounds?

_____

_____

_____

6. List the steps for standard application of any bandage to a limb.

A. _____

B. _____

C. _____

D. _____

E. _____

F. _____

G. _____

PHOTO MATCHING

Match the following bandages with the pictures.

A. Robert Jones bandage

B. Modified Robert Jones bandage

C. Ehmer sling

D. 90-90 Flexion sling

E. Velpeau sling

F. Carpal flexion sling

G. Hobbles

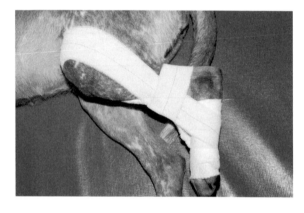

1. _____

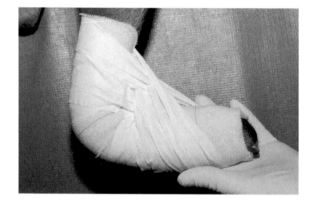

3. _____

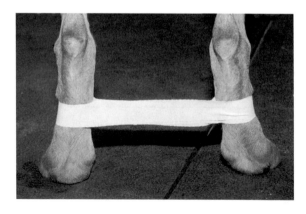

2. _____

4. _____

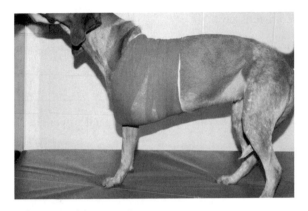

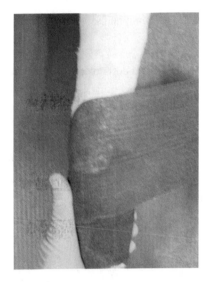

5. _____

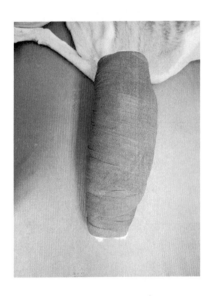

7. _____

6. _____

TRUE OR FALSE

Choose T (true) or F (false) for each statement below. If the answer is false, specify what makes it correct.

1. _____ During wound healing, the epithelium is usually visible on a wound in 4 to 5 days except with an incised wound, when the epithelium is usually visible immediately.

_____

2. _____ New epithelium is usually thick but very fragile initially.

_____

3. _____ Wound contraction helps to reduce the size of the wound and occurs along with epithelialization.

_____

Chapter **34** **Wound Healing, Wound Management, and Bandaging**

4. _____ Once a wound heals, it never regains the strength of normal tissue.

_____

5. _____ Infection and corticosteroids delay or stop wound repair.

_____

6. _____ Contaminated tissue becomes infected if the bacteria multiply to a critical number of organisms per gram
of tissue and then invade the tissue.

_____

7. _____ Movement in a healing wound is very beneficial; it helps strengthen the wound.

_____

8. _____ Water-soluble antibiotic ointments and antibiotic creams and powders may be applied and may be useful
in keeping the wound moist and reducing bacterial infection.

_____

9. _____ Honey and sugar are two substances used in a wound to help with débridement.

_____

10. _____ Bandages minimize postoperative edema around incisions and minimize exuberant granulation tissue
formation in open wounds on the entire limb of horses.

_____

11. _____ Leaving a wound open to dry and form a scab is a viable option in many cases.

_____

12. _____ Closure of decubital ulcers is usually very successful.

_____

13. _____ Degloving injuries require intensive management over a prolonged period of time.

_____

14. _____ Puncture wounds usually are small holes with extensive deep tissue damage and contain foreign material
and bacteria deep in the wound.

_____

15. _____ Burn wounds normally can be managed by primary closure.

_____

16. _____ Splints and casts should be checked daily in the hospital and weekly once an animal has been sent home.

_____

17. _____ When applying a splint, a bandage should cover the limb just above and below the ends of the splint.
This prevents pressure sores.

_____

18. _____ The following are indications for cast application in large animals: lower limb fractures, tendon lacerations, support postorthopedic surgery, and heel bulb lacerations.

_____

19. _____ Pressure sores can be caused by wrinkles or finger imprints on the initial layer of a cast.

_____

20. _____ In a modified Thomas splint, the traction should be maximal within the splint, so as not to create excessive pressure.

_____

MATCHING AND I.D.

Match the types of bandage material with its picture and then identify which layer it may be used in (some can be in more than one layer).

Possible layers of a bandage: bandage material:

1. Stirrups
2. Cast padding
3. Cling gauze
4. Vet Wrap
5. Elasticon

I. Primary layer
II. Secondary layer
III. Tertiary layer

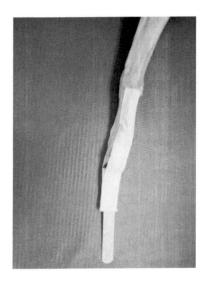

A. _____

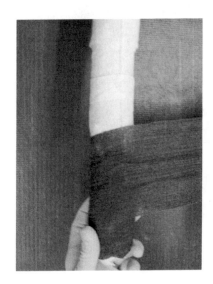

B. _____

Chapter **34 Wound Healing, Wound Management, and Bandaging**

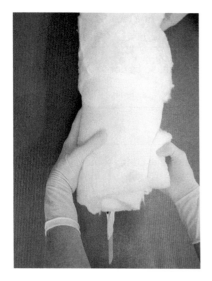

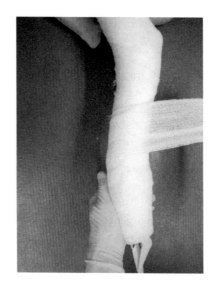

C. _____   D. _____

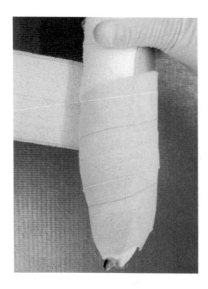

E. _____

SUPER CLUE

Answer each of the following questions by writing one letter of the answer on each line. The letters in boxes will form the answer to the Super Clue.

1. This is also known as healing by contraction and epithelialization.
2. This apparatus prevents quadriceps contracture after distal femoral fracture repair in young animals.
3. This phase of wound healing is characterized by the presence of neutrophils and monocytes.
4. This method of wound débridement involves trypsin products that dissolve necrotic tissue.
5. This device is used most frequently to provide maximum support/immobilization externally.
6. This is the most commonly used bandage for temporary immobilization of fractures distal to the elbow or stifle before surgery.
7. This phase of wound healing is characterized by an influx of neutrophils and monocytes.

8. These medications should not be added to wound lavage fluids.

9. This apparatus is placed after ventral coxofemoral luxation to prevent excessive abduction of the legs.

10. This phase of wound healing may last for several years.

11. This is another name for primary wound closure.

12. These bandages are indicated for granulating wounds that are minimally to moderately exudative.

13. These synthetic hormones depress all phases of wound healing.

14. Fibroblasts produce this material that matures into fibrous or scar tissue.

15. This is the most frequently used material for casts today.

16. This type of wound heals by reepithelialization and is a partial-thickness injury of the epidermis that exposed the deep dermis.

17. This is another name for exuberant granulation tissue in horses.

Super Clue: This apparatus helps to prevent animals from chewing their bandages and also prevents them from injuring their eyes, ears, or any other part of the head. _____

1. _ _ _ _ _ _   _ _ _ □ _ _ _ _ _   _ _ _ _ _ _ _

2. _ _ - _ _   _ □ _ _ _ _ _   _ _ _ _ _

3. _ _ _ _ □ _ _ _ _ _ _

4. _ _ □ _ _ _ _ _ _

5. _ □ _ _

6. _ _ _ _ _ □ _ _ _ _

7. □ _ _ _ _ _ _

8. _ _ _ _ _ □ _ _ _ _

9. _ _ _ _ _ _ _ _ _ □ _ _

10. _ _ _ _ _ □ _ _ _ _ _ _

11. _ _ _ _ _ _ □ _ _ _ _ _ _ _ _

12. _ _ □ _ _ _ _ _

13. _ _ □ _ _ _

14. _ _ □ _ _ _ _ _

15. _ _ _ _ _ _ □ _ _ _

16. _ _ _ □ _ _ _ _

17. _ □ _ _ _ _   _ _ _ _ _ _

Chapter **34** **Wound Healing, Wound Management, and Bandaging**

1. List, in order, the six steps taken in the application of any bandage. Assume that no wound is present. Include splint application as one of the steps.

   A. _____

   B. _____

   C. _____

   D. _____

   E. _____

   F. _____

2. What are the two most common causes of patient burns in an animal hospital?

   A. _____

   B. _____

3. Explain the difference between a Robert Jones and modified Robert Jones bandage and when to use each.

   A. Robert Jones _____

   _____

   B. Modified Robert Jones _____

   _____

4. Explain how to place a chest bandage for a bleeding wound.

   _____

   _____

   _____

   _____

5. When casting a bovine lower limb, what special technique is used to reduce pressure-sore formation at the dewclaws?

   _____

   _____

CROSSWORD PUZZLE

Across

2. A modified fibroblast present in granulation tissue that has characteristics of a muscle cell and is responsible for causing wound contraction
4. A _____ sling is a bandage used to hold the flexed forelimb against the chest, thus immobilizing the limb and preventing weight bearing
5. Wounds characterized by sharply incised edges with minimal tissue trauma
12. Metacarpal or metatarsal region of a horse's leg
15. Has a tonicity above that of living cells
17. The presence of microbes on the surface of an inanimate or living object
20. A _____ sling is a sling bandage configured around the hind limb to prevent weight bearing and hold the coxofemoral joint in adduction; useful after reduction of a coxofemoral luxation
21. A natural material that will absorb fluid; useful for placement on highly exudative wounds
22. _____ granulation tissue is an excessive proliferation of growth of granulation tissue in an open wound
23. A _____ ulcer is an open wound over a bony protuberance resulting from compression and necrosis of the skin and soft tissues over the bone; most common in thin, recumbent animals
24. Lying down

Down

1. A wound, typically of the limbs, where varying amounts of deep tissue (muscle, tendon, ligament, bone) and skin is torn away
3. A semipermeable dressing is impermeable to _____ but allows air transfer
6. Relating to the opposite side
7. Infection of the horny tissue of the hoof
8. Attracts fluid
9. Partial-thickness wounds of the epidermis with exposure of the deep dermis
10. Second-intention healing is healing of a wound by _____ and epithelialization
11. External _____ involves a rigid material (i.e., metal) used on the outside of a limb to join or maintain the ends together, such as a broken bone or cut tendon
13. First _____ healing is healing of a wound that is sutured
14. Removal of foreign materials, necrotic matter, and devitalized tissue from a wound or burn
16. Of or relating to the groin
18. Of or relating to the armpit
19. An _____ dressing is impermeable to air and fluid

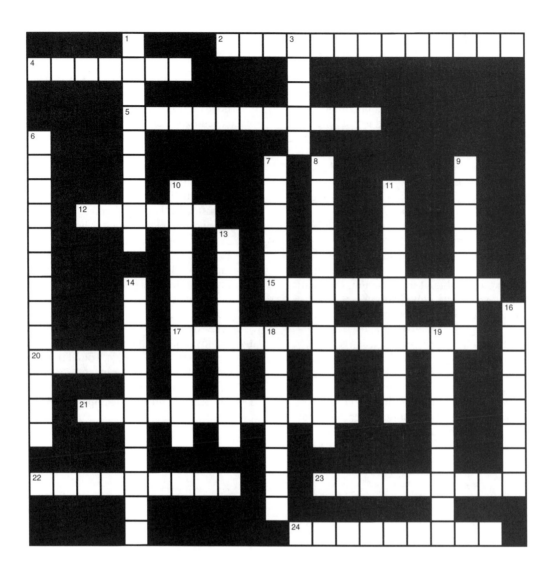

35 Toxicology

LEARNING OBJECTIVES

When you have completed this chapter, you will be able to:

1. Define common terms related to toxicology
2. Describe steps in managing of poison emergencies
3. Discuss initial management of patients with ocular and dermal toxic exposures
4. Describe procedures used in initial management of patients with oral toxic exposures
5. List common topical insecticides and describe signs of toxicity and initial treatment of affected patients
6. List common hazardous foods and household substances and describe signs of toxicity and initial treatment of affected patients
7. List common dangerous plants and describe signs of toxicity and initial treatment of affected patients
8. List common hazardous pesticides and describe signs of toxicity and initial treatment of affected patients
9. List common antifreeze products and describe signs of toxicity and initial treatment of affected patients
10. List common hazardous human medications and describe signs of toxicity and initial treatment of affected patients

MATCHING

1. _____ Subchronic toxicity
2. _____ Chronic toxicity
3. _____ Delayed toxicity
4. _____ Synergism
5. _____ Idiosyncratic reactions
6. _____ Antagonist
7. _____ Toxicology
8. _____ Poison
9. _____ Nephrotoxin
10. _____ Cathartic
11. _____ Toxicity
12. _____ LD 50
13. _____ Acute toxicity
14. _____ Hypersensitivity
15. _____ Subacute toxicity
16. _____ Hazard
17. _____ Zootoxin
18. _____ Immunotoxicants
19. _____ Teratogen
20. _____ Lethal dose
21. _____ Carcinogen
22. _____ Emesis
23. _____ Half-life

A. The study of poisons
B. Any substance that can interfere with the life processes of the cell
C. Immunologic responses and are results of previous sensitization to a chemical
D. Prolonged exposure to a toxicant for more than 3 months
E. Poisons that are produced by an animal
F. The dosage that is lethal to 50% of animals
G. A poison that causes cancer
H. A poison that causes birth defects
I. Is the amount of time needed for half of a substance to be eliminated from the body
J. Effects of a single or multiple dose during 24 hours
K. Are poisons that can affect cell-mediated immunity
L. Pesticides that are used to kill insects
M. Pesticides that are used to kill rats, mice, and other small mammal pests
N. Responses to toxicants that are not immediate and may not be manifested for several days
O. The probability that a chemical will cause harm
P. Abnormal and unexpected reactions to a chemical
Q. When two chemicals negate the effects of each other
R. The amount of a poison that results in toxic effects
S. Act of vomiting
T. Poisons that cause kidney damage or failure
U. The lowest dose that causes death of animals exposed to a poison
V. A substance that causes or assists with evacuation of feces through the gastrointestinal system

24. _____ Insecticides

25. _____ Rodenticides

26. _____ Hepatoxin

W. Repeated exposures to a poison from 1 to 3 months

X. Occurs when two chemicals have a combined effect when administered at the same time that is greater than either chemical alone

Y. Repeated exposure to a poison for up to 30 days

Z. Poisons that can cause liver damage or failure

FILL IN THE BLANK

1. A bufo toad's salivary glands contain bufotoxin. A bufo toad is an example of a _____.

2. The _____ is the amount of poison received by an animal divided by the animal's weight.

3. Corticosteroids have been associated with cleft palates in animals when the dam is given the medication during pregnancy. Corticosteroids are considered to be _____.

4. Acids are examples of _____ agents and can cause direct chemical damage to mucosal surfaces.

5. Bromethalin is found in some types of rat bait. Bromethalin is an example of a _____.

6. If a chemical causes damage to tissues that results in the expression of cancer, it is classified as a _____.

7. With any ocular exposures, the eyes should be _____ immediately.

8. If there is a topical exposure, the animal should be bathed with _____.

9. If an animal ingests a corrosive substance, _____ is contraindicated.

10. Hydrogen peroxide causes emesis through _____.

11. Syrup of ipecac causes emesis through gastric irritation and stimulation of the _____.

12. Apomorphine is a _____ acting emetic agent.

13. Activated charcoal adsorbs a toxicant and facilitates its removal from the body through _____.

14. During a _____ the stomach is gently flushed with warm water to help remove stomach contents.

15. _____ rodenticides compete with Vitamin K_1 and cause hemorrhaging through prevention of blood clotting.

16. The _____ is the test of choice to determine if there is a coagulation problem from exposures to anticoagulants.

17. Clinical signs associated with a bromethalin toxicosis involve the _____ system.

18. The oxidant damage caused by the toxic metabolite of acetaminophen causes _____.

19. Chocolate or dark brown colored blood is a common sign seen in _____ poisoning.

20. Facial or paw _____ is often seen in pets that have been poisoned by acetaminophen.

21. Methemoglobinemia results in blood that has poor _____.

22. With acetaminophen poisoning, _____ is possible because of the direct damage to the liver cells.

23. _____ directly binds with acetaminophen metabolites to enhance elimination and serves as a glutathione precursor.

24. Cats are deficient in _____ and therefore have a prolonged excretion rate of many medications.

MULTIPLE CHOICE

1. The plant below may cause kidney failure if ingested by a cat.
   a. Peace lily
   b. Poinsettia
   c. Easter lily
   d. Rose

2. Examples of emetic agents include:
   a. Mustard and salt mixture
   b. Rotten egg whites
   c. Hydrogen peroxide
   d. Salt mixed with sand

3. A cathartic:
   a. Helps guide the IV catheter
   b. Is another term for a laxative
   c. Causes animals to vomit
   d. Should always be used with animals that have diarrhea

4. Activated charcoal acts by:
   a. Binding to a substance and pulling it out of the system
   b. Causes the animal to vomit
   c. Binding to ulcers
   d. Blocking cholesterol

5. The dose for activated charcoal is:
   a. 10 mg/kg
   b. 100 mg/kg
   c. 1 to 3 g/kg
   d. 1000 g/lb

6. The following substances are contraindicated for using activated charcoal:
   a. Corrosive agents
   b. Ibuprofen
   c. Most heavy metals
   d. Acetaminophen
   e. Marijuana

7. Contraindications for inducing vomiting include:
   a. Ingestion of human medications
   b. Ingestion of petroleum distillates/hydrocarbons
   c. Animal that ingested poisonous plants
   d. Animal that ingested dangerous foods

8. Sorbitol is:
   a. A cathartic
   b. A type of activated charcoal
   c. Antidote for antifreeze poisoning
   d. An antifungal agent

9. Which of the following is true about anticoagulant rodenticides?
   a. Clinical signs include seizures and ataxia
   b. Antidote is atropine
   c. Antidote is vitamin K_1
   d. Clinical signs include seizures and tremors

10. Which of the following is true about bromethalin rodenticides?
    a. Is an uncoupler of the oxidative phosphorylation process
    b. Is an anticoagulant
    c. Atropine is the antidote
    d. Vitamin K_1 is the antidote

11. The way cholecalciferol causes damage is by:
    a. Causing a bleeding disorder
    b. Causes methemoglobinemia
    c. Causes liver failure
    d. Causes kidney failure

12. Which of the following is true about cholecalciferol rodenticide?
    a. Is an anticoagulant rodenticide
    b. Can be treated with pamidronate
    c. Causes increased calcium
    d. Causes decreased calcium

13. The antidote for bromethalin rodenticide poisoning is:
    a. Vitamin K_1
    b. Atropine
    c. Calcitonin
    d. There is no antidote

14. The toxic metabolite of acetaminophen is:
    a. N-acetyl-parabenzequinoneimine
    b. Acetaminophenol
    c. Salicylic acid
    d. Ibuprofen

15. In acetaminophen poisoning, the following are clinical signs:
    a. Anemia and pale mucous membranes
    b. Hepatoxicity
    c. Bright red mucous membranes
    d. Kidney failure

16. This medication is used in acetaminophen poisoning because it directly binds with acetaminophen metabolites to enhance elimination and serves as a glutathione precursor.
    a. N-acetylcysteine
    b. 5-FU
    c. Vitamin C
    d. Vitamin K_1

17. This medication is used in acetaminophen poisonings because it provides a reserve system for the reduction of methemoglobin back to hemoglobin.
    a. N-acetylcysteine
    b. 5-FU
    c. Vitamin C
    d. Vitamin K_1

18. This medication is often used to support the liver and to treat acetaminophen poisoning because it is considered a good source of glutathione and is used to treat hepatoxicity.
    a. SAM-e
    b. Vitamin C
    c. Acetaminophenol
    d. Fomepizole

19. Signs of an aspirin poisoning include:
    a. Fever
    b. Hyperpnea
    c. Vomiting
    d. Melena

20. The therapeutic dose of aspirin in dogs
    a. 10 to 20 mg/kg b.i.d.
    b. 1 to 2 mg/kg b.i.d.
    c. 100 mg/kg b.i.d.
    d. 0.5 mg/kg b.i.d.

21. Which of the following is a type of dangerous food?
    a. Almonds
    b. Macadamia nuts
    c. Carrots
    d. Green peppers

22. Ingestion of grapes/raisins has resulted in cases of:
    a. Kidney failure in dogs
    b. Alcohol poisoning in cats
    c. Liver failure
    d. Methemoglobinemia

23. Which sweetener has resulted in toxicity in dogs?
    a. Sugar
    b. Fructose
    c. Sucrose
    d. Xylitol

24. Activated charcoal is administered:
    a. Orally
    b. Subcutaneously
    c. Intravenously
    d. Intraocularly

25. The principle toxin in tobacco is:
    a. Persin
    b. Ricin
    c. Acetaminophen
    d. Nicotine

26. The following may cause a false-positive ethylene glycol test:
    a. Propylene glycol
    b. Saline
    c. Methanol
    d. Ethanol

27. The following statements are true concerning cats and ethylene glycol antifreeze.
    a. The EGT test is not sensitive enough for a dog.
    b. Cats are more sensitive to ethylene glycol than dogs.
    c. Cats are less sensitive to ethylene glycol than dogs.
    d. The only treatment for cats is fomepizole.

28. The following is true concerning chocolate and dogs:
    a. Milk chocolate is the most toxic type of chocolate.
    b. Unsweetened chocolate is the most toxic type of chocolate.
    c. Milk chocolate contains approximately 330 mg of methylxanthines per ounce.
    d. White chocolate is more dangerous than dark chocolate.

TRUE OR FALSE

Choose T (true) or F (false) for each statement below.

1. _____ Acetaminophen can be used safely in cats.

2. _____ Methemoglobinemia is a clinical sign seen in ibuprofen poisoning.

3. _____ Hepatoxicity is often seen in acetaminophen poisoning.

4. _____ Ibuprofen toxicity is dose dependent, and renal failure and gastric ulcerations are potential clinical signs of ibuprofen poisoning.

5. _____ N-acetylcysteine is used to treat ibuprofen poisoning.

6. _____ Vitamin C is the antidote for anticoagulant rodenticides.

7. _____ Activated charcoal helps adsorb poisons and helps to eliminate them through feces.

8. _____ Apomorphine is an emetic agent that should be used cautiously in cats because they potentially could have a paradoxical reaction.

9. _____ Emesis is most productive 24 hours after ingestion of a poisoning.

10. _____ Activated charcoal can be given repeatedly to help remove toxins, especially if there is enterohepatic recirculation.

11. _____ Aspirin has a therapeutic dose in cats.

12. _____ Easter lily and other members of the Lilium family have been shown to cause kidney failure in cats.

13. _____ Metaldehyde snail bait can cause seizures and tremors.

14. _____ The minimum lethal dose of 95% to 97% ethylene glycol is 4.4 to 6.6 ml/kg in dogs and 1.4 ml/kg in cats.

15. _____ Ethylene glycol may result in liver failure and stomach ulcerations.

16. _____ Fomepizole is the treatment of choice for ethylene glycol poisoning in cats, whereas ethanol is the only choice of treatment for dogs.

17. _____ Rhododendron species contain the toxic ingredient persin, which causes pulmonary edema.

18. _____ The toxic principle in castor beans is ricin.

19. _____ Cycasin is considered to be the toxic principle that is responsible for the hepatic and gastrointestinal signs seen with sago palm poisoning.

20. _____ The toxic principle in lilies that causes kidney failure is grayanotoxins.

21. _____ Mold toxins that induce muscle tremors and convulsions are termed tremorgenic mycotoxins.

22. _____ The toxic ingredients in chocolate are called methylxanthines.

23. _____ Dark chocolate is less toxic per weight than milk chocolate.

24. _____ Methylxanthines cause CNS depression, bradycardia, and sedation.

25. _____ The primary toxic principle of onions is n-propyl disulfide, which is thought to cause oxidative damage to erythrocytes, resulting in hemolysis.

26. _____ Macadamia nuts may cause tremors and seizures in dogs.

CALCULATIONS

1. A dog eats 12 oz of milk chocolate. The dog weighs 15 lb, and there are approximately 62 mg of methylxanthines per ounce of milk chocolate. What is the dosage ingested of methylxanthines? _____

2. A cat is accidentally given 500 mg of acetaminophen. What is the dosage ingested if the cat weighs

   11 lb? _____

3. A dog is supposed to be administered a loading dose of N-acetylcystine at 140 mg/kg. The dog weighs 90 lb. How

   many milligrams of N-acetylcysteine would the dog receive? _____

4. A dog gets into his owner's backpack and eats approximately 10 tablets of 200-mg ibuprofen. The dog weighs

   15 lb. What is the dosage? _____

5. A dog is being treated for ibuprofen poisoning and is to receive 3 μg/kg q8 h of misoprostol. The dog weighs 55 lb.
   How many micrograms would the dog receive in 24 hours? _____

6. A cat is given 2 ml of a topical flea treatment that contains 65% permethrin. If the cat weighs 9 lb, how many

   milligrams per kilogram of permethrin was the cat exposed to? _____

7. A dog chews up a weekly medication minder and ingests the following: 2 tablets of 25-mg diphenhydramine, 5
   tablets of 80-mg aspirin, and 7 of 500-mg acetaminophen. The dog weighs 79 lb. What is the dosage ingested of the
   three medications?

   A. Diphenhydramine _____

   B. Aspirin _____

   C. Acetaminophen _____

8. A 25-lb beagle mix eats 15 tablets of 200-mg ibuprofen. What is the dosage ingested? _____

9. A 10-lb miniature pinscher eats 10 cigarettes. If you assume each cigarette contains 30 mg of nicotine, what dosage

   has been ingested? _____

10. A 55-lb basset hound eats 8 oz of semisweet chocolate morsels. If you assume that 1 oz of semisweet chocolate

    contains 150 mg of methylxanthine per ounce, what is the dosage ingested? _____

11. You have 500 ml of 20% N-acetylcysteine and you need to make a 5% solution to treat a pet for acetaminophen

    poisoning. What volume do you need to add to the solution? _____

12. You have 1000 ml of 40% N-acetylcysteine and you need to make a 5% solution to treat a pet for ethylene glycol

    poisoning. What volume do you need to add to the first solution? _____

13. A ferret that weighs 3 lb eats a baggie of 200-mg ibuprofen; the estimated number of missing tablets is 23. What is

    the dosage that the ferret ingested? _____

14. A 65-lb bulldog eats a 1-oz (28-g) tube of 1% hydrocortisone cream. What is the dosage of hydrocortisone

    ingested? _____

15. A 9-lb cat is put on diazepam at 1 mg/kg bid. How many milligrams will the cat have if it is given the medication for 7 days?

MULTIPLE CHOICE

1. A cat is sprayed in the eyes and mouth with hair-spray by a child. The following would be necessary treatments:
   a. Emesis
   b. Activated charcoal
   c. Flush eyes thoroughly
   d. Gastric lavage

2. A pet rat ingests 1 oz of an anticoagulant rodenticide. The following treatment is contraindicated.
   a. Activated charcoal
   b. Vitamin K_1 therapy
   c. Emesis
   d. IV saline diuresis and mannitol therapy

3. A dog with a third degree heart murmur and epilepsy was accidentally given his owner's 500 mg naproxen medication. Which of the following is contraindicated for treatment?
   a. Activated charcoal
   b. GI protection medication administration
   c. Intravenous fluids
   d. Emesis

4. A cat was seen ingesting a large amount of ethylene glycol antifreeze. The following are treatment options:
   a. Fomepizole
   b. Ethanol
   c. Methanol
   d. Propylene glycol

5. A dog was seen ingesting ethylene glycol antifreeze and the EGT test was positive. The following are treatment options:
   a. Fomepizole
   b. Ethanol
   c. Methanol
   d. Propylene glycol

6. A dog was seen licking a corrosive bathroom cleaner. Which of the following is recommended for treatment?
   a. Emesis
   b. Dilution
   c. Activated charcoal
   d. Gastric lavage

7. In which species is emesis not contraindicated?
   a. Dogs
   b. Rabbits
   c. Mouse
   d. Guinea pig

8. Activated charcoal is considered ineffective or contraindicated with the following toxicants:
   a. Marijuana
   b. Ibuprofen
   c. Corrosive agents
   d. Naproxen

Match the following to the pictures:

A. Cycad palm
B. Foxglove
C. Day lily
D. Rhododendron
E. Lily-of-the-valley

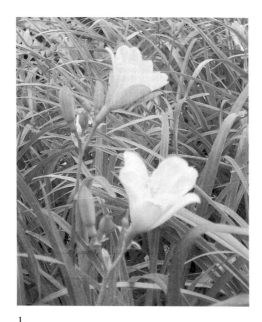

1. _____

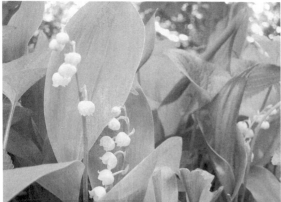

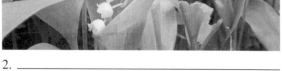

2. _____

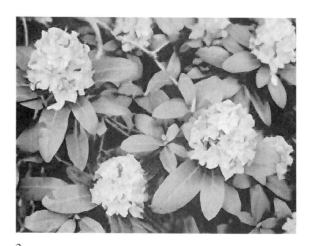

3. _____

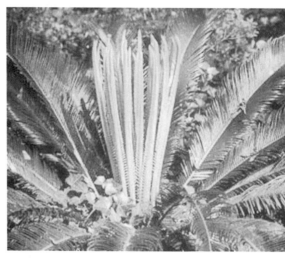

4. _____

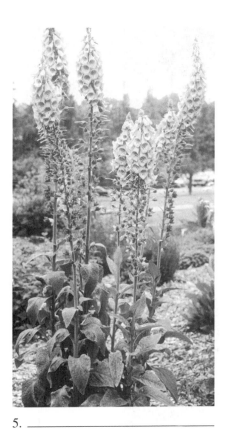

5. _____

CROSSWORD PUZZLE

Across

1. Medications that through their chemical effects increase the clearing of intestinal contents
2. Noxious or poisonous substance that is formed or elaborated during the metabolism and growth of certain microorganisms and some higher plant and animal species
4. Compound that is toxic to liver cells
7. Enterohepatic recirculation occurs with some compounds that are metabolized in the _____; the metabolites are emptied in the bile and are reabsorbed in the small intestines
9. Compounds whose water-based solutions have a sour taste, turn blue litmus paper red, and can combine with metals to form salts and yield hydrogen ions or protons when dissolved in water
11. Toxic or destructive to kidney cells
13. _____ antiinflammatory drugs are a large group of antiinflammatory agents that work by inhibiting the production of prostaglandins

Down

1. Highly reactive substance that causes obvious damage to living tissue
3. Any substance that when introduced into or applied to the body can interfere with the life processes of cells of the organism
4. Any of a large class of organic compounds containing only carbon and hydrogen; examples would be natural gas, propane, butane, kerosene, gasoline, and motor oil
5. _____ detergents are nonsoap surfactants that are in a positive state
6. The act of vomiting
7. Metabolic acidosis is a metabolic derangement of acid-base balance where the blood pH is abnormally _____
8. Any disease of toxic origin
10. Solid substance that attracts and holds a substance to its surface
12. Alkaline substances that produce hydroxide ions on contact with water

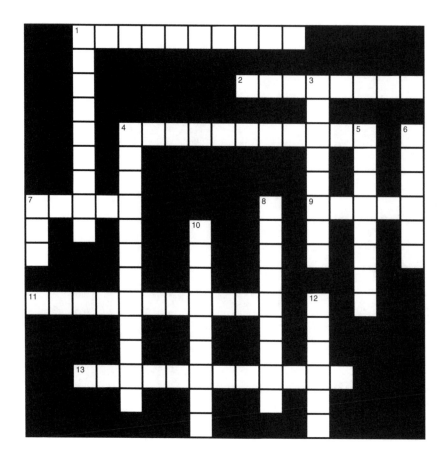

36 Veterinary Oncology

LEARNING OBJECTIVES

When you have completed this chapter, you will be able to:
1. Define oncology and explain mechanisms by which tumors cause clinical signs
2. Differentiate between malignant and benign tumors
3. List the classifications of tumors by tissue origin and provide examples of each
4. Describe methods used to stage and grade tumors based on their physical characteristics and microscopic features
5. List early warning signs of cancer in animals and discuss patient evaluation procedures in animals with suspected cancer
6. Differentiate between cytology and histopathology and state advantages and limitations for each diagnostic method
7. List and describe common methods used to obtain biopsy tissue and procedures for handling biopsy samples
8. Discuss considerations related to surgical treatment of cancer in dogs and cats
9. Discuss nursing considerations and safety concerns related to administration of the chemotherapeutic agent for treatment of cancer in dogs and cats
10. Describe the mechanism by which radiotherapy affects cancer cells and list potential adverse effects of radiation therapy

DEFINE

1. Acute radiation toxicity _____

_____

_____

2. Adjuvant therapy _____

_____

_____

3. Curative therapy _____

_____

_____

4. Cytotoxic _____

_____

_____

5. Ionizing radiation _____

_____

_____

387

6. Late phase radiation toxicity _____

_____

_____

7. Malignant _____

_____

_____

8. Metastasis _____

_____

_____

9. Mucositis _____

_____

_____

10. Multimodality therapy _____

_____

_____

11. Mutagen _____

_____

_____

12. Myelosuppression _____

_____

_____

13. Nadir of leukopenia _____

_____

_____

14. Neoplasm _____

_____

_____

15. Palliative therapy _____

_____

_____

16. Paraneoplastic syndrome _____

_____

_____

17. Radiation sensitizer _____

_____

_____

18. Tumor grade _____

_____

_____

19. Tumor stage _____

_____

_____

20. Vesicant _____

_____

_____

MATCHING

1. _____ Oncology
2. _____ Cancer
3. _____ Paraneoplastic syndrome
4. _____ Benign tumor
5. _____ Malignant tumor
6. _____ Metastasis
7. _____ Carcinoma
8. _____ Sarcomas
9. _____ TNM
10. _____ Carcinogenesis
11. _____ Doxorubicin
12. _____ Ultrasonography
13. _____ Cytology
14. _____ Histopathology
15. _____ Incisional biopsy
16. _____ Excisional biopsy
17. _____ Crysurgery
18. _____ Chemotherapy
19. _____ Carcinogens
20. _____ Radiation
21. _____ Desquamative dermatitis

A. Arise from mesenchymal tissues
B. Complete removal of a mass
C. Noninvasive technique
D. Arise from epithelial tissues
E. Study of cancer
F. Tumor staging system
G. Tumor, mass, neoplasia, or growth
H. Treatment of cancer using chemical agents
I. Aids in obtaining a clinical diagnosis
J. Cells do not destroy normal tissue
K. Used in treatment of cancer
L. Aids in obtaining a definitive diagnosis
M. Characterized by symptoms that occur at sites distant from the site of the primary tumor
N. Incision made into a mass
O. Loss of superficial layers of epithelium
P. Process of spreading to another location; lymph nodes, lungs, and liver
Q. Destroys the cell's DNA, which causes cell death
R. Process where normal cells transform into cancer cells
S. Complete tumor removal cannot be determined in this process
T. Causes DNA damage and ultimately leads to a second cancer
U. Cells can destroy local tissue

Chapter 36 Veterinary Oncology

1. A carcinoma may arise from which of the following?
   a. Mucous membrane
   b. Cartilage
   c. Bone
   d. Connective tissue

2. A sarcoma spreads via:
   a. Lymphatics
   b. Bloodstream
   c. Bone
   d. Epithelial tissue

3. High grade tumors will have:
   a. Normal cellular architecture
   b. Few mitotic figures
   c. Invasion of surrounding structures
   d. Well-differentiated cells

4. Upon a physical examination, what is a crucial element to evaluate in a patient that has cancer?
   a. Mucous membranes
   b. Body conditioning score
   c. Lymph nodes
   d. Heart rate

5. When working with any cancer patient, it is essential to obtain radiographs of the:
   a. Cranium
   b. Lymph nodes
   c. Thoracic cavity
   d. Vertebral column

6. When obtaining a blood sample on a cancer patient, the ideal vein is the:
   a. Femoral
   b. Cephalic
   c. Jugular
   d. Saphenous

7. What radiographic positions need to be performed to evaluate for metastasis?
   a. Ventral dorsal, right lateral
   b. Ventral dorsal, left lateral
   c. Ventral dorsal, right lateral, left lateral
   d. Ventral dorsal, right lateral, site of tumor

8. A common site of metastasis is:
   a. Lymph nodes
   b. Lungs
   c. Kidneys
   d. Brain

9. Cytology
   a. Differentiates neoplasia from inflammation or infection
   b. Provides information for staging of cancers
   c. Determines the best treatment needed for certain cancer types
   d. Noninvasive method of evaluating specific organs or masses

10. When performing a fine needle aspirate, the following items are required:
    a. 25-gauge needle, 3-cc syringe
    b. 25-gauge needle, 1-cc syringe
    c. 22-gauge needle, 12-cc syringe
    d. 22-gauge needle, 3-cc syringe

11. The most common needle size used for a bone marrow aspirate biopsy is:
    a. 18-gauge
    b. 20-gauge
    c. 22-gauge
    d. 25-gauge

12. A TruCut needle obtains which diameter of tissue?
    a. 0.1 to 0.15 cm
    b. 1 to 1.5 cm
    c. 2 to 2.5 cm
    d. 3 to 3.5 cm

13. Biopsy samples are placed in what percent of formalin?
    a. 1%
    b. 5%
    c. 10%
    d. 15%

14. The volume ratio of formalin to tissue for initial fixation is approximately:
    a. 1:10
    b. 10:1
    c. 0.1:1
    d. 1:100

15. The maximum thickness of a tissue that will allow for effective penetration of formalin is:
    a. 1 cm
    b. 2 cm
    c. 3 cm
    d. 4 cm

16. Once a sample has been fixed, the volume ratio of formalin to tissue is:
    a. 1:1
    b. 1:10
    c. 10:1
    d. 1:0.1

17. Cryosurgery can be used to freeze superficial cancers that are less than:
    a. 1 cm
    b. 2 cm
    c. 3 cm
    d. 4 cm

18. After treatment with a chemical agent, leucopenia may occur for _____ days.
    a. 0 to 6
    b. 1 to 7
    c. 8 to 15
    d. 16 to 20

19. Acute adverse effects of irradiation usually resolve in:
    a. 2 to 3 days
    b. 2 to 3 weeks
    c. 4 to 5 days
    d. 4 to 5 weeks

20. Chemotherapeutic agents usually are excreted from the body in the highest levels in _____ days.
    a. 3
    b. 5
    c. 7
    d. 10

SHORT ANSWER

1. A veterinary technician plays a vital role in _____, quality patient care, and client support.

2. Name four ways in which tumor growth can cause clinical signs.

    A. _____

    B. _____

    C. _____

    D. _____

3. List nine factors with carcinogen potential.

    A. _____

    B. _____

    C. _____

    D. _____

    E. _____

    F. _____

    G. _____

    H. _____

    I. _____

4. The chances of long-term control of any cancer are much greater if the tumor is diagnosed:

    _____

5. The two components of evaluating a dog or cat with the suspicion of cancer are to:

    A. _____

    B. _____

6. Any skin or subcutaneous mass should be measured and their location should be

_____.

7. Cystocentesis is contraindicated in cancer patients that _____

_____.

8. Every skin or subcutaneous sample identified during a physical examination should be evaluated by either:

   A. _____

   B. _____

9. Every mass that is removed must be _____, regardless of its location or gross appearance.

10. Individual tumors can exhibit significant cellular heterogeneity and may contain areas of:

    A. _____

    B. _____

    C. _____

    D. _____

11. All submitted tissue samples are examined to determine:

    A. _____

    B. _____

    C. _____

    D. _____

12. Common methods used to obtain biopsy tissue include:

    A. _____

    B. _____

    C. _____

13. The _____ is most commonly used for biopsy of cutaneous or subcutaneous masses.

14. Before any treatment is performed on a cancer patient, a veterinary technician should make sure that the

    animal has had _____

    _____.

15. _____ is used in systemic neoplastic disease.

16. Chemotherapy helps to increase the pet's _____.

17. Chemotherapeutic agents can harm cells within the body, especially those located in the:

A. _____

B. _____

C. _____

18. _____ is used for localized cancers.

19. _____ is evident with irradiation of the oral cavity.

20. Hair color changes are seen with _____.

21. List the components of metastasis.

A. _____

B. _____

C. _____

D. _____

22. In staging tumors, what do the letters TNM stand for?

A. T:_____

B. N:_____

C. M:_____

23. The American Veterinary Medical Association has adopted the early warning signs of cancer. List these signs.

A. _____

B. _____

C. _____

D. _____

E. _____

F. _____

G. _____

H. _____

I. _____

J. _____

24. When evaluating a dog or cat with the suspicion of cancer, history questions should include:

A. _____

B. _____

C. _____

D. _____

E. _____

F. _____

G. _____

25. The minimum data base for a patient with cancer should include:

A. _____

B. _____

C. _____

D. _____

26. List the methods in obtaining samples for cytology.

A. _____

B. _____

C. _____

D. _____

E. _____

27. The preferred sites for a bone marrow biopsy include:

A. _____

B. _____

C. _____

D. _____

28. When submitting a sample to the laboratory, what components need to be included on the sample record?

A. _____

B. _____

C. _____

D. _____

E. _____

F. _____

G. _____

29. After a diagnosis has been made, the veterinary technician's role includes supplying clients with information to help them understand the condition, treatment options, and other pertinent information. As a technician, list things that you can do to provide helpful information to clients.

A. _____

B. _____

C. _____

30. The three primary treatments for cancer are:

A. _____

B. _____

C. _____

31. Describe the proper way to prepare a large (greater than 20-cm diameter) biopsy specimen before placing it in formalin. Three specific points must be mentioned for full credit; do *not* include comments about the formalin-to-tissue ratio.

A. _____

B. _____

C. _____

32. An owner calls 10 days after her dog's last dose of a cancer-treatment drug to say the patient is not eating well and has diarrhea. What two critical pieces of information should you obtain from this client or from the patient's record for the veterinarian treating the patient?

A. _____

B. _____

33. Given the following sites/locations, name the type of cancer.

A. A bladder has transitional cells and cancers associated with the bladder are malignant. The tumor is

_____.

B. A cancer that is common in cats attacks the intestine where there are lymphatics and lymph nodes and the

cancer is malignant. The tumor is _____.

C. A cancer that attacks squamous cells and is malignant. The tumor is _____.

D. A cancer that attacks histiocytes and is found in young dogs and is considered benign. The tumor is

_____.

Signalment: 12-year-old male castrated golden retriever

History: Swollen left third eyelid and left-sided mucopurulent nasal discharge for 3 weeks

Physical examination: The dog was lethargic and seemed in pain. There was a mass involving the left third eyelid, with protrusion of the left eye from the socket (exophthalmos). The left mandibular lymph node was enlarged.

Diagnostic test results: Routine blood work, urinalysis, and chest and abdominal radiographs were normal. Fine-needle aspirates of the third eyelid mass and left mandibular lymph node revealed neoplastic mast cells. Malignant mast cells were also found on a bone marrow aspirate. A computed tomography scan was performed and showed a large mass involving the left orbit and left nasal cavity.

Definitive diagnosis: Systemic (metastatic) mast cell tumor.

Treatment and expected prognosis: The best single treatment for this dog was systemic chemotherapy because that was the only way to treat all of the different sites where he had mast cell tumor. However, his long-term prognosis was poor because of his advanced disease.

Outcome: This dog had an excellent response to lomustine chemotherapy; a complete remission was achieved within 5 days of starting therapy. Remission was maintained for 5 months, and during this time the dog enjoyed an excellent quality of life. The dog was eventually euthanized at 6 months when his cancer became progressive and his quality of life declined.

A. Why was chemotherapy chosen as a form of treatment instead of radiation therapy?

_____

_____

_____

B. What form of cancer is mast cell tumor? _____

C. Why was a fine needle aspirate performed? _____

CROSSWORD PUZZLE

Across

1. A process by which initiated cells that have damaged DNA are stimulated to grow into cancer
4. One of many diseases that are characterized by uncontrolled growth and spread of abnormal cells within the body
7. A _____ cancer is one that can invade and destroy surrounding normal tissues
8. A radiation _____ is a compound or agent that acts by any of a number of mechanisms to make cancer cells more susceptible to being killed by ionizing radiation
9. An agent or process that kills cells
11. A clinical assessment of how much cancer a patient has (volume of disease), and how much it has spread (two words)
15. The change that occurs in a normal cell as it becomes malignant
16. The _____ of leukopenia is the lowest circulating neutrophil count occurring after administration of a chemotherapy drug
18. _____ therapy is cancer treatment administered to relieve the symptoms and reduce the suffering caused by cancer
20. Acute radiation toxicity is the side effects caused by radiotherapy that occur between day one (the start of radiotherapy) and day _____
21. An agent or substance that may cause physical defects in a developing embryo when a pregnant female is exposed to that substance
22. An abnormal growth of tissue that may be benign or malignant

Down

2. A chemical or physical agent that causes permanent DNA injury and alteration within a cell
3. _____ radiation is radiation made by or arising from radiotherapy and x-ray machines, and radioactive substances
4. _____ therapy is cancer treatment whose purpose is to permanently control the tumor
5. A process by which normal cells are changed so that they have the potential to be able to form cancers
6. _____ therapy is cancer treatment that combines more than one form of therapy (e.g., surgery, radiotherapy, and chemotherapy)
9. Drug therapy for cancer
10. The process by which a malignant cancer spreads from the primary or original site to a distant location in the body
12. Inflammation of the mucous membranes lining the digestive tract from the mouth to the anus
13. Agent causing pain or inflammation at site of injection
14. A substance or agent that causes cancer in animals or people
17. An agent causing tissue destruction or necrosis on extravasation
19. A _____ cancer is one that may grow but does not invade surrounding normal tissues and does not spread (metastasize) to other parts of the body

Chapter **36** **Veterinary Oncology**

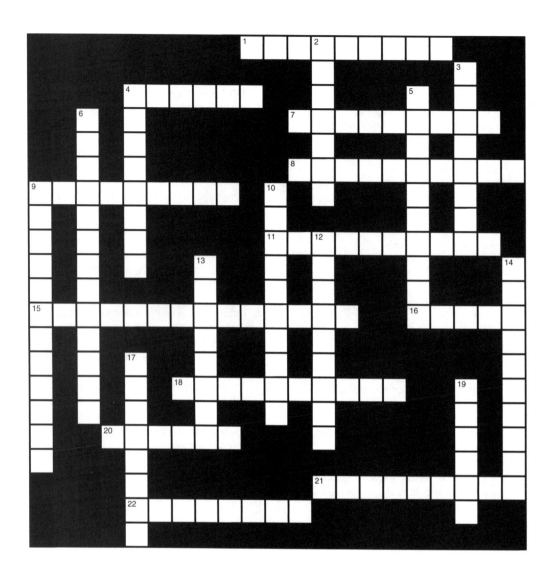

37 Geriatric and Hospice Care

LEARNING OBJECTIVES

When you have completed this chapter, you will be able to:
1. Describe the life stages of dogs and cats
2. List and describe the effects of aging on body systems
3. Discuss the importance of oral health in geriatric dogs and cats
4. List and describe common cardiac, respiratory, orthopedic, and kidney disorders of geriatric dogs and cats
5. List and describe common neoplastic and neurologic disorders of geriatric dogs and cats
6. List and describe common endocrine disorders of geriatric dogs and cats
7. Discuss components of hospice nursing care of geriatric dogs and cats
8. Discuss components of the physical examination of a geriatric horse
9. List and describe common disorders of geriatric horses
10. List and describe common chronic conditions that affect geriatric horses

DEFINE

Define the following terms.

1. Geriatric _____

_____

2. Hospice _____

_____

3. Incontinence _____

_____

4. Nasoesophageal tube _____

_____

5. Hirsutism _____

_____

6. Pediatric life stage _____

_____

7. Young adult life stage _____

_____

8. Mature adult life stage _____

_____

9. Senior life/adult life stage _____

_____

10. Halitosis _____

_____

MATCHING

Match the following elements of nursing care for the hospice patient.

1. _____ Pain management
2. _____ Decubital ulcers
3. _____ Subcutaneous fluids
4. _____ Bladder expression
5. _____ Urine scalding
6. _____ Appetite stimulants
7. _____ Feeding tubes
8. _____ Carts and slings
9. _____ Butterfly catheter
10. _____ Nasoesophageal tube

A. Assists in providing nutritional support
B. Supports hind limbs
C. Delivers a small amount of fluid
D. Antiinflammatory; NSAIDs
E. Pressure points on hips, tarsi, and elbows
F. Helps to maintain adequate hydration
G. Emptying urine from the bladder
H. Placed through the nasal cavity
I. Accompanies excessive urination
J. Increased appetite

FILL IN THE BLANK

Fill in the blank or complete the sentence.
1. It is important for the veterinary community to question owners closely regarding their pet's health status so that

_____.

2. Senior care should begin at the age of _____ years.

3. There are five tests/procedures that should be performed annually in geriatric dogs and cats. Blood and urine

tests screen for _____. Chest radiographs can be helpful in evaluating the

_____.

4. Halitosis, difficulty chewing, dropping food from the mouth, or excessive salivation should prompt an

_____.

5. Thickening of the heart valves may lead to

A. _____

B. _____

C. _____

6. Fatigue, exercise intolerance, collapse, or cough are suggestive of _____.

7. Collapsing trachea is a disorder of the _____ airway.

8. In geriatric patients, especially cats, chronic _____ is a common disease that may affect appetite and overall demeanor of the pet as the disease progresses.

9. Degenerative neurologic diseases and spinal cord problems may lead to difficulties with

_____.

10. With degenerative joint disease, _____ and _____ can help to improve the quality of life for the geriatric patient.

11. As a veterinary technician caring for a patient with an orthopedic disorder, it is critical to remember to

_____.

12. A geriatric cat that presents with an increase in heart rate, increased appetite, and weight loss is exhibiting signs of a

_____.

13. Diabetic animals require daily injections of _____.

14. Animals with diabetes are prone to urinary tract infections because glucose is a source of nutrition for

_____.

15. Tachycardia, tachypnea, elevated temperature, unwillingness to use a limb, and yelping when a limb is manipulated

can all be signs of _____.

16. Due to _____ of certain pain medications, routine blood work should be performed.

17. The three most common drugs used in geriatric pain management are:

A. _____

B. _____

C. _____

18. A recumbent patient should be turned every _____ hours to decrease the chances of decubital ulcers or bed sores.

19. Persistent anorexia, change in breathing rate or effort, pain that is not controlled by medication, or loss of interest in interacting with the owner may be indicators that the pet's health is declining and could be the deciding

factor in considering _____.

20. Geriatric horses are defined as greater than _____ years old.

21. List five common conditions of geriatric horses.

A. _____

B. _____

C. _____

D. _____

E. _____

22. The _____ is the most important element in good health practices of the geriatric equine because it aids the veterinary professional in evaluating the patient's physical condition.

23. Weight loss of a geriatric horse could be signs of dental, neoplasia, or _____ disorders.

24. Equine recurrent uveitis is also referred to as _____.

25. When a geriatric horse is no longer living a good quality life, _____ may be considered by the owner and/or recommended by the veterinarian.

MATCHING

Match the equine geriatric disorder with the definition.

1. _____ Arrhythmia
2. _____ Cushing
3. _____ Laminitis
4. _____ Heaves
5. _____ Melanoma
6. _____ Cataracts
7. _____ Neurologic
8. _____ Sinusitis
9. _____ Uveitis
10. _____ Wave mouth

A. Disorder of the hoof/foot
B. Associated with hirsutism
C. Moon blindness
D. Dental disorder
E. Atrial fibrillation
F. Unilateral nasal discharge
G. Tumor
H. Recurrent airway obstruction
I. Impairs vision
J. Ataxia and dragging the toe

MULTIPLE CHOICE

Choose the best choice.

1. Which of the following conditions is found in geriatric patients that have teeth of different lengths, preventing chewing action?
   a. Hooks
   b. Wave mouth
   c. Parrot mouth
   d. Points

2. Nasal discharge in the geriatric horse could signify:
   a. Upper respiratory infection
   b. Chronic sinus infection
   c. Tooth abscess
   d. Neoplasia

3. Hypertrophy of abdominal muscles may be evident in which of the following?
   a. Laminitis
   b. Heaves
   c. Anorexia
   d. Diarrhea

4. If a horse cannot move his or her nose toward the shoulder, it indicates:
   a. Face pain
   b. Neck pain
   c. Shoulder pain
   d. Back pain

5. Management of aged horses include hoof care (trimming) every:
   a. 2 to 3 weeks
   b. 4 to 5 weeks
   c. 6 to 7 weeks
   d. 8 to 9 weeks

6. Management of aged horses include having teeth floated every:
   a. 2 months
   b. 4 months
   c. 6 months
   d. 8 months

7. Horses with Cushing disease can develop other conditions because Cushing causes:
   a. Decreased appetite
   b. Immunosuppression
   c. Laminitis
   d. Muscle wasting

8. A horse with a condition called heaves is treated with steroids. A technician should be concerned with the possibility of:
   a. Arrhythmia
   b. Sinusitis
   c. Laminitis
   d. Uveitis

9. Renal failure or right dorsal colitis can result from:
   a. Founder
   b. NSAIDs
   c. Toxins
   d. Immunosuppression

10. General management of aged horses includes deworming every day or every _____ weeks.
    a. 2
    b. 4
    c. 6
    d. 8

CASE STUDY

Case Presentation 1

13-Year-Old Labrador Retriever

Hershey, a 13-year-old Labrador retriever, is brought into the clinic for difficulty using his hind legs. This has been a gradual onset, but is severe enough that he can no longer ambulate well on his own. The owner also reports a diminished appetite, and that Hershey is no longer getting up to urinate regularly. When he rises, he often has a puddle of urine on his bedding. Examination and diagnostic testing reveals severe arthritis in both hips and stifles. He appears to have good ambulation in his front limbs. No other systemic disease is found, and organ function appears within normal limits. He has extreme pain upon manipulation of the affected areas.

After discussion with the owner regarding Hershey's quality of life, it is decided to place him on nonsteroidal antiinflammatory medications to improve his comfort level. The owner purchases a sling to help Hershey move around better, and encourages him to go out and urinate every 4 to 6 hours by assisting him with ambulation. Soft, padded bedding is provided for him to rest comfortably on at home to prevent development of decubital ulcers. At a follow-up visit, Hershey still has difficulty walking, but is much more comfortable, and gets around well with his owner's assistance. The owner reports an improved appetite, and he is having less frequent urinary "accidents" in the house. With time, additional pain medications may be added if the discomfort begins to worsen. Serial urine cultures are performed for early diagnosis of urinary tract infections.

1. What could have been done to detect this condition earlier?

   _____

   _____

2. What are side effects of NSAIDs?

   A. _____

   B. _____

   C. _____

3. What will the owner watch for?

   A. _____

   B. _____

   C. _____

D. _____

E. _____

4. What tests/procedures should you as a technician be aware of in caring for a patient with this condition?

   A. _____

   B. _____

5. Why is it important for the canine to have soft padding to lie on?

_____

_____

_____

6. Why is it important to have the owner ensure the pet urinates on a regular basis?

_____

7. What additional pain medications are used for arthritis such as degenerative joint disease?

   A. _____

   B. _____

   C. _____

Case Presentation 2

32-Year-Old Quarter Horse

A 32-year-old quarter horse mare appeared depressed and inappetent, so the owner called her equine veterinarian and veterinary technician. On physical examination, the mare had poor body condition (body score 4/9), hirsutism, a wave mouth, and rings on the dorsal hoof wall of her front feet. Initial blood work was performed and no abnormalities were present. Samples were also submitted for ACTH, insulin, and dextrose. Samples were drawn three times in 1 day (AM, noon, PM) and dextrose testing was performed stallside using a dextrometer. Insulin levels were within normal limits, but dextrose was more than 200 mg/dl for each sample and ACTH levels were greater than 300 each sample. The mare was diagnosed with Cushing disease and treatment started (1 mg PO s.i.d. Pergolide). She was sedated with 2 mg detomidine and 1 mg butorphanol IV for a thorough dental float to correct the wave mouth. Radiographs were taken of her front feet, which showed chronic laminitic changes but minimal rotation of P3 (coffin bone). Her feet were in poor condition, so the farrier trimmed her feet and agreed to return every 4 weeks. Her diet was evaluated and her ration of Equine Senior was increased with ¼ cup corn oil added daily. The owner also clipped the mare and agreed to place a blanket on her in the winter. Within a week after starting pergolide treatment, the mare became much more active and bright. She nickered to everyone who came to her stall and ate readily, no longer dropping grain from her mouth. She began to play with the other horses again. After 3 months on her new diet, she was in better condition (grade 6/9) and the grateful owner was happy to have her beloved horse back.

1. On the physical examination, what were the clinical signs suggestive of Cushing disease?

   A. _____

   B. _____

   C. _____

   D. _____

404

2. What bone is associated with laminitis in horses?

_____

3. Why is it important for the horse to get regular foot care?

_____

4. What are other diseases and/or conditions that need to be discussed with the owner since the horse has been diagnosed with Cushing disease?

   A. _____

   B. _____

   C. _____

   D. _____

38 The Human-Animal Bond, Bereavement, and Euthanasia

LEARNING OBJECTIVES

When you have completed this chapter, you will be able to:
1. Discuss the aspects of strong attachments to animals
2. List and describe the stages of grief and the role of veterinary professionals in grief counseling
3. Discuss the impact of euthanasia and client grief on the members of the veterinary health care team
4. Discuss the legal and ethical issues related to euthanasia in animals
5. Describe the factors that owners consider when making decisions regarding euthanasia of their pet
6. Discuss the role of the veterinary health care team in counseling owners considering euthanasia of their pet
7. Describe considerations in scheduling of euthanasia appointments and preparing for unexpected events during euthanasia
8. List and describe acceptable methods of euthanasia in animals
9. List signs and symptoms of staff burnout
10. Discuss special considerations related to euthanasia of large animals

DEFINE

Define the following terms.

1. Anger _____

   _____

2. Barbiturate _____

   _____

3. Bargaining _____

   _____

4. Bereavement _____

   _____

5. Catharsis _____

   _____

6. Compassion _____

   _____

7. Denial _____

   _____

8. Depression _____

   _____

9. Drug Enforcement Agency (DEA) _____

_____

10. Grief process _____

_____

11. Resolution _____

_____

SHORT ANSWER

1. List two reasons for companion animals becoming a more important factor in people's support systems.

   A. _____

   B. _____

2. Due to the change in our modern society, fewer people live in rural areas. Therefore, approximately

   _____% of companion animals live inside the home.

3. Aside from companionship, pets provide adults and children stability, constancy, and security. List seven reasons why.

   A. _____

   B. _____

   C. _____

   D. _____

   E. _____

   F. _____

   G. _____

4. For the elderly, pets fulfill many needs including the following five:

   A. _____

   B. _____

   C. _____

   D. _____

   E. _____

5. What benefits do animals offer in therapy programs for people with physical and mental disabilities?

   A. _____

   B. _____

C. _____

D. _____

E. _____

F. _____

6. In the households that own at least one pet in the United States, about _____ of these owners classify their attachment to their pet as strong.

   A. 20%

   B. 35%

   C. 50%

   D. 65%

7. When the death of a pet occurs, the intensity of the loss is usually greatest in the following situation:

   A. Family pet

   B. Herding dog

   C. Hunting dog

   D. Assistance dog

8. Human-animal relationships have different levels of attachment. Think about your pets and your relationship with them. Describe some of the aspects of the relationships of people who form the closest attachment with their pet(s): **(There is no one correct answer.)**

   _____

   _____

   _____

   _____

9. Why would most pet owners not feel comfortable in mourning the death of their pet in a public way?

   A. _____

   B. _____

   C. _____

   D. _____

10. List a few of the considerations that an owner must think about when trying to make the decision to have their pet euthanized.

    A. _____

    B. _____

C. _____

D. _____

E. _____

11. Where should you place an IV catheter in preparing the animal for euthanasia and why?

_____

_____

TRUE OR FALSE

Choose T (true) or F (false) for each statement below.

1. _____ The breaking of the human-animal bond, in whatever way, is a significant event in the life of the pet owner. When an owner is faced with this loss, it is up to the veterinary staff to be unemotional when discussing this with the client.

2. _____ Helping a client deal with the grief of the loss of a pet is outside the realm of the veterinary professional.

3. _____ Most people feel pressured to be "back to normal" within a few days of their pet's death to avoid being labeled as neurotic, hysterical, or overly attached.

4. _____ It may be wise to recommend a professional counselor to a client who may be displaying signs of depression after the death of their pet.

5. _____ It is not a good idea to tell an owner that it's good to cry after the death of their pet.

6. _____ Making a suggestion as to how a client can help "memorialize" their pet is a positive way to help them during the stage of depression.

7. _____ It is not a bad idea to offer the client time to spend time with the body of their pet after euthanasia.

8. _____ As a veterinary professional, you may have to tell a client that it's time to get on with their life and to stop grieving.

9. _____ It is important for the veterinary professional to assure a client that what they are feeling is "normal" after the death of their pet.

10. _____ Once an owner who has lost a pet has gone through any one stage of grief, he/she will not return to that stage again.

11. _____ It may be important to restate a diagnosis, prognosis, and treatment plan when an owner is in the denial stage of grief.

12. _____ Advising a client who has just lost a pet to get a new animal as soon as possible is a good way to help them get over their loss.

13. _____ When an owner exhibits massive guilt, he/she is experiencing the anger stage of grief.

14. _____ Bereavement support is important in alleviating a client's anger.

15. _____ Irritability, change in sleep habits, and the inability to concentrate are symptoms of anger.

16. _____ Adults reach the stage of acceptance and resolution more quickly and easily than do children.

17. _____ When explaining the death of a pet to a child, it is best to use terms like "put to sleep" rather than using correct terminology.

18. _____ Having some children's books about the loss of a pet is a good way to help a child deal with the death of their own pet.

19. _____ Encouraging a client to choose an animal very close to their dead pet can be helpful.

20. _____ Veterinary professionals may go through the grief process with long-time patients who have died.

21. _____ It is not always in the common interest of the patient, client, and veterinarian that euthanasia is performed.

22. _____ The most important help that the veterinary team can give to a client is to provide information.

23. _____ It is helpful to answer the question "What would you do if he were your animal?" so that the owner can make the best decision for his/her pet.

410

24. _____ It is helpful for the client to be asked their reasons for choosing euthanasia when it may be apparent to you that it is for convenience.

25. _____ Discussing euthanasia with a client early on, when death may be a possibility for the pet, may help the client understand available options.

26. _____ It should be the veterinary professional who makes the decision whether the family should be present during euthanasia.

27. _____ Communication is the most important aspect of euthanasia to consider.

28. _____ Having a dedicated room in the veterinary practice, solely for euthanasia, is a good idea so that clients do not have to revisit that room when bringing in a new pet in the future.

29. _____ Do not burden your client with how payment for the euthanasia service before the process is done. Wait until about 2 weeks after the euthanasia to send a bill, or contact the owner by phone to find out when they want to come in to pay the bill.

30. _____ An intraperitoneal injection can be used for euthanasia because it works more quickly than injecting into a vein.

31. _____ Many clients need the assurance that their pet is really dead, especially if they are not present for the euthanasia.

32. _____ Euthanasia with the client present is less stressful to the veterinary staff than if the client was absent.

33. _____ It is best when a veterinary practice has a designated "team" to perform euthanasia.

34. _____ Shelter workers experience less stress over euthanasia because they are used to performing the procedure so frequently.

35. _____ Safety of personnel is of major importance when euthanizing large animals.

FILL IN THE BLANK

1. The acceptance stage of the grief process has also been called _____.

2. Clients experiencing the _____ stage of the grief process may have a change of appetite, withdraw from others, become irritable, and may have trouble sleeping.

3. The pet owner who starts to show you pictures from his recent vacation after being told that his pet cannot be saved after being hit by a car is experiencing the _____ stage of the grief process.

4. One way that a veterinary professional can help an angry client is to allow them to _____, or express their feelings.

5. The author, _____, worked extensively with dying persons and their families in the 1960s and wrote the book *On Death and Dying*.

6. Veterinary professionals may be tempted to become defensive or respond in like manner when the client is experiencing the _____ stage of the grief process.

7. As a general rule, children under the age of _____ do not really understand that death is final.

8. The client who tries to negotiate with God for miracles upon hearing the news that his pet is dying is experiencing the _____ stage of the grief process.

9. One definition of _____ is: ascribing human forms or attributes to a thing or being that is not human *(Webster's American Dictionary College Edition)*.

10. The depression stage has also been called _____.

Chapter **38** **The Human-Animal Bond, Bereavement, and Euthanasia**

CROSSWORD PUZZLE

Across

6. The quality of understanding the suffering of others and wanting to do something about it
7. The stage of grief experienced as conscious or unconscious attempts to control the situation or refute the loss
8. The stage during which there is no longer anger or depression but acceptance

Down

1. The actual grief; sorrow
2. The release of pent-up emotions with the result being alleviation of symptoms
3. The normal defense which serves to buffer an individual from some unbearable news or shock
4. The emotional process one experiences when anticipating or following the loss of an object of attachment
5. That stage of grief during which anger is the primary emotion expressed directly, indirectly, and specifically or generally

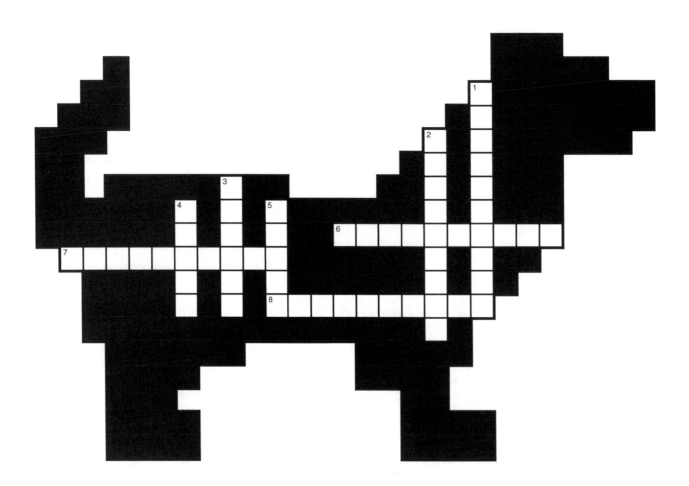

39 Necropsy

LEARNING OBJECTIVES

When you have completed this chapter, you will be able to:
1. Define necropsy and list indications for performing necropsy
2. Describe methods for evaluating and recording results of examination of lesions
3. List fixatives used for preservations of tissues and describe their uses
4. List equipment needed for performance of a typical necropsy
5. Describe procedures for collection of tissue samples for bacteriology and mycology evaluation
6. Describe the procedure for collection of segments of intestine and tissues for virus isolation
7. Describe the procedure for collection of tissues from suspect rabies samples
8. Discuss considerations related to shipping necropsy samples
9. List the steps in the necropsy procedure for small mammals
10. List variations on necropsy procedures applicable to large animals, laboratory animals, birds, and fetal and placental samples

MATCHING

Write the letter of the word which best fits each description in the appropriate space.

1. _____ Any abnormality in a tissue
2. _____ Sequence of events that leads to a disease
3. _____ The examination of a dead animal
4. _____ Microscopic pathologic changes seen in tissues
5. _____ The breakdown of tissues after death

A. Histopathology
B. Lesion
C. Pathogenesis
D. Autolysis
E. Necropsy

SHORT ANSWER

1. List four reasons to perform a necropsy.

   A. _____

   B. _____

   C. _____

   D. _____

2. If necessary when performing a necropsy, tissues may be collected for diagnostic techniques. List six possible diagnostic techniques that may be used.

   A. _____

   B. _____

   C. _____

   D. _____

E. _____

F. _____

3. List eight different criteria by which lesions should be described:

A. _____

B. _____

C. _____

D. _____

E. _____

F. _____

G. _____

H. _____

4. Which fixative is used for the storage of whole brains, bones, and intact spinal cords?

_____

5. Describe the steps which should be taken when working with chemical fixatives.

A. _____

B. _____

C. _____

6. List six different instruments required for most small animal necropsies.

A. _____

B. _____

C. _____

D. _____

E. _____

F. _____

TRUE OR FALSE

Choose T (true) or F (false) for each statement below.

1. _____ If an animal dies in a veterinary hospital, the veterinarian does not need the owner's permission to perform a necropsy.

2. _____ If a necropsy cannot be performed right away, the body should be refrigerated.

3. _____ The best fixative for tissues for histopathology is 10% ethyl alcohol.

4. _____ When submitting fixed tissues to a lab, ice should be used to prevent breakdown.

5. _____ If rabies is suspected, the head should be submitted to the lab for testing.

6. _____ The immediate covering over the brain is the meninges.

7. _____ A Stryker saw is used to open the abdomen.

8. _____ The thorax should be opened before opening the abdomen.

9. _____ In a cosmetic necropsy, the thoracic and abdominal organs are removed and the cavities are stuffed with paper and sutures closed.

MATCHING

Match the following terms.

1. _____ Abomasum
2. _____ Autolysis
3. _____ Gross pathology
4. _____ Pathogenesis
5. _____ In situ

A. Pathologic changes in tissue that are visible with the unaided eye
B. The self-digestion of tissues or cells
C. In its normal place, confined to the site of origin
D. The "true stomach" of the ruminant
E. Sequence of events that leads to or underlies a disease

SUPERCLUE

Fill in the blanks to solve the super clue in the center (hyphens have been given a space).

1. The large hole in the occipital bone through which the spinal cord exits the skull

2. Membranous sheet that attaches organs to the body wall

3. Location between the lungs that contains the trachea, esophagus, heart, nerves, lymphatic vessels, and major blood vessels

4. Bones that support the base of the tongue, the pharynx, and the larynx

5. The first segment of the small intestine after the stomach

6. The science and study of disease

7. Supportive mesenteries that arise from the greater and lesser curvatures of the stomach

8. Alterations or abnormalities in a tissue

Super Clue: Connective tissue layers that cover the brain and spinal cord

1. ___ ___ ___ ___ ___ ___ ___ ___ □ ___ ___ ___ ___ ___

2. ___ ___ ___ □ ___ ___ ___ ___ ___

3. ___ ___ ___ ___ ___ ___ ___ ___ □ ___ ___

4. ___ ___ ___ □ ___

5. ___ ___ ___ ___ ___ □ ___ ___

6. ___ ___ ___ ___ ___ ___ ___ □ ___

7. ___ ___ □ ___ ___ ___ ___

8. ___ ___ □ ___ ___ ___ ___

Super Clue: _____

CROSSWORD PUZZLE

Across

1. The middle layer of the heart and the main muscle layer responsible for contraction during systole
7. Prestomach chambers in a ruminant animal
10. The _____ nerve runs along the caudal aspect of the femur beneath the biceps
11. Connective tissue layers that cover the brain and spinal cord
16. The master endocrine gland; located in the brain
19. The second cervical vertebra
20. The foramen _____ is the large hole in the occipital bone through which the spinal cord exits the skull
21. The supportive mesenteries, which arise from the greater and lesser curvatures of the stomach
22. The self-digestion of tissues or cells by enzymes that are released by their own lysosomes

Down

2. The first cervical vertebra
3. _____ pathology refers to pathologic changes in tissue that are visible with the unaided eye
4. The bone in the neck region that supports the base of the tongue, the pharynx, and the larynx and aids the process of swallowing
5. The _____ is the person preparing a body for the necropsy
6. _____ is the examination of an animal, after it has died, to determine the abnormal and disease-related changes that occurred during its life
8. Hydronephrosis refers to dilation and distention of the _____ pelvis and calices usually caused by obstruction
9. Pathologic changes in tissue that are microscopic and can be seen with the use of a microscope
12. _____ are alterations or abnormalities in a tissue (pathologic changes) (e.g., wounds, sores, ulcers, tumors, cataracts, and any other tissue damage)
13. _____ is the sequence of events that leads to or underlies a disease
14. The thin, dome-shaped sheet of muscle that forms the boundary between the thoracic and abdominal cavities
15. The first segment of the small intestine after the stomach
17. _____ means in its normal place, confined to the site of origin (two words)
18. The interdigitations between the corium and hoof that serve as the attachment sites between the hoof and coffin bone

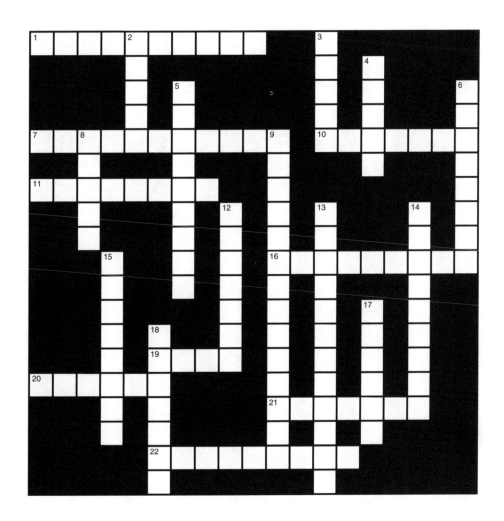